PRACTICAL
RADIOLOGY

A SYMPTOM-BASED APPROACH

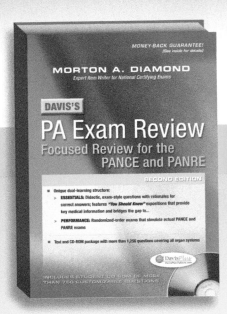
 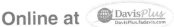
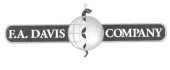

PRACTICAL RADIOLOGY

A SYMPTOM-BASED APPROACH

Edward C. Weber, DO
Radiologist, Imaging Center
Adjunct Professor of Anatomy and Cell Biology
Volunteer Clinical Professor of Radiology and Imaging Sciences
Indiana University School of Medicine
Fort Wayne, Indiana

Joel A. Vilensky, PhD
Professor, Anatomy and Cell Biology
Indiana University School of Medicine
Fort Wayne, Indiana

Alysa M. Fog, PA-C
Physician Assistant, Ortho Northeast
Fort Wayne, Indiana

F.A. Davis Company • Philadelphia

F. A. Davis Company
1915 Arch Street
Philadelphia, PA 19103
www.fadavis.com

Copyright © 2013 by F. A. Davis Company

Printed in the United States of America

Last digit indicates print number: 10 9 8 7 6

Acquisitions Editor: Andy McPhee
Developmental Editor: Jennifer Ajello
Manager of Content Development: George W. Lang
Design and Illustration Manager: Carolyn O'Brien

As new scientific information becomes available through basic and clinical research, recommended treatments and drug therapies undergo changes. The author(s) and publisher have done everything possible to make this book accurate, up to date, and in accord with accepted standards at the time of publication. The author(s), editors, and publisher are not responsible for errors or omissions or for consequences from application of the book, and make no warranty, expressed or implied, in regard to the contents of the book. Any practice described in this book should be applied by the reader in accordance with professional standards of care used in regard to the unique circumstances that may apply in each situation. The reader is advised always to check product information (package inserts) for changes and new information regarding dose and contraindications before administering any drug. Caution is especially urged when using new or infrequently ordered drugs.

Library of Congress Cataloging-in-Publication Data

Weber, Edward C., D.O.
  Practical radiology : a symptom-based approach / Edward C. Weber, Joel A. Vilensky, Alysa M. Fog.
    p. ; cm.
  Includes index.
  ISBN 978-0-8036-2832-8
  I. Vilensky, Joel A., 1951- II. Fog, Alysa M. III. Title.
  [DNLM: 1. Diagnostic Imaging. 2. Radiology. WN 180]

  616.07'54—dc23
                    2012035484

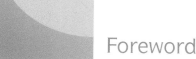

Foreword

The field of clinical medicine has become increasingly complex in recent decades and imaging is now an integral part of the diagnosis and management of most patients. It is very difficult for health care providers to understand all aspects of the wide menu of imaging studies that are available, including limitations and appropriate utilization. Dr. Edward Weber, Adjunct Professor of Anatomy and Cell Biology and Volunteer Clinical Professor of Radiology and Imaging Sciences at Indiana University School of Medicine–Fort Wayne, and his co-authors, have written this unique book to bridge the gap in knowledge about appropriate imaging.

The book begins with a discussion of various imaging modalities, including positioning and resulting images. Chapters 2–11 review the imaging of each anatomic region of the body. The book's organization is case-based, with clinical vignettes and clear descriptions of how imaging modalities may affect the work-up, diagnosis, and management of various disease presentations. Each chapter ends with a series of review questions.

The book has a unique emphasis on cost-effective medicine and the use of Appropriateness Criteria, such as those from the American College of Radiology (ACR), for proper use of imaging. With today's concerns about radiation exposure and the skyrocketing costs of health care, Dr. Weber's approach is particularly timely.

Chapter 12, "Clinical Practice Issues in Medical Imaging," is an excellent summary of topics that bridge all areas of imaging. There are outstanding discussions about how to deal with incidental findings, the ACR Appropriateness Criteria, and talking to patients about the risks and limitations of various imaging studies.

The target audience for *Practical Radiology: A Symptom-Based Approach* is physician assistant and nurse practitioner students. However, this clearly written and beautifully illustrated book would also be valuable to medical students, as well as residents and clinicians in a wide variety of specialties.

Valerie P. Jackson, MD, FACR
Eugene C. Klatte Professor and Chairman
Department of Radiology and Imaging Sciences
Indiana University School of Medicine

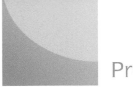

Preface

Practical Radiology: A Symptom-Based Approach is designed for mid-level clinicians, such as physician assistants and nurse practitioners, as well as primary care physicians. The book is organized by the clinical presentations of your patients and the medical imaging procedures you are likely to use while diagnosing or evaluating these conditions. We believe this patient-oriented approach provides a uniquely practical and useful radiology reference for the student and practicing medical provider.

APPROACH

Because this book will teach you how to use radiology as a clinical tool, the chapters are arranged by clinical presentation, generally with separate Modalities and Interpretation sections for each group of conditions. For each clinical problem we present the most appropriate imaging procedures for evaluation and diagnosis of your patients.

Practical Radiology also uniquely provides information about when it is unlikely that a radiologic study will change the diagnosis or treatment of your patient. In other words, we say when history, physical, or laboratory studies should be sufficient to diagnose a patient. We also emphasize instances when more costly radiologic procedures such as MRI are likely to be no more useful to diagnose your patient than less expensive procedures such as radiography. Our last chapter is also different from other radiology texts in that we discuss many of the issues facing the use of medical imaging in today's health care environment, such as radiation risk and the finding of unrelated abnormalities during radiologic procedures for specific clinical conditions. These are issues that influence how your use of medical imaging affects the care you provide.

FEATURES

Colored arrows on images. Within the many carefully selected radiologic images in the book, we use red arrows to indicate the pathology discussed in the text and blue to indicate normal anatomy. Students thus can easily recognize and learn how to interpret normal and pathologic structures and conditions.

Case Studies. Each clinical chapter begins with a case study that continues throughout the chapter, to help illustrate and create a real-world feel for how to recognize the most cost-effective and efficient modality, relative to a patient's condition, and how to interpret the associated radiologic images based on the modalities used.

Cost-Effective Medicine. These sections emphasize instances in which more costly radiographic procedures such as MRIs are unlikely to be more useful than less expensive procedures such as radiography.

Pediatric and Geriatric. Content especially pertinent to children and the elderly receives special attention in the book because treating these patients sometimes involves specialized radiologic approaches.

Patient Communication. These boxed elements help students learn how to communicate effectively with their patients and with teams of clinicians treating the patients.

Radiology Requisition Information. These tables illustrate how to concisely communicate important clinical data to radiologists.

Unique Glossary. A glossary is provided that not only includes boldface terms throughout the text and their definitions, but also a key that identifies the modalities to which the terms apply.

Chapter Review Questions. Each chapter concludes with several Chapter Review Questions, many with images from the chapter, to test knowledge of chapter content.

In all aspects of **Practical Radiology: A Symptom-Based Approach** we have striven to offer images and information of the highest quality possible, to present the most pedagogically effective content, and to provide a resource that all primary medical practitioners will find invaluable as they seek to provide the best patient care possible.

—*Edward C. Weber*
Joel A. Vilensky
Alysa M. Fog

About the Authors

Edward C. Weber has been in private practice as a radiologist for more than 30 years and has taught radiology to first- and second-year medical students at Indiana University School of Medicine in Fort Wayne (IUSM-FW) for almost 20 years. He guided the orientation of this book and provided most of the radiologic images and clinical information for it.

Joel A. Vilensky is an anatomist who has been teaching at IUSM-FW for more than 30 years. His role was primarily to ensure that all textual and graphic material presented in the book could be completely understood by students who have taken a course in medical anatomy and who have had some basic clinical experience.

Alysa M. Fog is a practicing PA who specializes in orthopedics. She ensured that the material was ideally presented for students and beginning medical professionals. Alysa also contributed much of the organization and clinical material for Chapter 2.

Contributors

Thanks to Peter Miller, MD; LCDR Kevin Preston, MD; and Keith Newbrough, MD for their generous contribution of images:

Peter Miller, MD, Indiana University School of Medicine

Chapter 1: Figure 1-3
Chapter 2: Figures 2-5, 2-12, 2-14, 2-28, 2-33, 2-36, 2-43, 2-47, 2-65, 2-67, 2-70, 2-76, 2-78
Chapter 3: Figures 3-3, 3-4, 3-5, 3-6, 3-7, 3-9, 3-11, 3-12, 3-28, 3-29
Chapter 4: Figures 4-1, 4-4, 4-5, 4-6, 4-7, 4-11, 4-13, 4-16, 4-18, 4-19, 4-20, 4-29, 4-33
Chapter 5: Figures 5-6, 5-13, 5-15, 5-17, 5-18, 5-19, 5-21, 5-22, 5-23, 5-24, 5-29, 5-30, 5-31, 5-33
Chapter 6: Figures 6-25, 6-43, 6-44
Chapter 8: Figures 8-1, 8-2, 8-3, 8-4, 8-6, 8-7, 8-9, 8-10, 8-11, 8-12, 8-13
Chapter 9: Figures 9-1, 9-2, 9-3, 9-4, 9-5, 9-10, 9-11, 9-17, 9-22, 9-24, 9-26, 9-27, 9-28, 9-29, 9-32
Chapter 10: Figures 10-15, 10-16, 10-17

LCDR Kevin Preston, MD, Indiana University School of Medicine

Chapter 2: Figures 2-35, 2-38, 2-39, 2-40, 2-41, 2-45, 2-56, 2-63, 2-79, 2-81, 2-83, 2-84
Chapter 6: Figures 6-5, 6-7, 6-12, 6-14, 6-18, 6-19, 6-21, 6-22, 6-23
Chapter 8: Figures 8-18, 8-20

Keith Newbrough, MD, Indiana University School of Medicine

Chapter 2: Figures 2-8, 2-9, 2-18, 2-29
Chapter 6: Figure 6-17
Chapter 7: Figure 7-5

Reviewers

Linda G. Allison, MD, MPH
Associate Professor, Pharmacy Practice
Belmont University School of Pharmacy
Nashville, Tennessee

Jesse A. Coale, PA-C
Assistant Professor
Physician Assistant Studies
College of Science, Health & the Liberal Arts
Philadelphia University
Philadelphia, Pennsylvania

Randy Danielsen, PhD, PA-C
Senior Vice-President
National Commission on Certification of Physician Assistants Foundation
Johns Creek, Georgia

Steve B. Fisher, MHA, PA-C
Senior Surgical Physician Assistant
Department of Neurosurgery, Kentucky Neuroscience Institute
University of Kentucky
Lexington Kentucky

Charlene Morris, MPAS, PA-C, DFAAPA
Family Medicine
Pamlico Medical Center, PA
Bayboro, North Carolina

Acknowledgments

This book originated in a spring 2010 meeting at a coffee shop near the Pennsylvania Turnpike between ECW and F.A. Davis Senior Acquisitions Editor, Andy McPhee. Andy showed immediate enthusiasm for the project, and we are grateful to him for that enthusiasm and his support and guidance throughout the project. We deeply appreciate the editing provided by our developmental editor, Jennifer Ajello, who managed this project. The book has a high level of consistency and organization because of her guidance. Liz Schaeffer ably guided the writing and assembly of ancillary materials available to instructors who adopt our book.

The medical images we present here offer superior clarity because of the skills and knowledge of Roberta Shadle, our graphic artist, who turned our raw images into the polished figures needed for the book. We are thankful to have had Roberta as part of our team.

Most of the clinical images in this book were acquired by ECW while in clinical practice at The Imaging Center, Fort Wayne, IN, and as consulting radiologist for The Medical Clinic of Big Sky in Big Sky, MT. However, in the outpatient setting in which ECW practices, appropriate images to accompany our text were not always available. Fortunately, many clinical images were provided by Peter Miller, MD, Lieutenant Commander Kevin Preston, MD, and Keith Newbrough, MD, while they were radiology residents at the Indiana University School of Medicine (p viii).

We are very grateful to Fen-Lei Chang, MD, for critically reviewing the chapter on brain imaging.

We extend our appreciation to Robert Conner, MD, and the technical staff at The Imaging Center, Fort Wayne, IN, for their support and their dedication to high-quality patient care.

We would also like to offer deep appreciation to the many scientists and engineers whose work has made possible the fantastic tools used in modern medical imaging. Furthermore, we acknowledge the commercial enterprises whose software and hardware make practical the analysis of the vast image datasets now produced in medical imaging facilities. ECW collected most of the clinical images for this book while using an advanced radiology workstation from Carestream Health, which provided the means for managing, viewing, and processing images from digital radiography, mammography, sonography, CT, and MRI.

We are very grateful to our spouses, Ellen Weber, Deborah Vilensky, and Daniel Fog, for their support of our efforts and toleration of our often spending more weekend time with each other than with them. We also acknowledge that two of the spouses have already been asking when we are going to begin our next project.

Finally, we would like to thank our students, who have taught us to shed our assumptions and years of experience and see radiology from the viewpoint of new immigrants to the strange and wonderful landscape of medical imaging.

Contents

1 MODALITIES OF MEDICAL IMAGING

RADIOGRAPHY

Radiography, discovered in 1895, is still the foundation of medical imaging. It is one type of imaging modality under the broader heading of radiology, which includes computed tomography (CT), magnetic resonance imaging (MRI), nuclear medicine (NM), and ultrasonography (sonography [US]).

Radiographic Densities

Radiography refers to the medical images that are the "shadows" projected onto a flat plane when x-rays pass through a patient. Similar to any shadow, they show the shape of the object causing the shadow. Figure 1-1 is a magnified small section of a chest radiograph. How many different anatomic structures do you see in this figure?

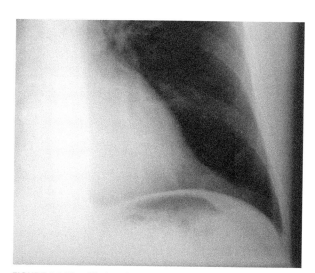

FIGURE 1-1 Magnified section of a PA chest radiograph.

The untrained eye and mind may only perceive several different structures. Careful and educated observation, however, reveals many more.

Radiographic shadows have different shades of gray that provide important information. These gray tones are referred to as radiographic densities. There are five radiographic densities, four biologic and one artificial/metallic density that is distinguishable from biologic calcium density (Table 1-1). You will see all four biologic densities if you look for them in Figure 1-1. It is normal to look at radiographs and just look at the shape of structures, but in order to fully comprehend the visual information in those images you must distinguish among radiographic densities.

The different shades of gray on a radiograph (radiographic densities) result from differences in the absorption and scattering of x-ray photons in their path from the x-ray source toward the digital x-ray detector. The degree to which x-rays are prevented from reaching the detector is referred to as radiographic attenuation. Different tissues attenuate the x-ray beam based upon the average atomic number and thickness of the tissue. These physical properties of tissue are also referred to as density, which can be confusing when radiographic density is often abbreviated as just "density."

Calcified tissue attenuates more of the beam than fat or water because it has a higher average atomic number, and therefore calcified tissue has a higher radiographic density than fatty tissue or fluid. The final shade of gray that you see in any one location on a film or on a monitor reflects the attenuation of the x-ray beam by all of the tissues along the path of the x-ray beam to that part of the image. The summation density at any particular point on a radiographic image thus reflects both the density and thickness of the

TABLE 1-1 Radiographic Densities and Associated Structures

Metal	Calcium (Bone)	Soft Tissue (Water)	Fat	Air (Gas)
Surgical clips, bullet fragments, orthopedic hardware	Cortical bone; medullary bone is summation of bone density and marrow (fat, soft issue density)	Muscle, tendons, solid organs such as liver, fluid-filled structures such as gallbladder	Subcutaneous fat, intermuscular and other deeper fat planes	Any collection of air or gas such as lungs, loop of bowel

Radiographic and fluoroscopic images are sometimes shown as a "negative" of the standard representation given above, so that metallic objects are black and air density is white.

intervening structures in the path of the x-ray beam at that anatomic position. There may of course be many overlapping structures that contribute to a particular summation density. Now look at Figure 1-2.

You may have noted the vertebral column initially (A in figure), but did you also notice the horizontal, very bright white lines representing the dense, compact bone of the vertebral body end-plates? These are brighter (more dense) than medullary bone in the remainder of the vertebral bodies. Medullary bone is not pure calcium density because marrow fat contributes to its summation density.

The first time that you looked at this figure, did you recognize correctly the border of the heart, or did you include epicardial fat as part of the heart shadow? Appreciating the lower radiographic density of epicardial fat allows you to accurately determine the border of the cardiac apex.

For an example of a summation density in Figure 1-2 look at the thick vertical band of very bright (white) density that is a summation density representing the descending aorta (B in figure) and other structures along the path of the x-ray beam. Note that the right side of the spine, visible through the heart shadow, is darker than the left side of the spine, visible through the heart shadow and the shadow of the aorta. You probably did not think, initially, that this image could show you the position or size of the descending aorta, but now you can ascertain that this patient has a normal left-sided aorta and it does not appear to be dilated.

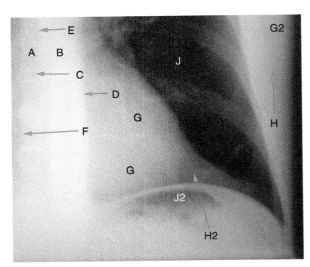

FIGURE 1-2 Same image as depicted in Figure 1-1 but labeled to highlight features visible if you look for subtle density differences. **(A)** Spine (calcium density); **(B)** Spine and aorta (calcium and soft tissue density); **(C)** arrow points to a disc space that is bordered by horizontal, very dense bone of vertebral endplates; **(D)** left border of spine and aorta; **(E)** right border of aorta; **(F)** right border of spine; **(G)** heart (soft tissue density); **G2)** muscle (soft tissue density); **(H)** fine dark stripe of intermuscular fat plane (fat density); **(H2)** epicardial fat pad (fat density); **(J)** lung (air density); **(J2)** air in gastric fundus (air density).

Untrained viewers just look at the shape of structures in radiographic images. However, by searching for subtle differences in radiographic density of different tissue, and appreciating summation densities, far more information can be discerned.

In later chapters, we will discuss the need for high quality radiography to show these shades of gray in specific clinical situations. Poor radiographs may fail to show important density differences. Even when radiographs are satisfactory, clinically important information that is visible may be overlooked if subtle differences in radiographic densities are not appreciated. For example, knee radiographs may not show a fracture but should not be interpreted as "negative" if the normal fat density deep to the quadriceps tendon is replaced by soft tissue or water density, perhaps indicating blood within the knee joint.

The interpretation of a radiograph and every other type of diagnostic image is an active rather than a passive process. You must look for normal anatomic structures and for evidence of pathology. In looking for the large number of important findings that may appear on a medical image, you must develop a consistent and thorough search pattern.

In radiography (and in CT), any edge that appears in an image is an interface between tissues that have different degrees of attenuation of the x-ray beam, such as the interface between air and soft tissue. When there is a horizontal edge between air and fluid in any medical image, it is called an **air-fluid level.** Identifying an air-fluid level on an image helps identify anatomic structures that contain air and fluid and the orientation or position of the patient when imaged. The search for abnormal air-fluid levels is often crucial in finding and in identifying pathology, such as the presence of gas and fluid (pus) in an abscess.

To improve the contrast resolution of an image, specific contrast materials (or "media" or "agents") may be administered to the patient. Contrast materials have a higher radiographic density than air, fat, or soft tissue, resulting in the visibility of structures that may not be seen on images without their use. (See section on Contrast Enhancement.)

COST-EFFECTIVE MEDICINE

High quality radiographs and interpretation provide diagnostic information that may avoid the need for more expensive cross-sectional imaging and may be critical in avoiding missed diagnoses.

Types of Resolution

Resolution refers to the ability to perceive two adjacent objects or points as being separate. Within radiology, the term is subdivided into *spatial, contrast,* and *temporal resolutions.*

The value of "sharp" images—that is, images with high spatial resolution—is obvious. Contrast resolution allows the differentiation among types of tissue. A third type of resolution may also be important: temporal resolution, the ability to image a structure during a very narrow window of time. As we discuss techniques and imaging protocols used to acquire clinically useful information, all three types of image resolution may be addressed, often with discussion of the strengths and weaknesses of different imaging modalities for different kinds of resolution.

COST-EFFECTIVE MEDICINE

These fundamental issues of spatial, contrast, and temporal resolutions are important in all imaging modalities. This is not a "technical" matter, it is a clinical issue. Does "X" imaging procedure have the temporal resolution that you need for a patient whose breath holding ability is limited? Does "Y" imaging procedure have the spatial resolution needed to see a very fine fracture of bone cortex? Does "Z" imaging procedure have the tissue contrast resolution to tell you if a tissue is edematous, although its size and shape are unchanged? Doing the ideal imaging procedure initially is less expensive than when a suboptimal procedure needs to be followed with additional studies.

Radiographic Projections

Note the apparent differences in the chest radiographs depicted in Figure 1-3. And yet they are the same patient! One cannot interpret radiographic images without understanding the various projections used.

Radiographic projections describe the relationship between the patient (body part) and the path of the x-ray beam. It is important to understand these projections in order to make sense of the anatomy shown and to understand why anatomic structures may appear differently in various projections.

PA/AP Views

In a PA projection, the path of the x-ray beam is from (the patient's) posterior to anterior (Fig. 1-4, left). In an AP projection, the path of the x-ray beam is from (the patient's) anterior to posterior (Fig. 1-4, right). Together, AP and PA projections are referred to as frontal views.

Because of the geometry of the diverging x-ray beam, anatomic structures may appear magnified, and this is often apparent when PA and AP projections are compared (Fig. 1-3). Those structures near the detector appear closer to true size than structures further from the detector (Fig. 1-4). The heart, an anterior structure in the thorax, is closer to the detector in the typical PA projection of an

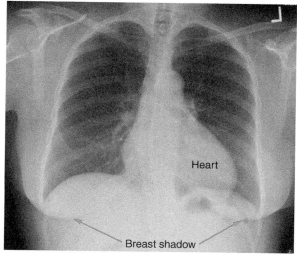

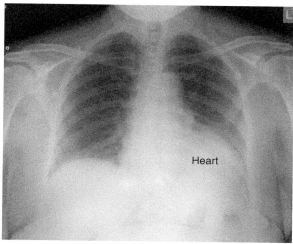

FIGURE 1-3 PA and AP chest radiographs of the same patient. The top image is a standing PA chest radiograph; the bottom image is an AP upright chest radiograph done in an ED using a portable x-ray machine.

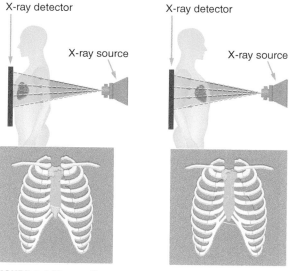

FIGURE 1-4 Diagram illustrating how PA and AP chest radiographs are done, with insets showing the relative representation of heart size on each.

upright patient and is thus more accurately depicted in a PA than in the AP projection (Figs. 1-3 and 1-4). In the portable AP radiograph shown in Figure 1-3, which was done on a semiupright patient in an emergency department (ED), the heart appears to be enlarged because of the geometric effect caused by the diverging beam.

Limitations of medical imaging, whether imposed by physics, imperfections of technology, or a variety of patient factors, such as metallic implants, and patient motion during imaging, can result in artifacts in a medical image. Countless times, a portable AP radiograph has been misinterpreted as showing cardiomegaly because of the geometric issue discussed above when in fact the heart was normal in size; therefore, never assume that a radiographic image perfectly represents "reality."

Lateral Views

In a lateral projection the path of the x-ray beam is from one side of the patient or body part to the other side. You may hear the phrase "true lateral," indicating that care was exercised in positioning the path of the x-ray beam in the coronal plane (Fig. 1-5). A "Left" or "Right" side marker is usually placed to indicate which side of the patient was closest to the detector. This is a different use of the markers than in frontal or oblique projections, in which the markers indicate the right or left side of the patient.

Oblique Views

There are many oblique projections that demonstrate anatomic features more clearly than in frontal or lateral projections. The designation of an oblique projection is based upon the orientation of the patient relative to the path of the x-ray beam. For example, for a right posterior oblique (RPO) projection, one may start with the patient oriented for an AP projection and then rotate the patient so that his or her right side is closer to the detector than the left side. It is understood that the x-ray beam passed from the left anterior aspect of the patient toward the right posterior aspect of the patient.

Figure 1-6 is an example of a common posterior oblique projection of the shoulder, described by Grashey

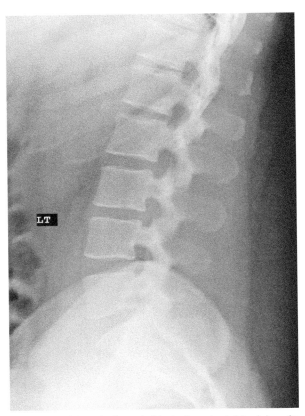

FIGURE 1-5 Left lateral radiograph of the lumbar spine. In lateral views the side indicator (LT) indicates the patient's side closest to the x-ray detector.

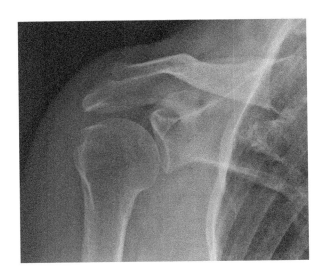

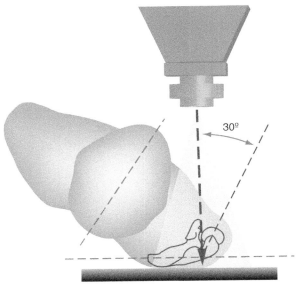

FIGURE 1-6 Grashey (oblique shoulder) view radiograph (top) and a schematic drawing of patient orientation for the Grashey view (bottom).

assução

in 1923, used for ideal visualization of the glenohumeral joint.

In Figure 1-6, the patient is rotated to his right in relation to the x-ray beam. The most important issue when viewing oblique images is that there is no uncertainty about which anatomic structures are on the right side of the patient and which are on the left side. In other words, if an oblique projection of the cervical spine clearly reveals cervical neuroforamina, the important issue is that there must be certainty as to whether these are the right or left neuroforamina. It does not matter if the oblique view was done as a right posterior oblique or a left anterior oblique, as long as an "R" marker indicates to the viewer which side of the image is the right side of the patient or an "L" marker indicates the left side of the patient.

Oblique radiographic projections may not only be angled in a left-to-right (or mediolateral) direction. There are also numerous special projections that use cranio-caudal (or its opposite) angulation, and in some cases an angle that is oblique in two planes. However, many of the numerous special radiographic projections, often done with highly creative patient positioning, are now performed rarely, if at all, because cross-sectional imaging has becomes the procedure of choice for viewing abnormalities that formerly presented a great challenge to demonstrate radiographically.

COST-EFFECTIVE MEDICINE
Good radiography including proper use of oblique and other special radiographic views can sometimes obviate the need for more expensive procedures. You will provide the best patient care if you use the simplest, safest, and least expensive medical imaging, such as radiography and ultrasonography (or no imaging), as appropriate to establish a diagnosis.

Viewing Radiographic Projections

The traditional practice of viewing radiographs is simple and consistent: For almost every body part, except those listed in the next paragraph, the radiograph is viewed as if the patient is looking at you. This is true for any AP, PA, or oblique projection.

The exceptions are these: Hands, wrists, and feet are viewed as if you are looking at your own. Forearms may be viewed either as if the patient is looking at you with elbows extended (anatomic position) or you are looking at your own forearms.

Examples of the first rule can be found by looking at Figure 1-3. These were done differently, one AP and the other PA, but both are printed the same way. The patient's left is to the viewer's right. The patient is looking at you.

Another example is the oblique view of a right shoulder (Fig. 1-6; Grashey view). Imagine that this patient was facing you and then turned toward his right but can still look at you out of the corner of his eye. An oblique view may be obtained in different ways, but that does not change how it is viewed (Fig. 1-7).

This standardized method of displaying radiographic images provides a consistency of anatomic identification and recognition that is essential to minimize confusion and error. It is the expectation that every radiographic image be properly marked with a Left or Right indicator to avoid a potentially serious error such as trying to drain fluid from the right hemithorax when it is the patient's left hemithorax that requires drainage. However, in the real world, the side markers may not be clearly seen, may be absent, or may be misplaced. In an emergency situation it is critical to have instant appreciation of which side of the patient has an emergent condition, rather than needing to search for the "R" or "L" identifiers.

The reason for standard image display that is independent from image acquisition can be explained through the following example: Imagine a patient is admitted to the ED and a portable AP chest radiograph is obtained. The next day, the patient is capable of standing for a PA chest radiograph. The patient's condition then worsens, and a portable AP chest radiograph is again obtained, this time in the intensive care unit (ICU). When evaluating this series of images and looking for changing or new radiographic findings, imagine viewing the series of images if they were viewed from the perspective of how they were done, rather than in a standard presentation. An abnormal pulmonary density might be in the side of the image toward the viewer's left in the first image, the right on the second image, and then back again toward the left. With multiple radiographic findings, viewing such a series of images would be very confusing.

A consistent appreciation of the patient's side of a radiologic finding (e.g., which knee is arthritic on bilateral knee radiographs) is far more important when viewing radiographs than how a radiograph was done (AP or PA).

The presentation of lateral views is more complex and less consistent than the other projections. A traditional practice has been to orient lateral radiographs to match the position of the patient when the radiograph was made. An alternate practice that provides a more consistent viewing experience when radiographs are viewed with cross-sectional images is to match the common presentation of sagittal CT and MRI images (Fig 1-8). These are, almost universally, shown as if the anterior aspect of the patient is to the viewer's left. This varies from the traditional practice of viewing sagittal ultrasound images, discussed later.

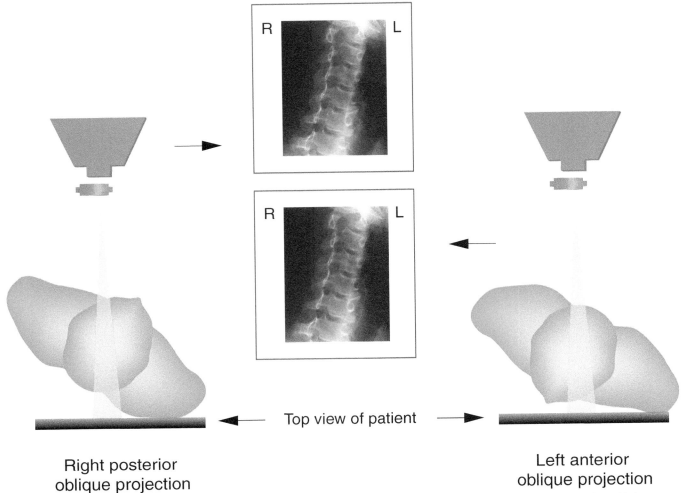

R   L

R   L

Top view of patient

Right posterior
oblique projection

Left anterior
oblique projection

FIGURE 1-7 Illustration of how right posterior oblique and left anterior oblique projections are done. The figure shows that the resulting radiographic images are viewed the same way—as if the patient was (obliquely) facing the viewer.

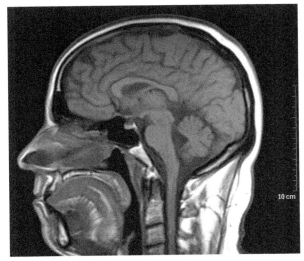

FIGURE 1-8 Sagittal MRI of the head and brain. Sagittal cross-sectional images, by convention, are presented as if the patient is facing the viewer's left.

Mammography presents an interesting issue with respect to how the images are shown. The original standard was for the images to be shown as mirror images with the anterior aspect of the right breast toward the viewer's left, and vice versa (Fig. 1-9). However, this standard is not consistently used among radiology practices.

Exceptions to standard radiology practices of viewing radiographs have always been common "in the clinic," often for logical reasons. For example, because at one time almost all spinal surgery involved a posterior approach, many spine surgeons viewed AP and PA spine films as if the patient was looking away from them—that is, they were looking at the back of the patient and the patient's right was to the viewer's right. The rationale for viewing spine radiographs this way has lessened with the increase in anterior approaches in spine surgery. Furthermore, such a practice results in left-right orientation of radiographs that are opposite that of CT and

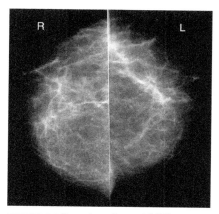

FIGURE 1-9 Normal cranio-caudal (CC) mammographic views; the anterior aspect of the right breast is typically toward the viewer's left and vice versa, but this is not always the case; thus, labeling of the right and left breasts is essential in mammograms. The lateral aspect of each breast is at the top of the image.

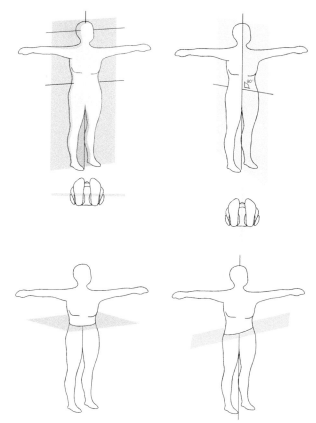

FIGURE 1-10 Anatomic planes. Purple, coronal; pink, sagittal; green, transverse (axial); orange, oblique. Cross-sectional images may be done in these conventional orthogonal anatomic planes here but may also be oriented in non-conventional multiple oblique planes.

MRI, which are often viewed along with those radiographs. Consistency of image orientation reduces the chance of error.

CROSS-SECTIONAL IMAGING, TOMOGRAPHY, AND BODY PLANES

It has always been a challenge to differentiate anatomic features shown within various patterns on radiographs because of the projection of "shadows" of overlapping anatomic structures. Overlapping results in the summation densities discussed earlier. By the middle of the twentieth century, an advanced radiographic technique called tomography was in widespread use to improve visualization of specific anatomic structures in radiographic images. Standard radiographic tomography is a technique that blurs out features in front of and behind an anatomic plane of clinical interest by linear motion of the x-ray tube and detector (in opposite directions) during the exposure; only structures in the focal plane appear sharp.

Thus, tomography could be considered a cross-sectional imaging technique because it clearly showed the structures in only one section or slice of the body. Cross-sectional imaging today, whether CT, MRI or ultrasound, similarly reveals slices or sections of the body. Originally, CT only showed axial (transverse) sections of the body. Subsequently, software was developed enabling sagittal, coronal, and oblique sections to be depicted (Fig. 1-10).

MRI was a multiplanar cross-sectional imaging technique from its first clinical use. Ultrasound examinations are a handheld technique that can display cross-sectional images in any plane.

Modern cross-sectional imaging has revolutionized medical diagnosis through the clear visualization of internal anatomy. But as with radiography, cross-sectional imaging involves making compromises and is subject to false positive and false negative results. These will be discussed with the individual cross-sectional imaging techniques.

COMPUTED TOMOGRAPHY: CROSS-SECTIONAL IMAGES AND RECONSTRUCTIONS

CT is an advanced computer-based form of tomography in which cross-sectional images are produced from the mathematical analysis of a large number of measurements. Through several generations of CT equipment, different arrangements and movements of x-ray tubes and detectors were developed. During each rotation of the x-ray tube and detector array, measurements of the attenuation of x-rays at millions of locations and angles in the axial plane are acquired (Fig. 1-11). The specific levels of gray used for each pixel of a displayed CT scan have a numerical value (Hounsfield number) ranging from −1,000 to +1,000, in which air is −1,000, water is 0, and compact bone is +1,000.

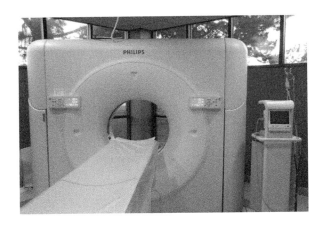

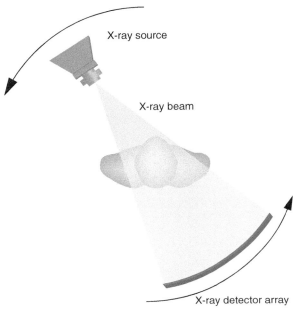

FIGURE 1-11 Illustration of basic CT scanner mechanisms with a photograph of a CT scanner.

Initially CT scanners were only able to acquire one axial section while the patient was motionless on a table, and then the patient table moved for each additional axial section, and so forth. More recent technology has resulted in the development of helical (spiral) scanners in which the patient table continuously moves during the CT scan. The most recent advance was the introduction of multidetector scanners that could acquire CT data from more than one slice simultaneously during each rotation of the x-ray tube and detector array. The first multidetector CT (MDCT) scanners were dual slice scanners. Progress has been rapid with the development of an increasing slice number on newer scanners. At this time, 64 slice scanners are common and the newest generation of scanners can image 256 or 320 slices in a single rotation. In addition, rotation speed has increased to where these many slices can be obtained in approximately $\frac{1}{3}$ of a second.

Inherent to the process of CT image acquisition are variables that must be set by the operator of the unit and that influence the duration of the scan, radiation exposure, and quality of the images. Furthermore, a large number of different image reconstructions are possible. The specific reconstruction algorithms used may be critical in determining what can be seen on the images. For example, the apparent density of an anatomic structure seen on CT can be misleading. Thicker reconstructed slices may have some advantages but may lead to an artifact called partial volume averaging, which results because each pixel (picture element) on the computer screen represents a voxel (volume element) of tissue (Fig. 1-12).

If a thickly reconstructed slice includes tissues of different CT densities, the apparent Hounsfield density measurement will be an average of all these tissues, and not an accurate measurement of any one of the individual anatomic structures included (partial volume averaging). A classic example would be the pulmonary nodule. A 5 mm thick slice that includes a 3 mm nodule and some normal lung tissue will not truly represent the density of the nodule.

Depending upon the relationship between visualized structures and the orientation of a cross-sectional image, geometric shapes of anatomic structures may be distorted. For example, as shown in Figure 1-13, a round tubular structure that runs obliquely to the long axis of the body will appear as an oval structure on a conventional axial scan. Additionally, a structure such as the splenic vein that meanders cranially and caudally as it traverses from the spleen in the extreme upper left abdominal quadrant to the portal vein in the upper right quadrant may pass into and out of a specific image section and might be misinterpreted as separate structures when viewed in a single slice. This is why radiologists must review a number of adjacent sections, and view CT scans in multiple planes, in order to be absolutely certain they are identifying an anatomic structure correctly.

You might be surprised to know that the spatial resolution (sharpness) of CT images is often not as good as that available in conventional radiography. But the contrast resolution for soft tissues is much better in CT.

Subsequent to the development of helical CT scanning, continued software and computer development resulted in the ability to reformat the CT image data so that sagittal, coronal, and oblique CT images could be viewed. Special image displays, such as maximum intensity projections (MIP; Fig. 1-14) and minimum intensity projections (MinIP; Fig. 1-15) are used to improve visualization of pathology. Very life-like three-dimensional representations (volume rendered or 3D displays) of anatomic regions or structures may also be produced (Fig. 1-16).

Because CT is a procedure that relies on ionizing radiation, the same intravenous (IV) iodinated contrast materials that are used in conventional radiography may be used in CT.

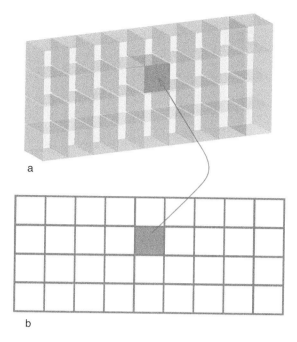

a

b

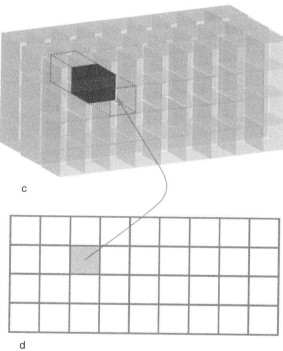

c

d

FIGURE 1-12 Partial volume averaging. Voxel (volume element) of tissue is represented as a pixel (picture element) on a computer screen (**A and B**) and how a CT or MR slice (**C**) that is thicker (acquired thickness or displayed thickness) than a structure of interest (e.g., tumor) may not accurately represent the tissue density or signal intensity on the 2D image (note differences in gray color in the lower two images) because of the averaging of all the tissue within the voxel that are represented by the pixel (**D**).

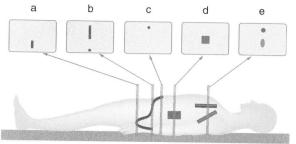

FIGURE 1-13 Schematic illustration of geometric distortion and/or possible misinterpretations in cross-sectional imaging. "Monitors" show projected axial images. (**A**) An axial "slice" may show only a small section of a tubular structure that meanders cranially and caudally. (**B**) Two sections of the same structure could give the false impression that the two are entirely different structures. (**C**) Cross-section of one end of a tubular structure. Note that the other end is not in the lowest slice so that a radiologist may have to follow such structure in serial images "down" and then back "up" again. (**D**) A rectangular structure in cross-section appears to be a square structure. (**E**) The round cross-section of a tubular structure appears as round only if the structure is perpendicular to the slice, while if the structure runs obliquely to the image slice, it appears as an ovoid structure.

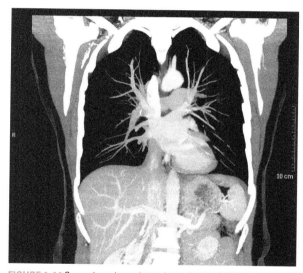

FIGURE 1-14 Coronal maximum intensity projection (MIP) of a chest CT.

The kinetics of the distribution of these agents must be considered when protocols are set up for contrast-enhanced CT studies. Thus, there are very specific protocols for contrast injection rates and timing between contrast injections and scanning for the imaging of various body regions. Another protocol issue relative to CT is the exposure to radiation. A typical CT scan exposes a patient to significantly more radiation than a standard radiographic study. But it should be noted that the exposure in a typical CT exam is about a third of the radiation a person receives from background radiation in a year. Nevertheless, as a primary care provider you need to be aware of patient radiation exposure concerns, especially if the patient is subjected to multiple CT scans or if the patient is a child (see Patient Safety section later in this chapter).

Axial CT images are presented as if the viewer is standing at the foot of the patient's bed; the patient's right is to viewer's left; the anterior aspect of the patient is toward the top of the image (Fig. 1-17). Coronal images are viewed the same way that the majority of radiographs are viewed; the images are oriented as though the patient is looking at you (Fig. 1-18).

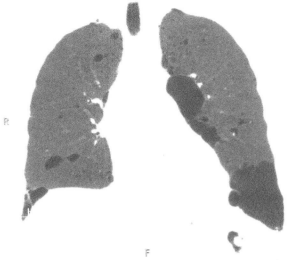

FIGURE 1-15 Coronal minimum intensity projection (MinIP) of a chest CT.

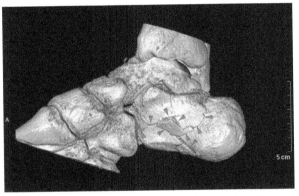

FIGURE 1-16 Three-dimensional volume-rendered display (CT) of the hindfoot showing multiple fractures of the calcaneus (red arrowheads).

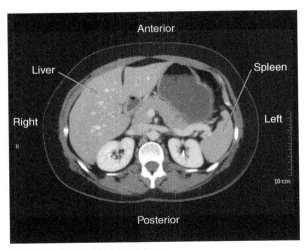

FIGURE 1-17 Axial CT of the abdomen.

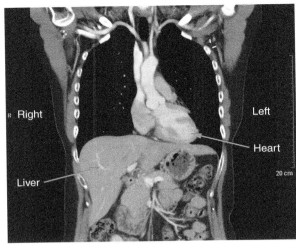

FIGURE 1-18 Coronal CT of the chest.

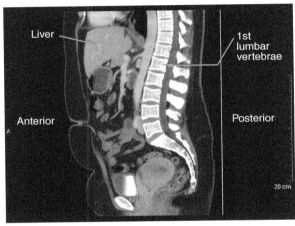

FIGURE 1-19 Sagittal CT of the abdomen.

Sagittal CT images are shown as though the patient is looking toward the viewer's left (Fig. 1-19).

CT is capable of capturing a much greater range of radiographic densities than can be appreciated by our visual system, which typically can differentiate about 16 shades of gray.

MRI also captures more than 16 levels of tissue signal intensity. Therefore, decisions must be made for the mapping of CT density levels and MR signal levels to the gray-scale values on an image used for viewing. These choices are referred to as windowing and leveling.

Because windowing and leveling in CT is a more important and clearly ordered process than in MRI, the following discussion will focus on CT. However, a similar process is followed when viewing MR scans.

The CT window is the range of densities that will be compressed into the shades of gray for viewing. In a narrow window CT image, only the CT densities within a limited range are assigned to various shades of gray, with tissues that have a CT density below that range depicted as black and tissue above that range depicted as white. The CT level refers to the mid density of the window. Narrow window CT images are perceived as high contrast, or very black and white, images. These images make conspicuous very slight differences in CT density among tissues but depict little contrast resolution for tissues outside the range chosen. A wide window CT image assigns broad ranges of CT density to each visible shade of gray but is perceived as a very low contrast, or very gray, image (Fig. 1-20).

MAGNETIC RESONANCE IMAGING

MRI does not involve patient exposure to ionizing radiation. MRI is based on the principle that protons may emit radio waves in the presence of strong magnetic fields and pulses of radiofrequency energy, neither of which have been shown to have significant biologic effects. Each set of images is the result of a series of radiofrequency pulses and variations in the magnetic field, known as a "pulse sequence." The physics of MRI is very complex and only a simplified description is provided here.

A typical MRI scanner looks grossly like a larger and thicker CT scanner (Fig. 1-21). Some MRI scanners, however, have different configurations, such as those open at the sides or vertically oriented. These "open" and "vertical" scanners may have some advantages for the claustrophobic patient but also may acquire images more slowly and may have reduced image quality compared with the closed scanners.

MRI scanners are often described by the strength of their primary magnet, typically 1.5 Tesla (unit of magnetic field strength). The primary magnetic field is modified by additional magnetic fields, resulting in varied magnetic field strengths or "gradients" that are used in the production of images. These fields affect the "spin" of hydrogen protons within the patient's body. Radiofrequency pulses are applied to these protons, which then emit radio waves (not that different from those received by your car radio) that are detected by antennas, called receiver coils. The output from those coils is used to create cross-sectional images. The specific gradient fields and radio pulses chosen for each set of images (known as a "pulse sequence") not only result in cross-sectional images in any chosen plane but also in the different appearance of tissues on the images.

The pulse sequences used in clinical MRI are quite varied, the most common of which are T1 or T2 spin echo, T1 or T2 fast spin echo, or T1 or T2* gradient echo sequences, as well as commonly used FLAIR and STIR sequences. Proprietary names for many pulse sequences available on MR scanners from different manufacturers are often referred to on radiology reports. However, sequences are often just referred to as either T1 or T2 sequences (or T1-weighted or T2-weighted) sequences.

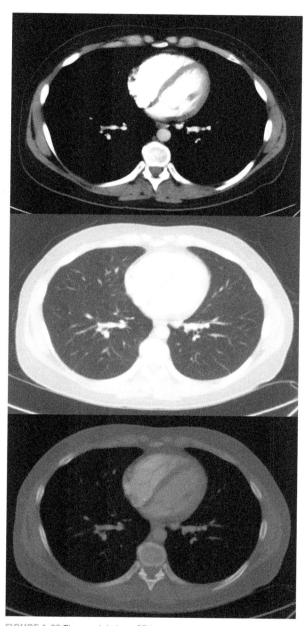

FIGURE 1-20 Three axial chest CT images using different window settings. The top image was made using a soft tissue window. In this image, the different soft tissue densities (note: muscles and intermuscular fat planes) and the bright contrast enhancement of blood in the heart are very conspicuous. The middle image was made using a lung window setting, in which lung markings, mainly pulmonary veins, are visible. The lower image was made using a bone window setting. With these window and level settings, you can see the distinction between marrow and cortical bone in the ribs.

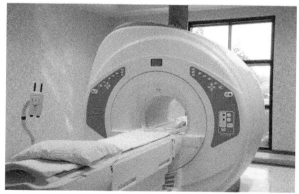

FIGURE 1-21 Photograph of a magnetic resonance (MR) scanner.

12

In T1 image sequences, fluid has low signal and appears dark on the image. Lipids and other specific tissues may have high signal and be bright (T1 hyperintensity). With contrast enhancement by a gadolinium-based contrast agent, tissue that contains the agent has high signal on T1-weighted images. In T2-weighted images, fluids (or tissue with high water content) have a high signal and appear bright (T2 hyperintensity) (Fig. 1-22 and Table 1.2). PD (proton density) sequences are neither T1 nor T2 weighted.

There are both T1 and T2 sequences that use a variety of techniques to suppress the MR signal from lipid, so that high signal from a lipid-containing tissue does not obscure high signal from adjacent high signal fluid or a gadolinium-enhanced tissue. These are referred to as fat suppressed ("FS") sequences.

MRI has intrinsically better soft tissue contrast resolution than CT. For that reason, there are many imaging examinations, such as internal derangement of the knee, in which MRI is vastly superior to CT. In other situations in which

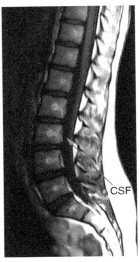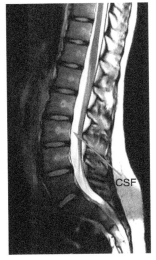

FIGURE 1-22 T1-weighted and T2-weighted axial MR lumbar spine images. Note that the cerebrospinal fluid (CSF) is hyperintense (bright) in T2 image and hypointense (dark) in T1 image.

TABLE 1-2 **Comparison of the Typical Appearance of Tissues on T1 and T2 MR Images***

Tissue Type	T1-Weighted Images	T2-Weighted Images
Fluid	Dark	Bright
Air	Black	Black
Muscle	Intermediate	Intermediate to dark
Tendon	Very dark	Very dark
Bone cortex	Black	Black
Bone marrow	Bright	Intermediate to bright
Fat	Very bright	Intermediate to bright
Gadolinium	Bright to very bright	No change from non-contrast (dark in high concentrations)

*Dark means low signal intensity, shown on images as darker shades of gray or black; bright means high signal intensity, shown on images as lighter shades of gray or white; intermediate signal intensity is assigned to an intermediate shade of gray on images.

either MRI or CT would be equally appropriate for diagnostic evaluation, but in which intravenous contrast administration (either iodinated- or gadolinium-based) is contraindicated by issues such as renal failure, unenhanced MRI is usually superior to unenhanced CT.

Because of the very strong magnetic fields associated with MRI, most metal objects should be removed from the patient before he or she enters the MRI room. Any other object that could also be affected by the magnet, such as credit cards, should also be removed. For surgically implanted (or otherwise embedded) metallic devices and objects, the issue becomes quite complicated, both with respect to safety and reduced image quality (because of the effect of such metal on the magnetic field). Do not make the assumption that because your patient has such an implanted metallic device he or she cannot undergo MRI. It depends upon the metals used, the shape of the objects, and the specific anatomic location involved. Many patients are given cards for their devices pertaining to MRI safety. Consult with the imaging facility you are referring the patient to in order to determine whether the patient can undergo MRI. A valuable resource to use is the web site www.MRIsafety.com.

MRI is an expensive diagnostic modality and may be difficult for the patient to undergo for psychological reasons, most notably claustrophobia. It has very high contrast resolution but is not the ideal imaging modality for every case. For example, compact bone has little or no MRI signal and therefore CT is better than MRI for cortical bone. The presentation of axial, sagittal, and coronal MR images is the same as in CT.

ULTRASOUND

Ultrasound was first developed for medical diagnostics in the middle of the twentieth century. In ultrasound, high frequency sound waves (1 to 30 MHz) are produced by a transducer, usually in contact with the skin. Pulses of sound waves are reflected back (echoed) to the transducer at interfaces between and within body tissues. Using an estimate of the speed of sound, the ultrasound unit places a dot (typically white) on the monitor screen at the locations that represent the positions from which each echo occurred. These dots create a cross-sectional image of the anatomy at the projected plane of the transducer on the body (Fig. 1-23).

A fluid-filled structure that contains no debris, precipitate, or cells will not have any interfaces within it to reflect sound. The fluid will be anechoic; on the image there will not be any echoes within a homogenous fluid collection. The echogenicity (level of gray or brightness on an ultrasound image) of soft tissue is described in relation to other tissues. Tissue that has the same echogenicity as the predominate

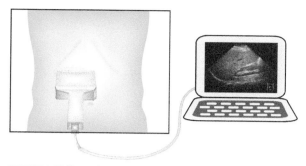

FIGURE 1-23 Illustration of ultrasound transducer on skin, with the blue material representing ultrasound gel, which acts to facilitate the transmission of the sound waves from the transducer to the skin.

tissue in an ultrasound image is isoechoic. Tissue that has fewer and weaker echoes is darker than a reference tissue and is considered hypoechoic. A tissue that has many strong echoes (bright) may be described as hyperechoic.

Because sound travels unimpeded through fluid, the echoes that are deep to a fluid collection (the "far side" in relation to the transducer) are brighter than in adjacent tissue. This is referred to as acoustic enhancement. A structure that blocks the transmission of the sound waves will cause an acoustic shadow (Fig. 1-24).

There is such a strong acoustic interface between tissue and air, and between soft tissue and bone, that diagnostic ultrasound is extremely limited when air-containing or osseous structures intervene in the field of view of an ultrasound transducer. It is not uncommon in an ultrasound report to state, for example, that a particular structure, such as the tail

of the pancreas, is not seen "because of bowel gas shadowing." In the chest or upper abdomen, acoustic shadows from the ribs may obscure underlying structures such as portions of the spleen or liver.

No study has clearly demonstrated any medical risks to a patient from an ultrasound exam. There has been some speculation that repeated ultrasound examinations during pregnancy may potentially harm the fetus, but again, this is unproven and unlikely because the sound waves used are very low power.

It is difficult to make generalized statements comparing the spatial and contrast resolution of ultrasound to radiography, CT, and MRI. The properties of tissues that result in echoes in ultrasound are different properties than those that cause attenuation of x-rays or produce signal in MRI.

Ultrasound images tend to be more difficult to interpret than CT, MRI, or radiography because the display of anatomic structures completely depends on the particular orientation and angulation of the transducer at any given moment during this generally "free hand" imaging modality. When examining the patient using a transducer, the examiner uses whatever transducer orientation maximizes the visualization of the structure of interest. Accordingly, ultrasound images rarely are oriented along strict anatomic planes (e.g., sagittal). Interpretation of ultrasound images, therefore, depends on the recognition of patterns of structures and is often very difficult for the novice (Fig. 1-25).

Most clinical ultrasound units used today are also equipped to visually identify, characterize, and quantify moving fluid, typically blood, based on Doppler principles. This allows differentiation among tubular structures based upon characteristics such as the direction and velocity of the fluid

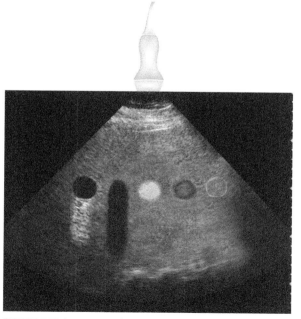

FIGURE 1-24 Appearance of common elements in ultrasound images. From left to right: acoustic enhancement posterior to an anechoic fluid-filled structure; acoustic shadowing; and hyperechoic, isoechoic, and hypoechoic structures.

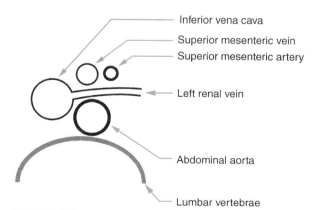

Inferior vena cava
Superior mesenteric vein
Superior mesenteric artery
Left renal vein
Abdominal aorta
Lumbar vertebrae

FIGURE 1-25 A common anatomic geometric pattern that illustrates how pattern recognition aids in the identification of anatomic structures on ultrasound images, even when spatial resolution and contrast resolution is limited. Specifically, in this case, note how the left renal vein passes anterior to the abdominal aorta to drain into the inferior vena cava, and the location of the superior mesenteric artery and vein anterior to that vein. This is a unique pattern that positively identified this set of structures.

flow. Abnormal flow can also be identified. For a simple example, the lack of blood flow in a painful testicle strongly suggests testicular torsion, which, if not surgically corrected, can lead to testicular infarction.

Recent model ultrasound units have become much better at producing higher resolution images than in the past and at the same time have become relatively inexpensive. These units are becoming increasing prevalent in emergency care departments, specialty clinics, and even in primary care settings. There have been some suggestions that the use of small ultrasound units may eventually be part of the routine physical examination. We will discuss the growing clinical application of ultrasound in many sections of this book.

As noted earlier, ultrasound images are not always oriented in strictly orthogonal (axial, coronal, sagittal) planes. Nevertheless, certain conventions of viewing ultrasound images are used. Ultrasound images that are close to being in the axial plane should be presented and viewed in the same orientation as described earlier for axial CT images. Images that are close to the sagittal plane are shown as if the viewer is looking at those sections from the right side of a supine patient, with the head end of the patient to the viewer's left and the foot end to the viewer's right (Fig. 1-26).

Ultrasound is a very "operator dependent" modality and successful results require varied degrees of skill, depending upon the clinical situation. Thus, while the identification of free fluid in the abdominal cavity after trauma may be very straightforward, the identification of a rotator cuff tear is much more difficult, requiring intensive training in musculoskeletal ultrasound. Furthermore, patient habitus has a strong effect on ultrasound image quality—the quality of ultrasound images may vary with the quantity of adipose tissue.

COST-EFFECTIVE MEDICINE
Ultrasound is often chosen by physicians seeking the least expensive imaging procedure for a particular clinical situation, and its use, when appropriate, provides significant savings compared with CT or MRI.

NUCLEAR MEDICINE

This discussion of nuclear medicine is limited to the most common procedures that are likely to be done on your patients. The fundamental imaging technique in nuclear medicine is scintigraphy, which is the creation of images that depend on the detection of the nuclear decay of elements that are distributed in body tissues via radiopharmaceuticals administered to the patient. Nuclear medicine is fundamentally different from other types of radiologic imaging because it emphasizes physiology rather than morphology. The images produced by nuclear medicine procedures have poor spatial resolution but can provide functional information about body tissues and organs that cannot be obtained any other way. Nuclear medicine images may be projectional or "planar," or may be cross-sectional images.

Prior to undergoing a nuclear medicine scan, the patient is injected with a radiopharmaceutical, which combines a radionuclide with a compound that has a biochemical affinity for the structure or process that is of interest. Once injected intravenously, the radionuclide emits radiation that can be detected by a device, commonly a gamma camera. Within the camera are crystals that detect the gamma radiation. When a gamma photon strikes the crystal, it emits light that is detected by photomultiplier tubes, which in turn are connected to a computer that produces a scintigraphic image (Fig.1-27).

The nuclear medicine scan depicts the regional distribution of radionuclide within the body. Either an increased or decreased uptake of the radionuclide compared with normal can indicate a disease process. In many cases, the time frame for tissue uptake of a radionuclide may provide important physiologic information.

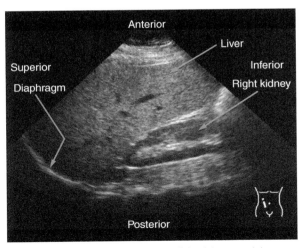

FIGURE 1-26 Sagittal ultrasound image of the right upper abdomen.

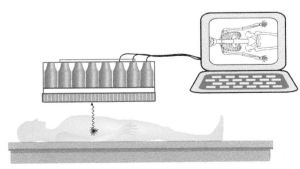

FIGURE 1-27 Schematic depiction of a nuclear medicine scanner.

The risks associated with nuclear medicine are quite small. The radiation exposure varies depending on the procedure but is typically less than that of a CT scan. Routine planar gamma camera images are displayed so that the viewer sees the subject from the same position as the gamma camera. An anterior view is thus presented as if the viewer is looking at the anterior of the patient; and a posterior view is displayed as if the viewer is looking at the posterior aspect of the patient (Fig. 1-28).

When the gamma camera acquires data from multiple positions, a cross-sectional representation of the distribution of scintillation events can be obtained. This is called single photon emission computed tomography (SPECT) imaging. Cross-sectional images in nuclear medicine are viewed the same way as CT and MRI (Fig. 1-29).

Positron emission tomography (PET) differs from typical nuclear medicine in its use of radioisotopes that emit

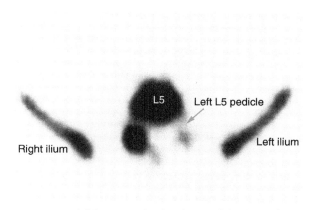

FIGURE 1-29 Axial cross-sectional nuclear medicine image from a SPECT radionuclide bone scan. Note the markedly asymmetric intense abnormal activity that is localized to the right posterior elements of L5.

positrons. The positrons travel only a very short distance before striking an electron, resulting in a pair of gamma rays being emitted in opposite directions. These are detected by the PET machine. The geometry of the gamma emission and the PET scanner result in cross-sectional representations of the radiopharmaceutical distribution. Currently, the primary PET radiopharmaceutical used is F-18-labeled fluorodeoxyglucose (FDG). The distribution of this agent depends on glucose metabolism and is primarily used to reveal the enhanced glucose metabolism in most cancers. Similar to typical nuclear medicine, PET images are generally relatively poor in spatial resolution (Fig. 1-30).

PET scans can be superimposed on CT scans done simultaneously. With PET-CT, the displayed cross-sectional images clearly depict foci of abnormal metabolic activity with high excellent anatomic localization. New scanners are now being introduced that can perform simultaneous PET and MR scans. PET scanning is at the forefront of the next fundamental way in which we will be examining patients in the future, known as molecular imaging.

INTERVENTIONAL RADIOLOGY

Interventional radiologists use image guidance to perform minimally invasive (non-surgical) procedures for diagnosis or treatment. Charles Theodore Dotter was instrumental in introducing numerous techniques of interventional radiology that are commonly done today. He published a report on the non-surgical treatment of severe arterial stenosis by the use of catheter angiography and balloon angioplasty in 1964. The medical world was introduced to the technique for percutaneously inserting a catheter into an artery by Seldinger in 1953.

Interventional radiology has expanded far beyond intra-arterial diagnostic studies and the restoration of arterial

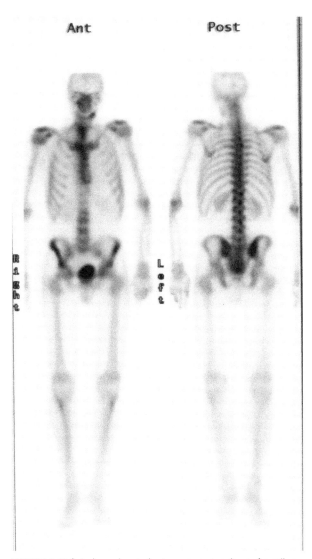

FIGURE 1-28 Anterior and posterior gamma camera views of a radionuclide bone scan.

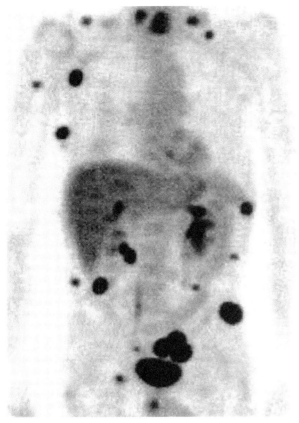

FIGURE 1-30 Anterior image from a PET scan; foci of increased activity suggest metastatic tumors.

patency with balloon angioplasty and stenting. Percutaneous (penetrating the skin surface with a needle, not a surgical incision) procedures have been developed to provide drainage of abscesses and to provide urinary drainage proximal to an obstructed urinary system. In 1981, one of the authors of this book published an article with Dr. Constantine Cope, "Percutaneous Biliary Bypass in Malignant Obstructions," which showed a better outcome for certain patients with malignant biliary obstruction when a minimally invasive procedure was used to establish biliary drainage than when surgery was performed. Interventional radiology has been instrumental to progress in providing medical care with progressively less discomfort and morbidity.

STRENGTHS AND WEAKNESSES OF IMAGING MODALITIES

Radiography is widely available, safe, and relatively inexpensive compared with cross-sectional imaging and has exquisitely high spatial resolution. High detail is critically important for some diagnoses. For example, the identification of the very fine calcifications in the breast that may indicate the presence of early breast cancer requires high spatial resolution that is not found in other modalities. The major weaknesses of radiography are the potentially misleading appearance of overlapping structures, which can be avoided with cross-sectional imaging, and the relatively poor soft tissue contrast resolution.

CT is cross-sectional, usually very rapid, easily tolerated by the patient, and can provide excellent soft tissue contrast resolution, especially with the use of intravenous contrast enhancement. CT is generally more expensive than radiography and exposes the patient to a higher dose of ionizing radiation.

MRI is cross-sectional, uses no ionizing radiation, and provides superb soft tissue contrast resolution. It may be a long procedure, difficult for claustrophobic patients, may not be safe for some patients, and is expensive.

Ultrasound is cross-sectional, uses no ionizing radiation, may provide excellent detail for certain tissues, and is relatively inexpensive. However, many body structures containing air, such as lung and much of the gastrointestinal (GI) tract, have such strongly echogenic interfaces that ultrasound exams are ineffective when these structures intervene. The surfaces of bone can be visualized with ultrasound, but the reflection of the beam is so great at the bone surface that viewing osseous structures with sonography is extremely limited.

CONTRAST ENHANCEMENT

Understanding the proper use of contrast-enhanced imaging is fundamental to radiology. The ideal use of various contrast agents may be required for diagnosis, but sometimes "contrast" (common clinical shorthand for administered contrast agents) can obscure a diagnostic finding, be medically contraindicated, or increase the risk of a procedure.

To increase radiographic density within the GI tract, various recipes of colloidal suspensions of barium sulfate are available. These are used for swallowing studies; examinations of the esophagus, stomach, and duodenum ("upper GI exam"); and examination of the small bowel. In CT of the abdomen and pelvis, dilute solutions of barium are used to opacify the lumen of bowel loops.

Iodinated contrast materials are used in radiography and in CT in order to increase the radiographic density of vessels, various tissues, and the lumen of the urinary system when the contrast agents are excreted. Iodinated contrast agents are most often administered intravenously. There is generally very little risk associated with the use of iodinated contrast agents. Severe allergic reactions are rare. Many patients who report that they have had a previous allergic reaction to such agents are mistaken, confusing common mild, transient physiologic reactions such as warmth or flushing with allergic-type reactions. If a patient has a documented history of true allergic or anaphylactoid reaction to previously administered IV contrast material, then consultation with a radiologist should be obtained before proceeding further with imaging. There are significant risks to the use of these contrast agents in patients with renal failure. Patients with insulin-dependent diabetes who have even mild decrease in renal function pose a special risk. Imaging departments/facilities all have specific policies that address this issue, such as requiring a serum creatinine be obtained on all diabetic patients prior to an elective procedure involving the IV injection of contrast material.

If you have any concerns about how a patient's significant or acute medical condition may impact the use of iodinated contrast agent, consultation with a radiologist is advised.

The gadolinium-based contrast agents used in MRI are generally considered to be quite safe. However, in 2010 the U.S. Food and Drug Administration issued a warning that these agents may pose a risk to patients with advanced renal failure. Some very ill patients with renal failure who had large doses and/or multiple doses of gadolinium-based contrast material (GBCM) within a short time frame developed a systemic illness called nephrogenic systemic fibrosis (NSF). However, recently established policies now widely used by imaging facilities governing the use of GBCM have virtually eliminated this risk. Therefore, the referring practitioner may be required to assess the renal status of patients prior to MRI.

Contrast enhancement of vessels in radiographic angiography, computed tomography angiography (CTA), and magnetic resonance angiography (MRA) is accomplished by the rapid injection of a contrast agent, followed by rapid acquisition of images before the contrast agent "leaks" out of the intravascular compartment.

The timing and pattern of the enhancement of normal and pathologic tissues, however, is a more complex subject. In the case of renal enhancement, active transport and concentration of contrast materials is involved. In central nervous system (CNS) imaging, it is the lack of blood-brain barrier in pathologic tissues that allows accumulation of contrast material in the interstitial space. This results in a change in a tissue's radiographic density (radiography and CT) or tissue's T1 intensity (MRI).

Generally, the degree of contrast enhancement usually varies with the vascularity of tissues. As a general principle, inflamed tissues that are hyperemic tend to display more intense enhancement than normal tissue in both CT and MRI. One can also differentiate viable tissue from necrotic debris by whether or not a tissue enhances.

An excellent example of the use of contrast enhancement in MRI is that post-operative contrast-enhancing epidural fibrosis (vascularized tissue) can be differentiated from a recurrent or new disc herniation (disc material with little or no vascularity) by the presence or absence of contrast enhancement after the administration of a gadolinium-based contrast agent during MRI.

THE RADIOLOGY WORKSTATION AND PACS SYSTEMS

The workstation at which medical images are interpreted and the electronic systems that distribute those images are now critically important components of diagnostic imaging. They are almost as critical as the CT, MR, and other scanners that acquire those images. You need to understand the issues involved with this part of the "imaging train" just as you must understand the basics of ultrasound or CT scanning.

When you receive patient images from a radiology facility, the images will likely include software that will enable you to page through the sets of images that have been prepared for such viewing. You will not usually be provided with the entire imaging dataset that radiologists and radiology technologists use at much more advanced computer stations, which can manipulate the image datasets to produce advanced reconstructions such as the 3D image shown in Figure 1-16.

Many imaging studies done today produce an astonishingly large number of sections. For example, with multidetector CT scanners capable of capturing cross-sectional images as thin as 0.5 mm, scanning of a patient's chest, abdomen, and pelvis in a trauma case can result in hundreds or even thousands of images. From the original thin axial slices or "dataset," a set of thicker axial images is typically prepared for viewing by software that sums the data from the original images into the thick slices. Similar sets of reconstructed coronal and sagittal images are prepared. These are the sets of images that are scrolled through at terminals or that you will typically scroll through on your computer if you have received images through a network or on disk.

Digital imaging data may sometimes be evaluated by software in addition to being evaluated by a radiologist, a process that is called "computer aided detection" (CAD). This is most widely used now in mammography. CAD systems place marks on mammographic images that the software "flags" as potentially significant. There is no doubt that the use of CAD improves interpretation of mammograms. Early breast cancers are detected sooner with CAD than without. However, it is not yet entirely clear whether the use of CAD has made a significant difference in the stage at which breast cancers have been diagnosed by screening, or if there is a statistically significant improvement in final patient outcome when CAD is used in mammography screening. The use of CAD in breast diagnosis, chest imaging interpretation, and other areas will continue to be refined and will increase in importance.

The archiving and distribution of medical images (and reports) is now in the domain of picture archiving and communication systems (PACS) and the information technology (IT) staff. The management of the distribution of images by the IT staff and design of PACS system must deal with the conflict between concern for confidentiality of patient information and accessibility to images by various health care providers. Distribution of medical images on the internet, even in "the cloud," increases access to images but must be done with careful controls to protect privacy.

The widespread access to images via PACS and the internet, when coupled with modern communications systems, facilitates consultation between you and the radiologists who are engaged in their role in the care of your patients.

THE RADIOLOGY REQUISITION AND THE RADIOLOGY REPORT

The radiology requisition or "order" is an important clinical tool. The proper use of this tool may be critical in determining the most ideal imaging protocol. These protocols require the kind of clinical history and clinical impression that the patient is rarely able to provide while in the imaging department or facility. Therefore, you should include history, findings on physical exam, relevant laboratory findings, and clinical diagnosis on every imaging order. Important diagnostic imaging findings can often be subtle or uncertain. Providing appropriate clinical information to the radiologist can mean the difference between establishing a correct diagnosis and having an important piece of information lost because of poor communication between medical practitioners. It is patient outcome that always matters most. When filling out an imaging order, one should remember that one does not provide information "for the radiologist" so much as provide information to the radiologist "for the patient." Within the subsequent chapters of this book we provide tables showing the types of patient information that should be provided to the radiologist on the imaging requisition. These tables are divided up into two columns: (1) specification of imaging procedure ordered and (2) the concise clinical data relevant to the procedure, using common medical abbreviations that can make this process simple and quick.

This book provides foundational knowledge useful in deciding which imaging procedure will be most appropriate in various clinical situations. However, the ideal procedure for your patient can vary with technologic changes, locally available equipment and advances in the practice of diagnostic radiology. One of the roles and responsibilities of the radiologist is to consult with you about imaging on your patients. Take advantage of that.

When ordering specific procedures, it is important to use proper terminology for those exams that utilize various contrast enhancing techniques. When the phrase "CT with contrast" or "MRI with contrast" is used, it is usually understood to mean that a study is done with an intravenous injection of contrast material, whether iodinated contrast agents in CT or gadolinium-based contrast agents in MRI. Intra-arterial injections of iodinated contrast agents through catheters are invasive angiographic examinations and are very different from a "CT scan with contrast" even though the agent used may be the same or very nearly the same in both exams. When a vascular study is needed and the diagnosis can be determined without invasive catheter angiography (still the "gold standard" of vascular imaging) it is important that you specify a "CT angiogram" or "MR angiogram" be done, not just a CT or MRI "with contrast." For the imaging of joints, whether a radiographic, CT, or MR arthrogram is done, contrast agents are injected directly into a joint for optimum visualization of structures. Arthrography is far superior to routine imaging for many joint conditions (see Chapter 2). You must be specific in requesting an arthrogram when needed. For example, request an "MR shoulder arthrogram" rather than an "MRI of the shoulder with contrast."

Just as it is critical that the referring medical practitioner thoroughly communicate patient details along with the imaging requisition, it is also critical that the radiology report effectively communicates the diagnostic information revealed by the imaging studies performed on the patient.

An ideal radiology report should contain four basic sections: demographics, clinical information, descriptive information, and diagnostic conclusion.

<u>Demographics</u>: includes patient identifiers (name, sex, age, etc.); facility name and location; referring practitioner; and basic type of imaging examination performed.

<u>Clinical Information</u>: contains a short summary of the clinical information provided by the referring practitioner and, if available, the International Statistical Classification of Diseases and Related Health Problems Codes (ICD-9) for the patient's condition.

<u>Descriptive Information</u>: includes a description of the specific imaging studies performed, including use of any contrast media and any patient reaction; description of radiologic findings using appropriate anatomic and pathologic terminology; listings of any limitations of the findings associated with the sensitivity and specificity of the imaging procedures; and details of comparisons with any available previous radiologic studies.

<u>Diagnostic Conclusion</u>: contains as precise a diagnosis as possible with a differential diagnosis; lists any recommendations for additional studies. Some radiologic findings, such as fractures, are definitive. Others may only suggest a diagnosis that

requires confirmation by either correlation with clinical and laboratory data, additional testing, or biopsy.

Because the final radiology report is the definitive means of communication between the radiologist and the referring practitioner, it should be clearly written with minimal or no typographical errors. It must also follow any appropriate state or federal regulations (e.g., for mammography reporting). Finally, the report must be transmitted by optimal means to the referring practitioner in a very timely manner.

When appropriate (e.g., an emergency situation), a radiologist should provide a preliminary report by personal direct communication, in addition to the formal report.

HOW SAFE IS MEDICAL IMAGING?

The risk of harm from radiation is related to an individual's absorbed dose, although there is debate about the exact mathematical relationship. The dose is expressed in millisieverts (mSv). Yearly background radiation exposure in the United States is approximately 6.2 mSv and is greater for individuals living at high elevations. Smoking adds approximately 2.8 mSv per year. A single PA chest radiograph exposes the patient to 0.02 mSv. CT of the head exposes the patient to 2 mSv.

Abdominal CT exposure has been estimated at 8 mSv, but this is quite variable with the protocol used, and many scans are now being done with protocols that reduce this exposure. The most recent generation of scanners are incorporating advanced techniques to further reduce the radiation dose.

A discussion of the risk of cancer from radiation exposure is found in Chapter 12.

Ultrasound exams have never shown deleterious biologic effects, although there is a theoretical risk (never proven) that prenatal ultrasound exams could pose a very small risk to the fetus. Therefore, prenatal ultrasound exams should only be done for specific medical indications. In the adult, there is simply no risk from diagnostic ultrasound.

The magnetic fields and RF pulses used in clinical MRI cause no biologically significant tissue changes; MRI poses no medical risk. However, caution is needed when a patient has embedded metallic objects, as discussed in the MR section earlier.

The intravenous injection of iodinated contrast agents is associated with the risk of nephrotoxicity and very low risks of significant reactions, discussed in the previous section on Contrast Enhancement. Transient subjective sensations of heat and flushing are quite common and are not significant. Mild allergic-type reactions, such as urticaria, may occur in a small percentage of patients. The fatality rate from reaction to iodinated contrast agents, predominately anaphylactoid reactions, is in the range of 1:70,000 to 1:100,000.

The rare risk of NSF caused by the use of gadolinium-based contrast media (GBCM) in patients with renal failure was discussed in the Contrast Enhancement section earlier. Acute allergic-type reactions to GBCM are rare—less than 1% of injections. Only a small fraction of these are severe. The mortality rate from acute reactions to GBCM is so low that it has been hard to calculate, but most likely it is similar to the rate cited earlier for intravenous iodinated contrast agents.

Only about 1% to 2% of patients who undergo interventional radiologic procedures, such as catheter angiography, suffer a serious complication that may require further intervention or hospitalization. For common procedures such as image guided breast biopsies, the incidence rate of significant complications is well under 1%.

Chapter Review

Chapter Review Questions

1. Which of the following is not correct about the summation density at a particular point on a radiograph?

   A. The thickness of all of the structures along the path of the x-ray affects the density

   B. The x-ray attenuation (mean atomic number) of tissues along the path of the x-ray beam to that point affects the resulting radiographic density

   C. Overlap of structures anywhere along the path of the x-ray beam to that point, whether or not they are actually physically related, affect the radiographic density at that point

   D. It is typically presented on a radiology report as a Hounsfield number

   E. If the point is along the esophagus, it may be increased through the ingestion of a barium solution

2. In an AP projection of the chest:

   A. the heart is likely to appear enlarged compared with a PA projection.

   B. cardiac size is likely to appear reduced compared with a PA projection.

   C. the lungs are likely to appear more dense compared with a PA projection.

   D. the lungs are likely to appear less dense compared with a PA projection.

   E. contrast resolution of the vertebral column is likely to be better than in a PA projection.

3. Which of the following is incorrect about viewing radiologic images?

   A. Axial CT images are presented as if the viewer is standing at the foot of the patient's bed and the patient is lying in a supine position

   B. Sagittal MR images are shown as if the patient is looking toward the viewer's left

   C. Radiographic chest images are viewed as if the viewer is looking at the back of the patient

   D. Sagittal ultrasound images are viewed as if the viewer is looking at the right side of the patient, with the head end of the patient toward the viewer's left

   E. An axial nuclear medicine image is viewed the same way as an axial CT image

4. In CT:

   A. Thin sections are more likely to result in partial volume averaging errors than thicker sections

   B. Patients are typically exposed to less ionizing radiation than in a normal chest radiograph

   C. Images from subsequent axial sections are used to make a mammogram

   D. Gadolinium is used as a contrast agent

   E. Special images such as MIPs may be produced

5. In MRI:

   A. Images are created by projection of multiple laser beams of light through the body

   B. A T2-weighted image typically shows fluids as bright (high signal intensity)

   C. Multiple MRI scans within a short period have been shown to increase the risk of cancer

   D. Cost is typically less than CT

   E. Patients usually feel more comfortable than undergoing CT because MRI is a faster procedure

6. If a patient has an implanted metallic device, you may need to consult with the radiologist about safety issues before scheduling the patient to undergo:

   A. CT

   B. MRI

   C. Ultrasound

   D. Radionuclide bone scan

   E. Chest x-ray

7. You have a patient whom you suspect has a facial fracture more extensive than a simple nasal fracture. The best imaging modality to confirm your diagnosis and clearly show the position of the fracture fragments is most likely to be:

   A. MRI.

   B. ultrasound.

   C. maxillofacial CT.

   D. nuclear medicine.

   E. radiography.

8. "Bowel gas shadowing" is associated with:

   A. MRI.

   B. ultrasound.

   C. CT.

   D. nuclear medicine.

   E. radiography.

2 SHOULDER, PELVIS, AND LIMBS

CASE STUDY

A 55-year-old male sees you in clinic with a chief complaint of shoulder pain. Patient history reveals a recent lifting injury, but upon further questioning, the patient admits to mild chronic discomfort in the shoulder. Physical exam shows questionable mild weakness of abduction and a full range of motion. No neck maneuvers elicit or worsen the pain and there are no sensory findings to suggest radiculopathy. No other joint is symptomatic. You order radiography of the shoulder.

EXTREMITIES

FUNDAMENTALS OF MUSCULOSKELETAL IMAGING

When musculoskeletal imaging is referred to radiology, the imaging process starts with the information that you detail on the imaging requisition (Table 2-1). Proper attention to this part of the process benefits the patient by increasing the sensitivity of detection of subtle abnormalities by the radiologist. Relevant clinical information leads to clinically appropriate recommendations and may result in a report that focuses on, or emphasizes, your current clinical concern while minimizing the sometimes lengthy reporting on findings that are not clinically significant.

In acute trauma cases the requisition should indicate the mechanism of injury and findings on physical exam, such as point tenderness. In chronic conditions, history and findings on physical exam, such as the location (medial or lateral) of joint line tenderness, positive McMurray test for meniscus tear, and important laboratory results such as elevated sedimentation rate, must be included. It seems obvious to state, but important to emphasize, that many radiologic findings can be subtle, equivocal, or confusing. Better patient care occurs when the clinical care provider communicates with the radiologist about a specific clinical concern.

Patients do not always provide ideal medical histories when undergoing diagnostic testing. For example, a patient with an apparent orthopedic problem may not think to tell Radiology that she has a history of breast cancer. Should the radiologist see some subtle bone changes on radiographs, or equivocal bone marrow signal changes on MRI, your efforts to provide relevant medical history could be critical in whether or not a subtle metastatic lesion is perceived. You do not provide such important relevant medical history "for the radiologist." You do so for the benefit of the patient.

The relative value of different imaging modalities in musculoskeletal imaging is presented in Table 2-2.

Almost all of the joints of the upper and lower limbs are synovial joints and therefore sites for the development of osteoarthritis (degenerative joint disease; DJD) or inflammatory joint disease (most commonly, rheumatoid arthritis; RA). The frequency of DJD and RA differs markedly at different joints. For example, DJD is relatively common in the hip and knee joints but uncommon in the shoulder joint. Regardless of the site, each condition has its own set of radiologic correlates (Table 2-3 and Table 2-4).

The features of DJD are very apparent radiographically. Loose joint bodies related to arthritis may be seen on radiographs, although when clinical findings suggest joint bodies and radiographs are normal, CT, MRI, or MR **arthrography** should be considered. (See Patient Communication Box 2-1.)

In the later stages of RA, joints become grossly deformed (subluxed) and eventually can become fused. In addition to clinical findings, laboratory evidence for RA, such as rheumatoid factor, are important for correlation with radiographic findings.

Fractures are identified on radiography as a break of cortical bone. The continuation of a fracture through trabecular bone does not contribute significantly to the linear radiolucency of a fracture visible on radiographs; radiographs essentially show only a cortical discontinuity.

 All fractures near growth plates in the immature skeleton must be characterized by the **Salter-Harris classification** system because prognosis and treatment decisions are dependent upon this organization of these fractures (Fig. 2-1). Of the nine types of Salter-Harris fractures, the first five are the most important:

Type I fractures are through the physis (growth plate).
Type II fractures are through the metaphysis and the physis.

TABLE 2-1 Sample Musculoskeletal Radiology Requisition Information

Modality	Body Region	Clinical Data/History
Radiography	Right hand	Hyperextension injury, point tenderness at third MCP joint
MRI (w/o contrast)	Left ankle	Inversion sprain 3 months ago with progressive pain; R/O peroneal tear
CT	Left wrist	Fall on outstretched hand, pain in snuff-box; radiographs negative; R/O scaphoid fx
MRI (contrast if needed)	Right foot	Diabetic patient; progressive foot pain, high sedimentation rate, borderline leukocytosis; Charcot foot vs. osteomyelitis
MR arthrography	Left knee	Medial meniscus surgery (posterior horn) 3 years ago; medial pain due to recent injury; positive McMurray; R/O recurrent tear

Type III fractures are through the physis and the epiphysis.
Type IV fractures involve the metaphysis, physis, and epiphysis.
Type V fractures are crush or compression injuries of the growth plate.

The variability in appearance of growth plates in children and adolescents may require consultation with a radiologist or reference material to avoid confusion when there is an "apparent" fracture, just as in the case of normal anatomic variants. In young patients especially, routine radiography of the contralateral side "for comparison" exposes a patient to excess ionizing radiation and should be avoided.

TABLE 2-3 Radiologic Features of Degenerative Joint Disease (DJD)

Feature	Definition	Modality
Reduction in "joint space"	Radiolucency of articular cartilage causes radiographic appearance of a "joint space." With degeneration of the articular cartilage in DJD, this joint space appears to be reduced, leading to bone on bone contact.	Radiography, weight bearing views for appropriate joints (joint space narrowing seen on CT; cartilage seen on MRI. But CT and MRI usually not needed for diagnosis of DJD)
Osteophyte (spur)	A bony projection (spur) that forms along the margin of an affected joint resulting from compensatory osteoblastic activity	Radiography
Sclerosis of subchondral bone	Increase in density of the cortical and trabecular bone immediately deep to the articular cartilage also resulting from compensatory osteoblastic activity	Radiography
Loose osteo-cartilaginous joint bodies	Degeneration-related fragments of bone or cartilage that freely float within the joint	Radiography and CT if calcified cartilage or bone. (MRI—variable detection)
Subchondral cysts	Radiolucencies beneath the cortex that are probably from intravasation of joint fluid through cartilage and cortical defects	Radiography and CT (seen well on MRI done for complications of DJD or other reason, such ACL tear)

COST-EFFECTIVE MEDICINE

Radiography, with its extremely high spatial resolution, is fundamental to the initial, and perhaps definitive, imaging evaluation of musculoskeletal trauma and disease. There has been a growing tendency in musculoskeletal diagnosis

TABLE 2-2 Radiologic Modalities and Musculoskeletal Imaging*

	Radiography	CT	MRI	Radionuclide Bone Scan
Cortical bone	Excellent, but problems with overlapping structures	Very good; cross-sectional images can overcome issue of overlapping structures	Fair to poor	Excellent sensitivity, but poor specificity
Medullary bone/bone marrow process	Not high sensitivity, but high specificity, i.e., for bone tumors	Fair to good	Good to excellent for edema, infiltrative processes	Excellent sensitivity, but poor specificity
Soft tissue calcifications	Very good	Excellent	Fair to poor	Positive during active deposition of calcium
Cartilage/joint space	Good; joint spaces can be evaluated during weight bearing	Good with arthrography	Good	
Ligaments	Poor without, but good with arthrography	Poor without, but good with arthrography	Good without, excellent with arthrography	
Tendons and muscles	Poor	Poor to fair	Very good to excellent	

*Ultrasound can be very poor to excellent for almost all the listed structures; however, because this modality is so user-dependent and so influenced by body habitus, it is impossible to make generalizations and so is not included in the table.

to bypass radiography in favor of cross-sectional imaging. However, for many clinical conditions, radiography can be definitive or can add visual perspective on a musculoskeletal problem that is as valuable as or even more valuable than cross-sectional imaging, such as MRI. As an example, important soft tissue calcifications may be obvious in radiographs but not apparent in MRI. Fine cortical erosions, important in diagnosis of joint disease, are best seen on radiographs. Certainly, radiography is usually more cost-effective than CT or MRI. Radiography is the mandatory initial imaging procedure for almost all disease of bone and joints.

Radiography, which is so fundamental in the diagnosis of musculoskeletal disease involving bones and joints, usually has little or no value in evaluating soft tissue masses. For confirmation of clinical suspicion that a soft tissue mass or focal swelling is a cystic lesion (such as a ganglion cyst) or simple subcutaneous lipoma, ultrasonography may be sufficient. However, other soft tissue masses, especially those suspicious for sarcomas, should be evaluated with MRI without and with contrast enhancement.

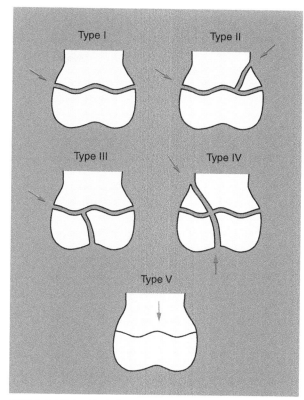

FIGURE 2-1 Salter-Harris fracture classification

TABLE 2-4 **Radiologic Correlates of Rheumatoid Arthritis (RA)**

Synovitis	Inflammation of synovial membrane, usually with joint effusion	MRI (contrast enhanced)
Juxta-articular bone demineralization	Decrease in bone density in the subchondral bone (unlike sclerosis of subchondral bone with DJD)	Radiography
Reduction in "joint space"	Loss of articular cartilage as in DJD but tends to occur uniformly in joint, whereas in DJD the joint space reduction is typically asymmetric	Radiography
Joint deformation	Loss of typical joint architecture with eventual fusion	Radiography

SHOULDER AND ARM

Trauma and Acute Pain

Acute post-trauma pain of the shoulder or arm is usually due to fracture and/or dislocation of the glenohumeral joint, acromioclavicular (AC) injury, rotator cuff tear, or proximal biceps tendon rupture. Diagnosis of the cause of acute shoulder or arm pain can usually be made by history, physical exam, and radiography. The physical exam is most important for ensuring that that the pain is indeed originating from the shoulder and not being referred to the site (e.g., radicular in origin) and for guiding the decision as to which imaging studies to request (or for determining that no imaging is needed).

Modalities

If your clinical exam of the acute shoulder patient suggests humeral head or glenoid fracture or glenohumeral dislocation, then a shoulder trauma radiographic series should be requested. The specific images that are associated with this series vary somewhat among practices but ideally consist of an AP shoulder with internal rotation view; a **scapular Y** view (lateral scapular) (Fig. 2-2); a **Grashey** view (posterior oblique with external rotation), which we mentioned and

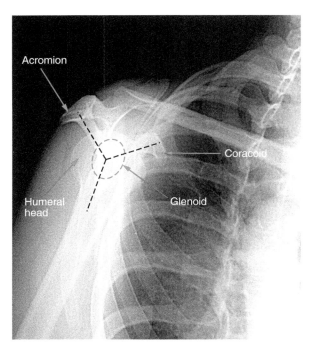

FIGURE 2-2 Normal Y view radiograph of the shoulder. Note that the humeral head overlies the glenoid. The Y is formed by the coracoid, acromion, and body of the scapula (dashed line).

showed in Chapter 1 (see Fig. 1-6); and an axillary view, which is shown in Figure 2-3. Although the first three of these views are taken in the erect position and use postures that generally can be tolerated even by the acutely injured patient, the axillary view requires arm abduction and may be precluded by the patient's pain.

Dislocation of the glenohumeral joint is a very common injury and can usually be appreciated in the frontal projection, but the geometric relationship between the dislocated humeral head and the glenoid fossa can be seen best on an axillary or Y view radiography. In a significant percentage of shoulder dislocations, a tear of the glenoid labrum occurs.

COST-EFFECTIVE MEDICINE

If there is significant clinical concern about a labral tear after shoulder dislocation, obtaining an MRI shortly after injury while post-traumatic fluid remains in the joint may avoid the subsequent need for MRI arthrography (a more expensive and invasive procedure that requires the injection of contrast media directly into the joint) by taking advantage of the post-traumatic joint fluid (Fig. 2-4).

Figure 2-4 shows this effect in that there is excess bright joint fluid, which is presumably blood, in the joint cavity in a patient shortly after shoulder trauma. Similarly, it may be reasonable with patients older than 40 years to obtain an MRI because there is a high incidence of rotator cuff tear after shoulder dislocation in this age group.

Glenoid fractures sometimes are associated with humeral head dislocations. An anteroinferior glenoid articular fracture is known as a Bankart fracture and may be visible on AP or axillary views. CT may also be needed for complex and displaced glenoid fractures.

If your clinical exam leads you to suspect that your patient has a humeral shaft fracture rather than an injury to the shoulder joint proper, AP and lateral humeral radiographs should be obtained. If your clinical exam indicates a clavicle fracture, then only AP views of the clavicle are generally needed. If a clavicular fracture needs additional evaluation, a 45-degree cephalic tilt AP radiograph can be ordered.

If pain, tenderness, and deformity are directly overlying the AC joint, an AC series of radiographs, consisting of PA views with and without weight-bearing (weights in the hand), should be requested in order to evaluate stability of the AC joint. Weight-bearing accentuates widening of an AC

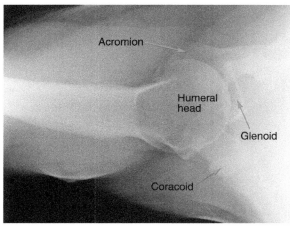

FIGURE 2-3 Normal axillary radiograph of the shoulder

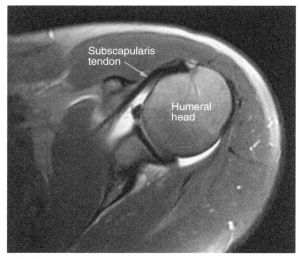

FIGURE 2-4 Axial T2 MRI of the shoulder. Note very bright intra-articular fluid, presumably a hemarthrosis when seen shortly after trauma.

joint with an advanced injury, resulting in the appearance of a "shoulder separation."

When a patient presents with acute shoulder pain and x-rays are normal, you should determine whether there is weakness associated with the shoulder pain. This would then suggest rotator cuff injury and an MRI should be requested. Patients with rotator cuff tears may also have tears of the tendon of the long head of the biceps.

Scapular fractures are unusual injuries and typically occur as a result of a high impact blow to the posterior shoulder such as in a motor vehicle accident (MVA). AP, Grashey, and scapular Y views are used to assess the scapula for fractures.

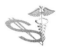 **COST-EFFECTIVE MEDICINE**
A CT scan improves the assessment of scapular fractures but is not usually necessary.

Interpretation

Figure 2-5 demonstrates a fracture of the anatomic neck of the humerus that is by definition intra-articular and often associated with fractures of the articular surface of the humeral head. In contrast, the fracture of the surgical neck of the humerus shown in Figure 2-6, which is similar to more distal humeral shaft fractures, does not disrupt the integrity the shoulder joint.

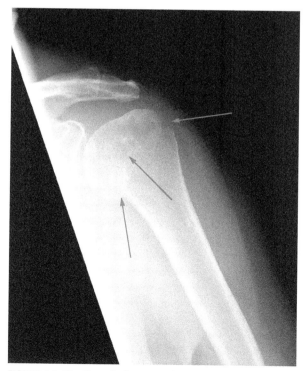

FIGURE 2-5 AP radiograph of an anatomic neck fracture (arrows) of the humerus. Note the abrupt step-off of the medial cortex of the humeral head caused by the fracture.

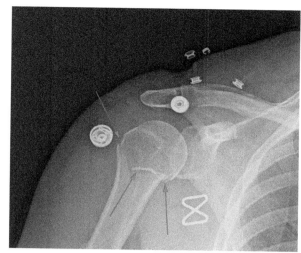

FIGURE 2-6 AP radiograph of a surgical neck fracture (arrows) of the humerus. Note the metallic objects that are patient gown clips.

Proximal humerus fractures are most commonly seen in the elderly after a fall. Fractures of the proximal humerus are classified by the location of the fracture line(s) and degree of displacement. Typically, if a single fragment is separated less than 1 cm from its anatomic position and has less than a 45-degree angulation, the injury can be treated non-surgically with immobilization. However, more displaced and angulated or comminuted fractures are likely to require surgery.

Surgical treatment of proximal humeral fractures is very dependent on the general health of the patient. Non-surgical treatment may be the best approach in elderly, infirm patients even in cases of multiple humeral head fractures.

Shoulder dislocations are classified as anterior or posterior depending on the displaced position of the humeral head relative to the glenoid fossa and typically just need to be reduced. Anterior dislocations are far more common, and occur when there is a force applied to the arm while it is abducted and externally rotated, resulting in a subcoracoid appearance of the humeral head on AP radiographs as seen in Figure 2-7. Figure 2-8 shows the radiographic appearance of a posterior dislocation, which occurs when there is a blow to the arm while it is in internal rotation and adduction and is most common in football players and in epileptic patients.

In cases similar to that shown in Figure 2-9 in which dislocation is complicated by a fracture (in this case a Bankart fracture), surgical treatment is likely needed based on the amount of displacement of the fractures.

Another fracture associated with glenohumeral dislocations is a compression fracture of the posterolateral aspect of the humeral head. This is known as a Hill-Sachs lesion and is a common deformity of the proximal humerus seen on radiographs of a shoulder that has suffered a previous anterior dislocation.

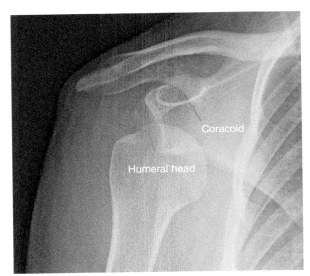

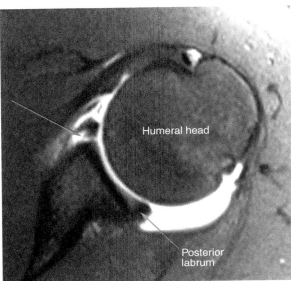

FIGURE 2-7 **Top:** AP radiograph of an anterior shoulder dislocation. Note the subcoracoid position of the humeral head (blue arrow). **Bottom:** Axial T1 MRI from shoulder MR arthrogram done 1 month later showing the anterior labral tear (red arrow) that presumably occurred when the humeral head impacted on the anterior labrum while dislocating anteriorly.

Clavicular fractures are classified by location as distal, middle, or medial, with distal fractures being the most common; most can be treated non-surgically, which would be the case for the mid-clavicular fracture shown in Figure 2-10.

AC joint separations are identified by the altered relationship between the distal clavicle and the acromion. AC injuries are classified based on severity, ranging from a sprain of the associated ligaments in which anatomic relationships are maintained to cases similar to that shown in Figure 2-11, in which there is severe disruption of all components of the joint including the coracoclavicular ligaments. If the latter ligaments rupture, surgical repair may be required.

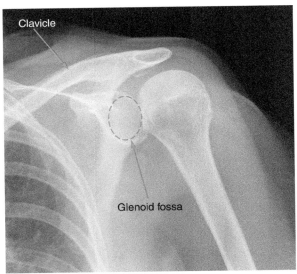

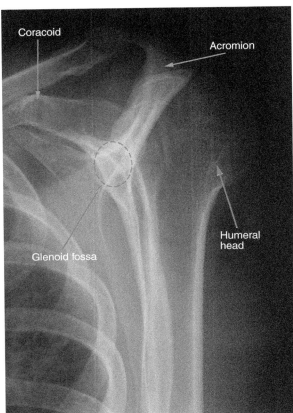

FIGURE 2-8 AP **(top)** and Y view **(bottom)** radiographs of posterior shoulder dislocation.

Most acute rotator cuff tears occur in tendons that are weakened by chronic tendinopathy. The interpretation of MRI for rotator cuff tears is discussed later in the section on chronic problems of the shoulder.

Scapular fractures are usually minimally displaced and do not need surgical treatment. Surgery is recommended only when the glenoid surface is disrupted.

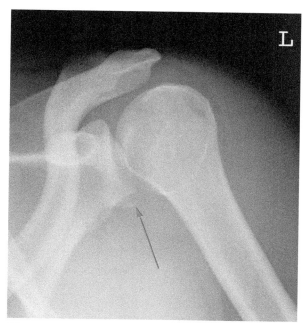

FIGURE 2-9 Grashey view shoulder radiograph, Bankart fracture. Note displaced fracture fragment of the glenoid rim (arrow).

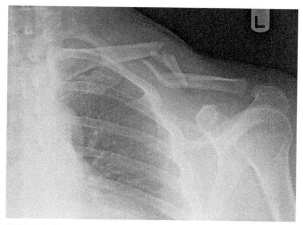

FIGURE 2-10 AP radiograph of clavicle fracture.

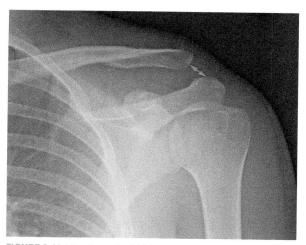

FIGURE 2-11 AP radiograph of AC joint separation. Note depression of acromion in relation to the distal end of the clavicle (and widened acromio-clavicular space; double-headed arrow).

Chronic Conditions of the Shoulder Including Soft Tissue Masses

Chronic conditions of the shoulder and upper arm include AC and glenohumeral joint arthritis (most commonly DJD), shoulder impingement, chronic rotator cuff tear, avascular necrosis of the humeral head, and bone tumors. A thorough history and physical exam is required for diagnosis and to guide the imaging evaluation.

Modalities

As with any musculoskeletal problem, the initial imaging examination for chronic shoulder pain is radiography, typically an AP with internal rotation, Grashey view, Y view, or outlet view (shoulder radiograph similar to Y view angled to best show the supraspinatus outlet—the space formed by the coracoacromial arch superiorly and shoulder joint proper inferiorly).

Patients with shoulder impingement usually show no weakness of the rotator cuff and full range of motion, but pain upon elevation and internal rotation. Shoulder impingement is primarily diagnosed clinically, although the presence of spurs (causing tendonitis of the rotator cuff tendons) on radiographs can be seen with impingement syndrome.

Pain is usually the presenting symptom of patients with arthritis of the shoulder. Chronic pain on the superior aspect of the shoulder with or without crepitation can be related to acromioclavicular joint DJD. This can be seen on AP and Grashey radiographic views. Often DJD of the AC joint can be a finding on radiographs even though patients do not complain of pain in that location. Chronic pain that is felt "deep" in the shoulder joint or in the anterior and lateral shoulder with crepitation and sometimes decreased motion can be related to glenohumeral joint DJD.

Chronic pain of the shoulder with gradual decrease of strength and sometimes range of motion can be associated with a rotator cuff tear. If AP, Grashey, axillary, and scapular Y views look normal in a patient with chronic, persistent pain that has not been relieved by conservative treatment, MRI should be considered. If a patient with subacute or chronic shoulder symptoms has clinical findings of a possible labral tear, MR shoulder arthrography is a far better procedure than routine shoulder MRI. In addition, patients who have had prior rotator cuff surgery and have recurrent symptoms should have shoulder MR arthrography, rather than routine shoulder MRI. There is no significant risk associated with shoulder arthrography, aside from the very small risk of allergic reaction to contrast agents.

Patients may have a rotator cuff or proximal biceps tendon tear even though they do not appear to be very weak or have a reduced range of motion. Many patients who undergo MRI for chronic shoulder pain are found to have rotator cuff tears.

If you suspect a patient has a rotator cuff tear but is one who cannot undergo MRI (perhaps because of a pacemaker; see Chapter 1), then an ultrasound of the shoulder is often done where the expertise is available. Ultrasound exams are technically demanding in obese patients. Radiographic arthrography may also show whether there is a full thickness tear of the rotator cuff, but may not show the width of the tear; more complete evaluation can be obtained with CT arthrography of the shoulder.

Patients with chronic pain who have history of sickle cell disease, previous trauma, alcoholism, chronic steroid use, or radiotherapy for cancer should get an MRI to evaluate for possible avascular necrosis of the humeral head.

Patients with persistent pain in the upper humeral area should get AP humeral radiographs. Most bone tumors can be seen on radiographs. A bone biopsy may proceed directly from the radiographic findings of bone tumor. If the radiographic findings are not characteristic of a benign tumor, MRI is often done to evaluate bone tumors further before biopsy.

Soft tissue masses of the upper arm with or without pain can usually be diagnosed by history and examination. If there is any question about the identity of the mass, MRI or ultrasound should be done.

Bone scans may be indicated when there is suspected metastatic disease to the shoulder underlying new symptoms in an oncologic patient.

Interpretation

When interpreting radiographs of the shoulder it is important to evaluate all features on all views. As exemplified by the AP view depicted in Figure 2-12, this view is excellent for visualizing osteophytes at the AC joint. In this case, the spur is located at the inferior margin of the joint and is likely impinging upon the patient's underlying supraspinatus

tendon; this patient may suffer chronic degeneration of the tendon that may lead to a full thickness rotator cuff tear.

A slightly modified scapular Y view, done with caudal angulation, is good for evaluating the morphology of the acromion. This may be important in planning surgical treatment for impingement syndrome.

Figure 2-13 demonstrates how calcific tendonitis, in this case of the supraspinatus tendon, may be seen radiographically (such patients may be treated with oral anti-inflammatory medications and/or with steroid injections).

COST-EFFECTIVE MEDICINE
Radiographs of the shoulder are necessary and usually definitive for glenohumeral joint osteoarthritis (DJD) based on the characteristic features as presented in Table 2-1 and demonstrated in the Grashey view shown in Figure 2-14. When radiography reveals advanced glenohumeral joint DJD, MRI is only needed for pre-operative evaluation if the patient is a candidate for arthroplasty.

CASE UPDATE
The radiographs that you ordered on your 55-year-old patient with shoulder pain reveal narrowing of the glenohumeral joint space, mild sclerosis of the glenoid articular surface, and a marginal spur projecting caudally from the articular surface of the humeral head. There is no severe AC joint disease; no large undersurface spur of the AC joint is present. There are no soft tissue calcifications related to the rotator cuff tendons. Before ordering MRI, you need to decide whether such additional imaging would alter current management of the patient.

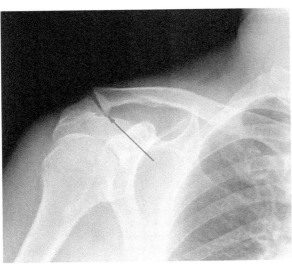

FIGURE 2-12 AP radiograph showing degenerative arthropathy of the AC joint with inferior marginal spur of the clavicle (arrow).

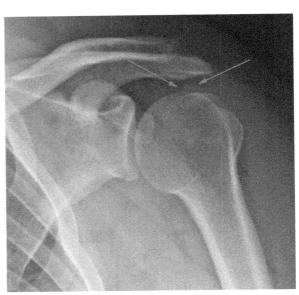

FIGURE 2-13 Grashey view shoulder radiograph demonstrating calcification in the distal supraspinatus tendon (arrows).

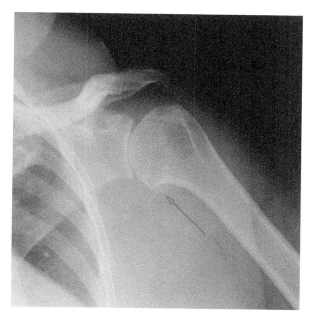

FIGURE 2-14 Grashey view shoulder radiograph demonstrating gleno-humeral joint DJD. Note marginal osteophyte of the humeral head (arrow) and the narrowed glenohumeral joint space (compare with the normal glenohumeral joint space in Fig. 2-13).

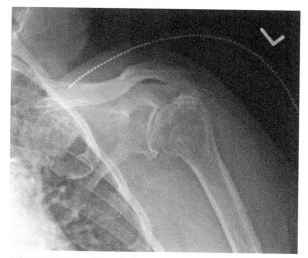

FIGURE 2-15 AP radiograph showing close apposition of the humeral head and undersurface of the acromion process, with sclerotic bone (dashed circle) that indicates chronic tear of the supraspinatus.

On AP and Grashey views it is important to note the distance between the acromion and humerus. If the distance is abnormally small and the humeral head looks to be migrating toward the acromion; this is evidence of rotator cuff arthropathy.

 COST-EFFECTIVE MEDICINE
When the humeral head impinges on the undersurface of the acromion process, the diagnosis of a full thickness rotator cuff tear is established radiographically. When the inferior margin of the acromion process is severely eroded by such impingement, full thickness rotator cuff tear is chronic and the patient may no longer be a candidate for rotator cuff repair. Therefore, further imaging with MRI may not be needed because the diagnosis of chronic rotator cuff tear has been established radiographically, as is the case for the patient depicted in Figure 2-15. Older patients with chronic rotator cuff tears are often not candidates for rotator cuff repair. Shoulder MRI should only be done when it will change patient outcome, and there is little to be gained for a patient who is not a candidate for surgery.

Tears of the rotator cuff are usually reported as partial thickness or full thickness tears. Partial thickness tears can usually be treated non-surgically. Figure 2-16 shows an MRI of a patient with a full thickness tear who will likely require surgical repair for functional improvement and pain reduction. This study shows no severe supraspinatus muscle atrophy, which if present would indicate that the full thickness tear is chronic and might be a contraindication for surgery.

COST-EFFECTIVE MEDICINE
In patients without advanced radiographic findings of chronic rotator cuff tear, MRI should be done for suspected rotator cuff tear only if the patient would be a candidate for surgical repair.

If there is radiographic evidence of collapse of the humeral head without history of recent trauma, this is indicative of avascular necrosis and MRI is not needed. Patients who describe chronic pain of the shoulder with radiographs that may look normal but who have known risk factors for avascular necrosis (e.g., chronic use of steroids) should be considered for MRI. All cases of avascular necrosis should be referred to a surgeon.

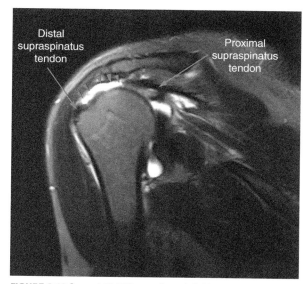

FIGURE 2-16 Coronal T2 MRI revealing a full thickness supraspinatus tear (arrowheads).

ELBOW AND FOREARM

Trauma and Acute Pain

Elbow trauma may result in fractures and dislocations of the distal humerus or forearm and distal biceps tears. During an examination of the elbow after trauma, palpate and look for swelling throughout the limb because associated fractures could have occurred.

Modalities

Radiography is always the initial imaging modality for elbow trauma, consisting of AP and lateral projections and usually an oblique projection optimized for showing the radial head. Radial head fractures are often very subtle or radiographically occult. Therefore, careful positioning and technique are important for optimum visualization of the elbow fat pads, displacement of which indicates the presence of a joint effusion. In the trauma setting, such a finding may indicate a hemarthrosis, strong evidence for intra-articular fracture that may not be visible on initial radiographs. In some cases, CT scanning can be very valuable in revealing geometric deformity caused by fractures around the elbow.

With distal biceps rupture, patients will report a sudden, painful tearing sensation in the cubital fossa and weakness with flexion. Usually there is tenderness and ecchymosis over the cubital fossa and distal upper arm. Sometimes a defect is palpable in that area, but often the tendon cannot be palpated because the muscle belly has retracted, which implies that there is a complete rupture of the tendon. Radiography of the elbow is recommended to rule out bone injury, even when the primary diagnostic consideration is a tendon tear. MRI is often done to evaluate suspected distal biceps tendon tears, especially if the diagnosis is not clinically certain.

Interpretation

An elbow dislocation is an emergency and needs to be reduced immediately by a specialist, if available, because of the neurovascular structures that traverse the joint and because the longer the elbow remains dislocated, the more difficult reduction becomes. About 90% of these dislocations are posterolateral, as is the case for the patient shown in Figure 2-17. Reduction of the elbow always requires IV sedation. After reduction is done, AP and lateral post-reduction radiographs are always obtained. At that time the elbow can be reevaluated for associated fractures (e.g., radial head, coronoid process) and to determine if surgery is needed. These associated fractures are sometimes not visible pre-operatively on radiographs, and CT may be done as part of the pre-operative evaluation.

Distal humerus fractures can be seen on AP and lateral views of the elbow. These fractures can be described as

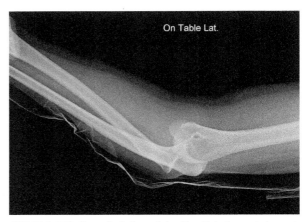

FIGURE 2-17 Radiograph of elbow dislocation. Note the posterior position of the radial head in relation to the distal humerus. There is overlap of the proximal ulna with the distal humerus. These patients are usually in severe pain and cannot extend the elbow, and it is commonly impossible to obtain a true AP or true lateral view.

intercondylar (involves fractures through the intra-articular surface), transcondylar, or supracondylar.

 Supracondylar fractures are most commonly seen in children, as is apparent by the unfused physes evident in Figure 2-18.

If any of these fractures appear to be stable and non-displaced, they can be treated non-surgically with splinting. Most commonly, however, these fractures are unstable, comminuted, and/or intra-articular and need to be referred for surgical treatment.

CT scanning may be useful in demonstrating a fine, non-displaced (radiographically occult) intra-articular fracture that is suspected because of joint effusion or hemarthrosis. In adults this is usually a non-displaced radial head fracture. In pediatric patients it is more likely to be a fracture of the distal humerus.

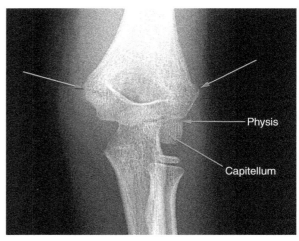

FIGURE 2-18 AP radiographs of a pediatric supracondylar fracture (arrows).

Elbow joint effusion or hemarthrosis, which is associated with intra-articular elbow fracture, is indicated by the presence of displaced periarticular fat pads on lateral radiographs. In Figure 2-19, a long arrow shows the posterior elbow fat pad; visibility of this fat pad indicates the presence of an effusion or hemarthrosis. Also shown in the figure is the anterior elbow fat pad, which is abnormal when it is elevated, and you can clearly see its inferior margin (short arrow).

CT volume rendered (3D) displays can be very helpful in depicting the spatial relationships caused by displaced fractures, as shown in Figure 2-20, which depicts an adolescent

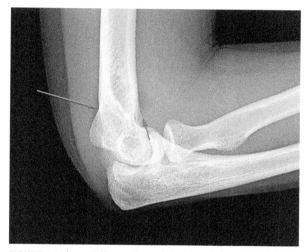

FIGURE 2-19 Lateral elbow radiograph showing displacement of the anterior and posterior fat pads. Whenever the posterior fat pad (long arrow) is visible, there is excess fluid in the joint. The anterior fat pad is abnormal when it is elevated and one can clearly see its inferior margin (short arrow).

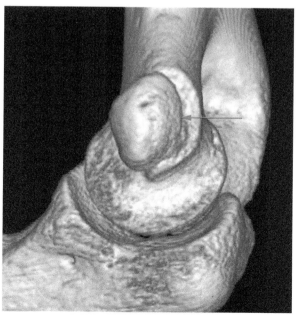

FIGURE 2-20 Volume rendered CT reconstruction showing a displaced epicondyle (arrow) after fracture through the physis (Salter-Harris classification I).

who suffered a Salter-Harris type I fracture through the physis of the medial epicondyle.

Olecranon fractures (Fig. 2-21) are usually displaced fractures and require surgery.

Sometimes olecranon fractures are associated with a dislocation of the radial head, which necessitates surgical referral. Displaced radial and ulnar shaft fractures in the adult must be reduced. After reduction, these fractures, and non-displaced fractures of the radial and ulnar shafts, undergo surgical fixation.

 Children usually do not need surgical treatment if their fractures are non-displaced or if closed reduction results in good alignment. Usually the closed reduction attempt should be done in an emergency department under IV sedation by an orthopedic specialist.

AP and lateral views of a patient with a suspected distal biceps rupture will usually be normal. Sometimes an avulsion fracture can be seen at the radial tuberosity.

 COST-EFFECTIVE MEDICINE
These patients usually do not need an MRI or ultrasound because clinical evaluation provides sufficient evidence to make this diagnosis.

However, if the diagnosis is questionable, an MRI, as shown in Figure 2-22, can demonstrate partial tears and the degree of retraction of complete tears.

When radiography reveals fractures of the shafts of the radius and ulna, it is important to evaluate the geometric

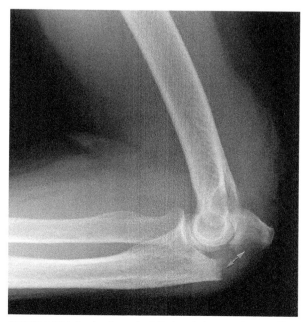

FIGURE 2-21 Lateral radiograph of displaced olecranon fracture. Note the gap between fracture fragments (double-headed arrow).

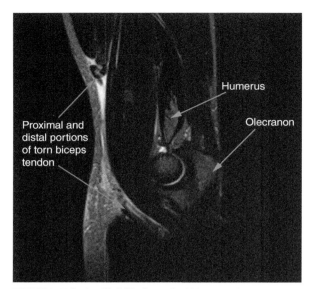

FIGURE 2-22 Sagittal T2 MRI of torn distal biceps tendon.

relationship between the radial head and the capitellum of the humerus because radio-capitellar dislocation may occur with forearm fractures.

Chronic Conditions of the Elbow

Chronic conditions of the elbow include DJD, rheumatoid arthritis, medial and lateral epicondylitis (golfer's and tennis elbow), and ligament tears or tendonitis. Patients with DJD of the elbow will have a history of persistent chronic pain and may have a history of prior trauma or RA. They may describe their pain as popping or grinding or complain of decreased range of motion and/or locking.

Modalities

AP and lateral radiographs are sufficient for an initial evaluation in cases of chronic elbow pain.

Medial and lateral epicondylitis are most commonly diagnosed by history and physical exam, but AP and lateral radiographs should be done to rule out any other possible elbow pathology, especially when symptoms do not respond to conservative medical treatment. If your patient does not respond to medical treatment for epicondylitis, you should consider alternative diagnoses, such as more advanced tears of the common flexor and extensor tendons or collateral ligament tears that can be demonstrated on MRI.

The ulnar (medial) collateral ligament (UCL) is the most commonly torn elbow ligament, typically seen in baseball pitchers. Onset of symptoms can be acute, with the athlete experiencing a pop and medial elbow pain. However, most commonly, patients will have a gradual onset of pain especially with throwing. Radial (lateral) collateral ligament tears

are less common. AP and lateral radiographs should be done first to rule out any other elbow pathology. MR elbow arthrography (MRI done with intra-articular injection of contrast material) is usually the best way to diagnose a collateral ligament tear.

Routine elbow MRI, without arthrography, can demonstrate epicondylitis, tendon tears, and bone disease such as aseptic necrosis. Elbow ultrasonography is considered to be an alternative to MRI, but the high level of expertise needed for this procedure is not widely available.

Interpretation

DJD of the elbow (radiographic findings of DJD are presented in Table 2.3) is generally treated conservatively but may be referred to an orthopedic specialist if the patient wishes to discuss joint replacement. Sometimes loose osteocartilaginous joint bodies can also be seen radiographically. When clinical findings suggest joint bodies and radiographs are normal, either MRI or MR arthrography should be considered.

There is an overlap in the symptoms between epicondylitis, chronic tears of collateral ligaments, and tears of the common flexor and extensor tendons. For example, the patient shown in Figure 2-23 had symptoms of epicondylitis but MRI showed intra-tendon fluid signal interpreted as a partial tear of her common flexor tendon.

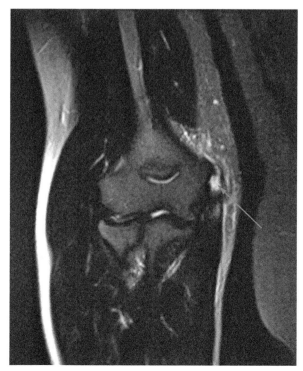

FIGURE 2-23 Coronal T2 MRI showing fluid signal (arrow) within a tear of the common flexor tendon.

Acute or chronic tears of collateral ligaments of the elbow result in joint instability and laxity on physical exam. Sometimes an avulsion fracture can be seen of the medial epicondyle on radiographs, which is functionally a tear of the UCL. UCL tears or tendonitis will most commonly have normal AP and lateral radiographs and will typically be treated conservatively, although they may be repaired in some patients, especially athletes. Elbow MR arthrography will demonstrate discontinuity in a torn collateral ligament as shown in Figure 2-24.

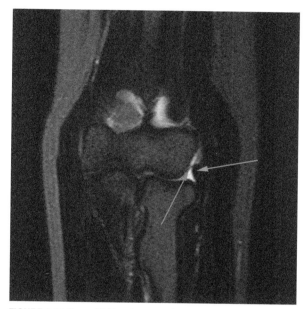

FIGURE 2-24 Coronal MR arthrogram showing tear (red arrow) of the radial collateral ligament (blue arrow).

WRIST AND HAND

Acute Pain and Trauma

Modalities

Radiography should be performed on any patient who presents with pain, swelling, bruising, or deformity in the wrist, hand, or fingers after an injury. Standard radiographs are PA, PA oblique (lateral rotation), and lateral views of the hand and/or wrist.

Supplementary radiographic views of the wrist (e.g., special scaphoid views and/or PA views done with ulnar and radial deviation) are often done when there is clinical suspicion of wrist injury that is not demonstrated on routine radiographic projections.

A significant number of non-displaced scaphoid fractures are radiographically occult. Even if a fracture is not apparent on a radiograph but the patient is tender over the scaphoid ("anatomic snuff-box") with or without swelling, the wrist needs to be immobilized immediately. Repeated and delayed

(1–2 weeks) radiographs or immediate CT or MRI should be done in cases in which there is a discrepancy between positive findings on physical examination and "negative" initial radiographs.

Wrist symptoms that are not explained by radiographic findings are often evaluated further with MRI. When there is pain on the ulnar side of the joint leading to suspicion of tear of the triangular fibrocartilage, CT or MR arthrography is recommended. This procedure is also commonly performed for suspicion of scapholunate ligament tear and the ulnar impaction syndrome, in which a long ulna (positive ulnar variance) impinges on the lunate.

COST-EFFECTIVE MEDICINE

Cross-sectional imaging is rarely needed for acute hand injury, with one exception: Gamekeeper's (skier's) thumb involves a tear of the ulnar collateral ligament of the first metacarpophalangeal joint and may require MRI for definitive diagnosis when surgical repair is being considered.

Interpretation

In the most common distal radius fracture (Colles fracture), there is dorsal angulation of the distal fragment as shown by the red line in Figure 2-25. Mildly angulated fractures may be treated with closed reduction and casting. If the angulation cannot be corrected to an acceptable position, then the patient should see an orthopedic surgeon. Post-reduction radiographs must always be obtained to ensure adequate reduction.

Fractures angulated more than 20 degrees, comminuted fractures, and fractures that result in significant shortening of the radius may require open (surgical) reduction. Associated fracture of the ulnar styloid process increases the likelihood of instability. A Smith fracture, with volar angulation of the distal radial fragment, is also known as a reverse Colles fracture. Figure 2-26 shows an intra-articular fracture of the distal radius. Such fractures typically require surgery because

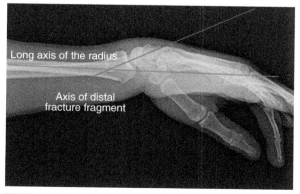

FIGURE 2-25 Lateral radiograph of a Colles fracture; lines drawn to measure the dorsal angulation of the distal radial fragment.

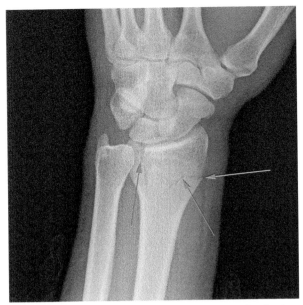

FIGURE 2-26 AP radiograph showing a comminuted distal radius fracture (arrows) with fracture line on the ulnar side that extends to the articular surface.

even mild deformity of the articular surface may lead to early osteoarthritis of the radiocarpal joint.

When intra-articular fractures are shown radiographically, CT is often done to evaluate any deformity of the articular cortex.

 Pediatric patients often suffer incomplete or "buckle" fractures as shown in the frontal and lateral radiographs found in Figure 2-27. Very young patients may even suffer a "plastic bowing deformation" injury of bone in which the injured bone is literally bent. When one side of a long bone in a young patient bends and the opposite side clearly fractures, the injury is commonly referred to as a greenstick fracture.

In the patient depicted in Figure 2-28 (top), who has pain in her anatomic snuff-box, there is no radiographic evidence of a scaphoid fracture, but the fracture is apparent on the MRI shown in Figure 2-28 (bottom).

Soft tissue injuries of the wrist are extremely complex and require orthopedic referral. Disruption of intrinsic ligaments may result in a variety of carpal dislocations that may be apparent on radiographs. For example, the grossly widened scapholunate space evident in Figure 2-29 indicates tearing of the scapholunate ligament. CT or MR wrist arthrography

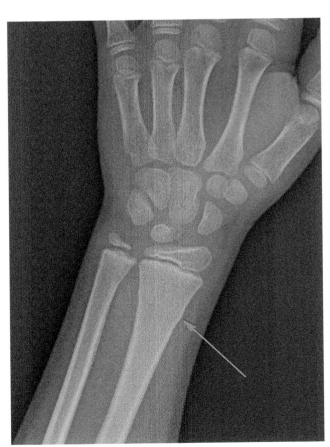

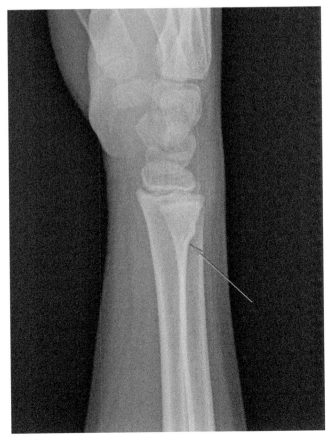

FIGURE 2-27 PA and Lateral radiographs reveal a buckle (torus) fracture in 8-year old-patient (arrows).

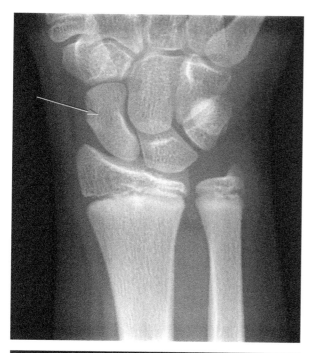

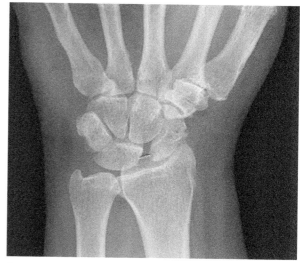

FIGURE 2-29 PA radiograph that shows a widened scapholunate space (double-headed arrow).

may be used to show tears of various wrist ligaments and the triangular fibrocartilage complex (TFCC). As shown in Figure 2-30, tears appear as a contrast-filled discontinuity of what is normally a continuous hypointense structure.

Metacarpal fractures of the hand (Fig. 2-31) typically occur in the shaft or neck of the metacarpal. If there is significant displacement, angulation, and/or shortening of the metacarpal, open reduction and internal fixation may be needed. A fracture of the distal fifth metacarpal shaft with volar angulation of the distal fragment is known as a Boxer's fracture.

Dislocation of the interphalangeal joints (Fig. 2-32) is obvious on physical exam, but radiographs are needed to check for fractures and to determine the orientation of the

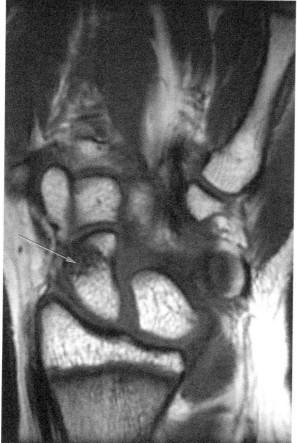

FIGURE 2-28 **Top:** PA radiograph that shows no visible fracture of the scaphoid (arrow). **Bottom:** Coronal T1 MRI done just a few days later that reveals a fracture of the mid-scaphoid (arrow).

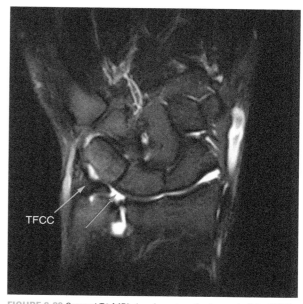

FIGURE 2-30 Coronal T1 MRI showing a tear (red arrow) of the TFCC.

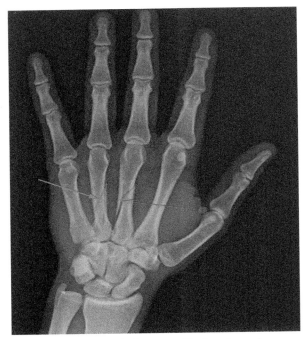

FIGURE 2-31 PA radiograph of metacarpal fractures (arrows).

dislocation. The dislocation should be reduced and post-reduction films should be obtained.

Chronic Conditions Including Soft Tissue Masses

It is likely that late subacute to chronic conditions of the hand and wrist are the result of acute trauma in which the pathology

is unrecognized immediately and symptoms persist or worsen weeks or months after the episode of trauma. Therefore, in many cases the distinction between acute and chronic may be arbitrary, with overlapping symptomatology and radiologic correlates.

Modalities

As in all bone and joint disease, radiography is required as an initial evaluation in chronic wrist/hand pain. Kienbock's disease, avascular necrosis of the lunate, may be evident on radiographs. Degenerative and inflammatory arthritis of the wrist and hand is usually diagnosed definitively with plain radiography. Radiography is also fundamental in the characterization of bone tumors of the hand (e.g., an enchondroma).

If you only need confirmation of the presence of suspected ganglion cysts, ultrasonography is the procedure of choice.

Interpretation

Osteoarthritis (DJD) in the hand and wrist joints shows the usual radiographic features described in Table 2-3. More advanced cases of DJD and inflammatory forms of DJD may show significant erosive/cystic bone changes. DJD is commonly found in the first carpometacarpal joints (Fig. 2-33), first metacarpophalangeal joints, and distal interphalangeal (IP) joints of the fingers. Proximal IP joints may also be involved.

The distribution of affected joints in RA is different than in DJD; that is, there is more involvement of metacarpophalangeal, mid-carpal, and radiocarpal joints. As demonstrated in Figure 2-34, the erosion of articular cartilage can be

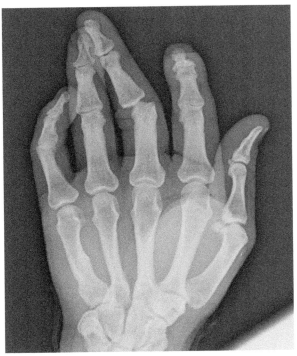

FIGURE 2-32 PA radiograph of dislocated PIP joint of the third finger.

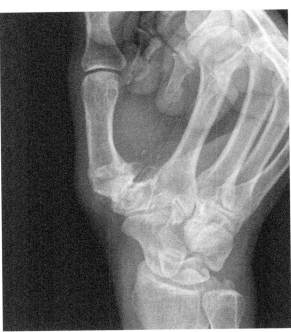

FIGURE 2-33 PA radiograph that shows DJD of the first carpometacarpal joint, with large marginal spurs (arrows).

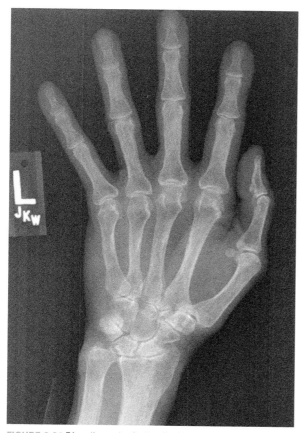

FIGURE 2-34 PA radiograph of a hand with RA. Note interphalangeal joint space narrowing without osteophytes.

striking, with considerable loss of joint space but no marginal osteophytes.

With other less common arthropathies, such as psoriatic arthritis, the hand and wrist may also be involved. The pattern and appearance of an arthropathy in the hand and wrist may lead to a radiology report that suggests one of these other entities. The clinical information you provide on a radiology requisition that is relevant to possible systemic arthropathy will greatly improve the chance of the radiologist providing a specific diagnosis.

Ganglion cysts are visible on ultrasound or MRI as simple or loculated fluid collections, usually very closely related to tendons. Chronic ligament or TFCC tears are no different than acute tears but may be associated with secondary degenerative bone and joint changes.

PELVIS, HIP, AND THIGH

Trauma and Acute Pain
Modalities

Patients who suffer high impact trauma to the pelvic region, whether they complain of pelvic pain or not, should always get an AP pelvis radiograph because of the potential damage

to pelvic visceral and neurovascular structures caused by displaced pelvic fractures. The AP pelvis radiograph may also show hip and acetabular fractures and hip dislocations. If hip fracture or dislocation is suspected, a hip radiograph should also be specifically requested, as this is centered over the hip, not the midline as is done for pelvis radiography. CT scans of the pelvis are highly recommended if the initial AP pelvis shows disruption of the pelvic ring or if radiographs are negative but the pelvis feels unstable on examination. CT scans are often requested by surgeons for surgical planning.

In the rural clinic setting in which CT scanning is not immediately available, oblique AP and inlet/outlet angled radiographs are often very helpful in identifying fractures not apparent in the AP projection. With fractures of the osseous ring around the obturator foramen, oblique radiographs can show displacement of fractures that seem non-displaced in the AP projection.

Elderly patients who present after a fall with hip or groin pain, inability to bear weight, apparently shortened limb, and rotated thigh (most often externally rotated) usually have a hip fracture. AP and frog leg or cross-table lateral radiographs should be obtained, although pain may preclude the frog leg view. If radiographs are normal but there is high suspicion of hip fracture, a limited view MRI of the hip, or CT scan, should be considered, because non-displaced fractures of the hip may not be visible on radiographs. These patients may often still bear weight (but painfully). They may have point tenderness in the buttocks, groin, or anterior pelvis.

Patients who present with pain, swelling, and/or deformity of the thigh, especially after a high impact trauma, should get AP and lateral femoral radiographs for suspected fracture of the femoral shaft, in addition to AP pelvis/hip radiographs.

Interpretation

Hip dislocations, as seen on AP pelvis radiographs (Fig. 2-35), need to be reduced as soon as possible because of the chance of osteonecrosis of the femoral head. CT is highly recommended for evaluation of suspected acetabular fracture. Acetabular fractures require attendance by an orthopedic surgeon; the displaced acetabular fracture apparent in Figure 2-36 would likely be surgically reduced.

Hip fractures in the elderly typically occur in the femoral neck (Fig. 2-37) or around the trochanteric area (usually intertrochanteric or subtrochanteric; Fig. 2-38). Hip fractures need to be surgically treated typically by fixation or arthroplasty. Young patients with femoral neck fractures need to be treated quickly and surgically because of the chance of osteonecrosis of the femoral head (i.e., most of the vascular supply to the femoral head ascends along the femoral neck and the arteries may become disrupted over time if the fracture is not stabilized).

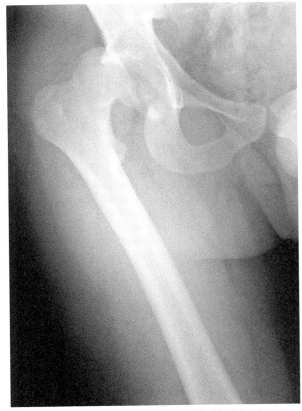

FIGURE 2-35 AP radiograph showing a posterior hip dislocation.

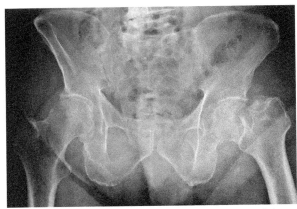

FIGURE 2-37 AP radiograph of a fracture of the neck of the left femur. Compare the normal right femoral neck with the shortened left femoral neck, and note the medial displacement of the left femoral head in relation to the trochanters. The oblique dark bands overlying the proximal femurs are caused by skin folds.

specialty care whether non-displaced or displaced because internal fixation is needed.

 Hip spica cast treatment for femoral shaft fractures can be done in children younger than 6 years.

Chronic Conditions Including Soft Tissue Masses

Chronic conditions of the pelvis, hip, and thigh include arthritis, stress fractures, labral tears, and avascular necrosis of the femoral head. In the hip, DJD is far more common

When a pelvic radiograph shows isolated and limited pubic rami fractures, as is the case in Figure 2-39, and the patient exam does not reveal pelvic instability, the patient can be treated non-surgically.

Abnormal widening of the pubic symphysis (more than 2 cm) that is visible on AP radiographs (Fig. 2-40) suggests pelvic ring disruption or instability. A CT scan can be ordered for further evaluation of the pelvis, but usually once the widened pubic symphysis is seen the patient should be referred to an orthopedic specialist for internal or external fixation.

Femoral shaft fractures, such as the severe comminuted fracture shown in Figure 2-41, should also have orthopedic

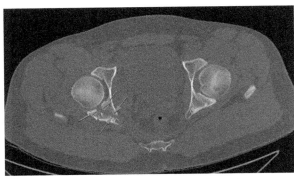

FIGURE 2-36 CT scan of a fractured acetabulum (arrows).

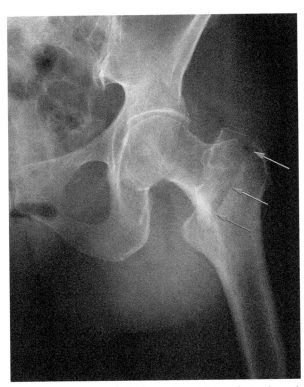

FIGURE 2-38 AP radiograph of an intertrochanteric femoral fracture (arrows).

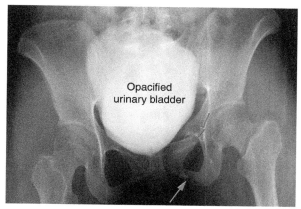

FIGURE 2-39 AP radiograph of pubic rami fractures (arrows) done after contrast-enhanced CT on patient who was in MVA. Distended bladder could be secondary to urethral injury.

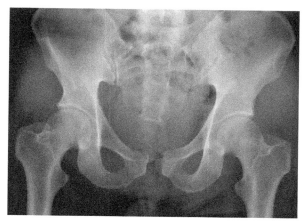

FIGURE 2-40 AP radiograph that shows a widened pubic symphysis.

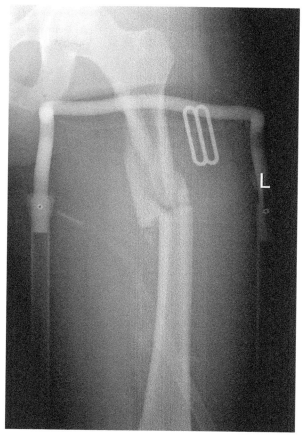

FIGURE 2-41 AP radiograph of comminuted femoral shaft fracture; note overlying immobilization device.

than inflammatory disease, such as rheumatoid arthritis. Patients with DJD will describe chronic hip and groin pain, especially when they walk. The pain may radiate down their thigh to the knee. They also state that they have decreased range of motion (many will commonly say they cannot bring their leg up to tie shoes or to put on socks).

Modalities

AP pelvis, AP hip, and frog leg position lateral hip radiographs should be requested to evaluate the hip.

If an older patient does not have radiographic evidence of hip joint DJD and conservative therapy does not alleviate pelvic or hip pain, an MRI of the hip should be requested to look for stress fractures. If the patient is not a candidate for MRI, a radionuclide bone scan should be done. Femoral neck stress fractures should also be suspected in young patients with chronic groin or pelvic pain who have been undergoing rigorous athletic training. As with elderly patients, an MRI needs to be requested; this exam is actually more critical in young patients because these stress fractures can result in avascular necrosis and the need for subsequent arthroplasty—something

to be avoided in young people because joint replacements may only last for 10 to 20 years. Patients with chronic pain who have a history of sickle cell disease, old trauma, alcoholism, chronic steroid use, or radiation from cancer therapy should have an MRI to evaluate for avascular necrosis of the femoral head. The MRI should be of both hips because avascular necrosis is often bilateral and can be asymptomatic.

 Pediatric causes of chronic hip pain include slipped capital femoral epiphysis, diagnosed radiographically, and Legg-Calve-Perthes disease, usually also diagnosed with radiography, but MRI may be needed for definitive diagnosis.

Patients with persistent thigh or hip pain should get femoral as well as same hip radiographs to rule out bone lesions. If such lesions are suspected based on these radiographs or strongly suspected on clinical grounds even with normal radiographs, further evaluation should be done by MRI. However, when the clinical presentation reveals pain mostly at night in an adolescent or young adult (mostly males) and suggests osteoid osteoma, then CT is recommended after initial radiographic evaluation.

Labral tears of the acetabulum may result from trauma to the hip but may also have no apparent direct cause. These patients will have persistent groin pain and may report a "catching or locking" of the hip. On physical exam their motion is good but there will be pain at the extremes of motion. AP and lateral radiographs of the hip cannot reveal labral damage but should be done to rule out other pathology. An MRI arthrogram should be then requested.

Superficial soft tissue masses that clinically are likely to be simple benign lipomas can be evaluated with ultrasound. However, for most soft tissue masses, MRI is the procedure of choice. It is recommended to order such an exam "with contrast enhancement as needed" so that the radiologist has the option to obtain contrast-enhanced MR image sequences if the finding of potentially malignant soft tissue mass requires those additional images.

Interpretation

Osteoarthritis of the hip (Fig. 2-42) is initially treated conservatively, but when conservative treatment fails, then the patient is referred to an orthopedic surgeon for possible hip replacement. In Figure 2-42 note the typical (see Table 2-3) loss of "joint space," subchondral sclerosis, and the present of subchondral cystic changes in the acetabulum and femoral head.

In stress fractures, usually MRI will show a linear fracture line surrounded by bone marrow edema (Fig. 2-43). Most stress fractures can be treated non-surgically but patients with femoral neck stress fractures, especially young patients, need to be referred to a specialist for possible internal fixation.

In avascular necrosis of the femoral head, radiographs may show a subtle curvilinear lucency just beneath the cortex of the articular surface. On MRI, there is a characteristic curvilinear

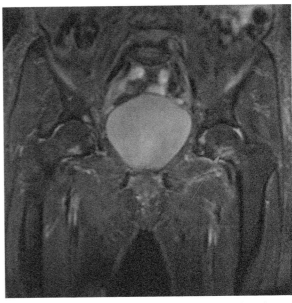

FIGURE 2-43 Coronal T2 MRI showing stress fracture of the femoral neck (arrow).

hypointense line that demarcates the devascularized segment of bone (Fig. 2-44). Associated bone marrow edema will be hypointense on T1 and hyperintense on T2 MR sequences.

 Pediatric avascular necrosis of the femoral head, typically seen in children ages 4 to 10 (Legg-Calve-Perthes disease), has radiographic findings essentially the same as found in adults with avascular necrosis of the femoral head.

In advanced avascular necrosis, radiographs will show sclerosis and/or collapse of the femoral head. These patients need to be referred to an orthopedic surgeon for likely partial or complete joint replacement.

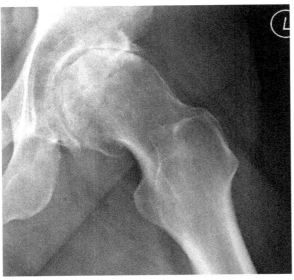

FIGURE 2-42 AP radiograph of the left hip done with the leg abducted and externally rotated (also called "frog position" lateral) showing advanced DJD. Note loss of articular cartilage space ("joint space") sclerosis and subchondral cystic changes in the acetabulum and femoral head, and osteophytes along the inferior margin of the joint.

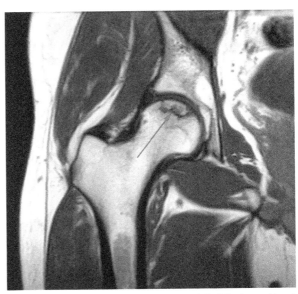

FIGURE 2-44 Coronal T2 MRI demonstrating AVN of the femoral head, characterized by the hypointense subarticular line (arrow).

A cause of subacute to chronic hip pain that is unique to adolescents, usually obese males, is a slipped capital femoral epiphysis, which is shown in Figure 2-45. Note in the figure that the femoral head appears to have slipped inferiorly relative to the femoral neck.

Labral tears of the acetabulum, such as the one revealed by MRI in the patient shown in Figure 2-46, can be treated conservatively if they are minimally symptomatic. However, more symptomatic labral tears are usually repaired surgically.

Bone tumors of the femur may or may not be symptomatic, and, as shown by Figure 2-47, can involve both lytic and blastic lesions. Radiographs of bone tumors should be interpreted by a radiologist or an orthopedic surgeon with experience in musculoskeletal oncology. Further imaging is not always needed, but MRI is often done for suspected malignant bone tumors to evaluate extent, to narrow the differential diagnosis based on imaging features, and to see if there is an associated soft tissue mass.

KNEE AND LOWER LEG
Acute Pain and Trauma
Modalities

Patients who can bear weight after knee trauma, have no focal tenderness, and show no clinical sign of knee joint effusion may not need any imaging. However, with severe pain, inability to

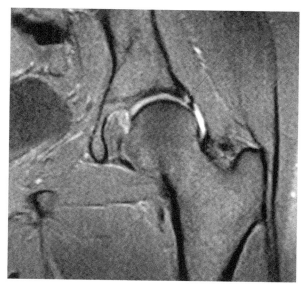

FIGURE 2-46 MR arthrogram showing torn acetabular labrum (arrow).

bear weight, focal tenderness upon palpation, bruising, soft tissue swelling, or clinical suspicion of joint effusion/hemarthrosis, imaging is appropriate.

Initial imaging should include AP, AP oblique, and lateral radiographs to determine if there are fractures of the distal

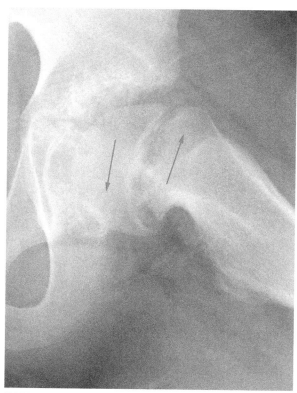

FIGURE 2-45 AP radiograph showing slipped capital femoral epiphysis; the metaphysis has "slid" upward and lateral to the femoral capital epiphysis.

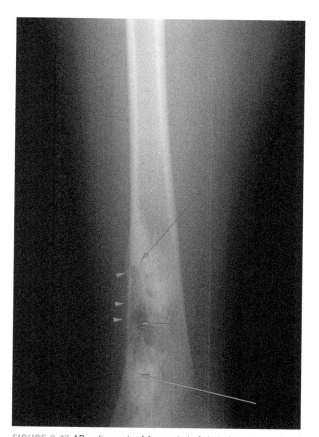

FIGURE 2-47 AP radiograph of femoral shaft lytic (short arrow) and blastic (long arrows) bone tumor with periosteal new bone, also called periosteal reaction (arrowheads).

femur, patella, or proximal tibia. If the patient can bear weight and is able to bend the knee, a merchant view (knee flexed with the beam directed through the knee from superior to inferior), which reveals patella alignment and fracture, is also recommended.

If the patient complains of pain and tenderness in the lower leg with or without bruising and swelling, you should request AP and lateral tibia/fibula radiographs.

Patients who have negative radiographs for fractures may need an MRI based on their mechanism of injury and physical exam findings in order to reveal acute tearing of the menisci and/or the ligaments of the knee. These patients typically report a twisting type of injury with or without feeling and/or hearing a "pop." They likely will have difficulty bearing weight and will have joint effusion. Such patients often complain of instability of the knee (associated mostly with anterior cruciate ligament [ACL] tears) or locking or catching in the knee (associated mostly with meniscal tears). Patients sometimes will report all these symptoms, suggesting both ligamentous and meniscal tears.

A medial collateral ligament (MCL) injury or tear is the result of a valgus force applied to the knee, whereas a lateral collateral ligament (LCL) injury or tear results from a varus force to the knee. Isolated LCL injuries are less common than MCL injuries. Injuries to these ligaments can occur in isolation or in association with meniscal and/or cruciate ligament tears.

The ACL is the primary stabilizing ligament of the knee. Patients who tear this ligament often have had a twisting or hyperextension injury. They may complain of instability afterward and will have swelling. An anterior drawer or Lachman test is used to assess the integrity of the ACL.

A Merchant view will reveal patellar dislocation, often the result of a twisting injury. After reduction, Merchant images are also required to check for proper alignment. Sometimes, in young patients, an MRI may need to be considered to evaluate the soft tissue structures that maintain patellar alignment (primarily the medial patellofemoral ligament), especially if the patient has had several episodes of patellar dislocations/subluxations. These patients present with medial pain from a torn medial patellofemoral ligament, but their patella alignment may appear normal due to spontaneous reduction.

Patients who have fallen on their flexed knee and cannot extend it against resistance (or at all), with tenderness and/or swelling around the quadriceps tendon, probably have partial or complete rupture of that tendon. Patients who cannot extend their knee at all and have swelling and tenderness over the patellar tendon probably have a patellar tendon rupture. Radiographs should still be done to rule out fracture, but

usually physical exam is sufficient to make this diagnosis. However, when there is clinical uncertainty or suspicion of partial tear of these tendons, MRI should be considered.

Tibial plateau fractures usually occur after high impact trauma or a fall from a height. Patients will have knee pain and will be unable to bear weight. There is usually a significant amount of swelling due to hemarthrosis. AP, AP oblique, and lateral radiographs should be done. Even structurally significant fractures, such as those of the tibial plateau, may be radiographically occult, so secondary signs of fracture such as a joint effusion or hemarthrosis are important to appreciate.

Supracondylar femor fractures can occur after a high-impact trauma and in osteoporotic elderly patients after a fall.

These patients are unable to bear weight and have swelling and pain around the knee. With displaced and/or severely angulated fractures, visible deformity is seen. AP and lateral radiographs of the distal femur are appropriate. Tibial and fibula shaft fractures are associated with major trauma to the lower leg. Swelling and/or deformities can be seen. AP and lateral radiographs should be done, and it is important to view the entire length of tibia and fibula because associated fractures can occur distal or proximal to the primary fracture.

Interpretation

Knee dislocations (anterior, posterior, or lateral; Fig. 2-48) are an emergency situation because of the chance of neurovascular trauma and need to be reduced as soon as possible. After reduction, a post-reduction radiograph is needed to evaluate for fractures. Usually with knee dislocations at least three of the four ligaments are torn (usually the ACL, posterior cruciate [PCL], and LCL). Therefore, these patients require further examination with MRI and will eventually need surgery to repair these ligaments. In these patients, MRA of the knee should be done along with MRI to evaluate the integrity of the popliteal artery. Alternative imaging of the popliteal artery is via CTA or catheter angiography.

MCL and LCL injuries can be best viewed on the coronal sequences in MRI (Fig. 2-49). Whether an MCL injury is a sprain or tear, these are almost always treated non-surgically with therapy and bracing.

MCL injuries may be associated with other internal derangements. In O'Donaghue's terrible (unhappy) triad, MRI reveals MCL, ACL, and medial meniscus tears. These occur in injured athletes when there is a blow to the lateral side of the knee when the foot is fixed to the ground and the leg is externally rotated.

ACL injuries commonly occur as an isolated internal derangement of the knee after trauma. Radiographs are

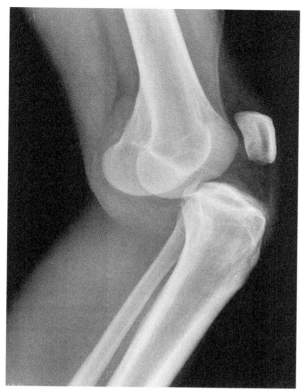

FIGURE 2-48 Lateral radiograph of anterior knee dislocation.

typically normal in ACL and PCL tears, but the presence of a Segond fracture (fracture of the lateral rim of the lateral tibial plateau; Fig. 2-50 top) is highly suspicious for ACL tear. ACL tears can be appreciated on axial, sagittal (Fig. 2-50 bottom), and coronal MRI sequences. ACL tears in young and active patients almost always need to be surgically repaired because

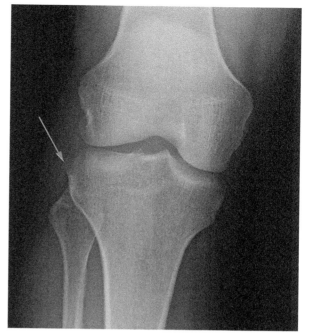

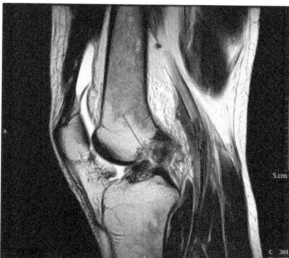

FIGURE 2-50 AP radiograph **(top)** showing a displaced fragment (arrow) of a Segond fracture that correlates highly with the presence of an ACL tear. Sagittal T2 MRI **(bottom)** of torn ACL in the same patient (arrow).

the instability increases the risk of developing DJD. Isolated PCL injuries are rare and most often treated non-surgically, with therapy and bracing. Surgery may be needed for patients who have failed non-surgical treatment if they are young and very athletic.

Traumatic meniscal tears usually result from a twisting injury to the knee. Sometimes these patients may feel or hear a pop. There is typically swelling and stiffness 2 to 3 days from the injury. They may report locking or catching in the knee. Radiographs are usually normal. As shown by the arrow in Figure 2-51, a meniscus tear is best seen on coronal and sagittal MRI views as a linear hyperintensity within a meniscus

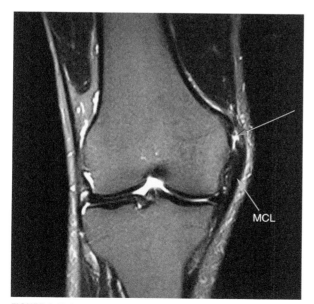

FIGURE 2-49 Coronal T2 MRI that shows a tear (arrow) of the MCL.

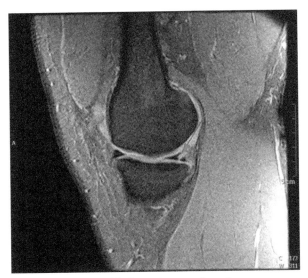

FIGURE 2-51 Sagittal MRI of a meniscus tear (arrow).

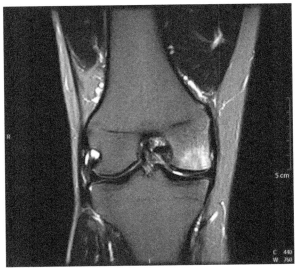

FIGURE 2-53 Coronal T2 MRI done after acute knee trauma showing region of high signal (bright) in the medial femoral condyle that indicates bone marrow edema secondary to trabecular microfracture (bone bruise).

that extends to the joint surface. A portion of the meniscus may be displaced from its normal location, typically producing the "bucket handle" type of meniscus tear shown in Figure 2-52, and which is associated with "locking" of the knee. In young patients the meniscus can be repaired because there is usually still a good blood supply. In patients age 30 and older the meniscus is just shaved back to remove the loose fragment that causes the pain and mechanical symptoms.

MRI can also reveal bone bruising (region of trabecular microfracture) that can occur after trauma. As shown in Figure 2-53, a bone bruise is revealed by T2 hyperintensity in the bone marrow space. Bone bruising does not require surgical treatment but may explain the presence of severe pain, and the pattern of bone bruising may reveal the mechanism of injury.

Joints effusions in the knee are often present after an injury and may represent hemarthrosis. Effusions are

hyperintense on T2 MRI, as is shown by the bottom image in Figure 2-54. The presence of a large knee joint effusion increases suspicion of acute internal derangement after trauma and may lead to detection of an otherwise subtle or unclear radiologic finding. Fluid–fluid levels on horizontal beam lateral radiographs, as in the radiograph presented as the upper image in Figure 2-54, or on MRI (lower image) indicate the presence of a lipohemarthrosis. In addition to blood in the joint, there is lipid from bone marrow, indicating the presence of an intra-articular fracture, which might be radiographically occult.

Patellar fractures that are not displaced or minimally displaced and are not comminuted usually do not need surgery and are treated with an immobilizer with non–weight-bearing for about 6 weeks. Significantly displaced or comminuted fractures, as shown in the Merchant view of the knee presented as Figure 2-55, require surgery.

It is important, however, when looking for a patella fracture not to mistake the normal variation of a bipartite patella for a fracture. The radiolucency that separates segments of the bipartite patella are usually well marginated by corticated bone, unlike fractures (Fig. 2-56). If corticated margins of a bipartite patella are not conspicuous, absence of overlying soft tissue swelling and absence of joint effusion/hemarthrosis support a diagnosis of this common normal variant, rather than fracture.

Lateral radiographs may show a high riding patella ("patella alta") that results from a tear of the patellar tendon or a developmentally long tendon. The patella may be in a low position if the quadriceps tendon is torn ("patella baja"). Ideal lateral knee radiographs usually show these tendons well. However, when there is a great deal of post-trauma soft

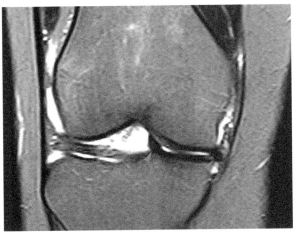

FIGURE 2-52 Coronal T2 MRI of a meniscus with bucket handle tear. Arrows point to separated fragments of the meniscus.

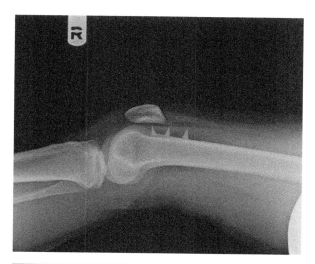

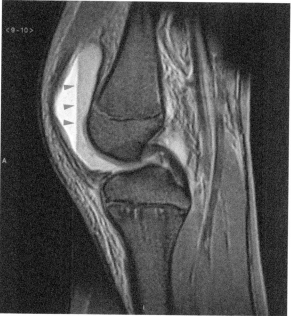

FIGURE 2-54 Lateral radiograph **(top)** and sagittal MRI **(bottom)** demonstrating a lipohemarthrosis. Arrowheads indicate the fluid-fluid level between the bloody effusion and the lipid floating above it. This fluid-fluid level was of course horizontal in the patient who was supine during the MRI procedure.

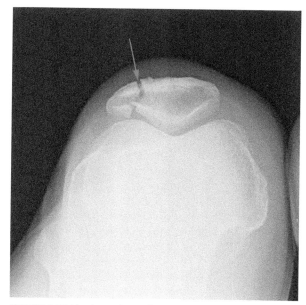

FIGURE 2-55 Merchant view radiograph of a patella with an acute fracture (arrow).

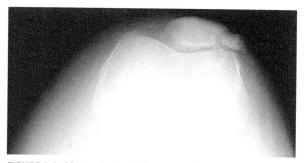

FIGURE 2-56 Merchant view of bipartite patella.

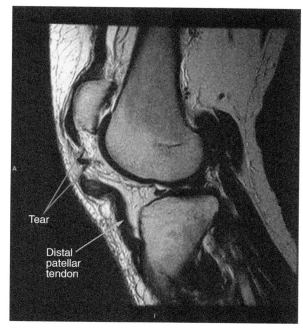

FIGURE 2-57 Sagittal T2 MRI of a torn patellar tendon (red arrows).

tissue swelling, these tendons may not be clearly seen, and a sagittal knee MRI similar to that shown in Figure 2-57 may be needed if the clinical diagnosis is uncertain.

Tibial plateau fractures may be seen on radiographs as radiolucencies extending to the tibial articular surface or as areas of step-off or depression of the articular surface, as indicated by the red arrow in Figure 2-58. Non-displaced fractures can be treated non-surgically, but comminuted and displaced fractures need internal fixation.

These fractures may also be occult on radiographs. A helpful radiographic sign of a clinically suspected but radiographically occult tibial plateau fracture is evident on a lateral radiograph done with a horizontal x-ray beam

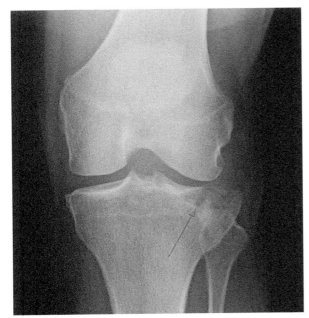

FIGURE 2-58 AP radiograph of a tibial plateau fracture (arrow).

Isolated fractures of the fibula can be seen on AP and lateral radiographs and can be treated non-surgically. If a proximal fibular fracture is seen, make sure that there is not a related fracture in the distal tibia at the ankle. Long bone radiographs must always include the entire length of the injured bone.

("cross-table lateral"). Blood and lipids from bone marrow may escape into the joint and form a fluid–fluid level, indicating a lipohemarthrosis as shown in Figure 2-54. A CT scan (Fig. 2-59) is appropriate for further diagnosis and surgical planning for tibial plateau fractures.

Tibial shaft fractures in adults require internal fixation.

 Non-displaced tibial shaft fractures in children can be treated with casting as would be the case for the patient depicted in Figure 2-60.

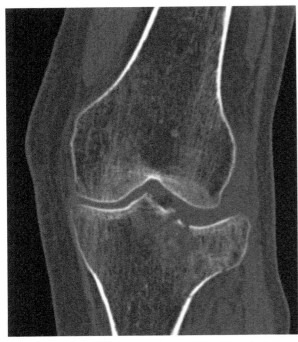

FIGURE 2-59 Coronal CT reconstruction of a tibial plateau fracture.

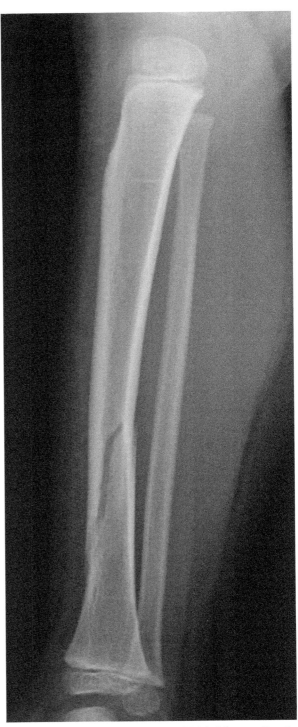

FIGURE 2-60 AP radiograph of a pediatric tibial shaft fracture. Note the open growth plates.

Chronic Knee and Lower Leg Pain

Chronic knee pain is usually the result of arthritis (DJD, RA); osteochondral lesion, which is a form of aseptic osteonecrosis; patellofemoral syndrome; stress fractures; non-acute meniscal tears, and Osgood-Schlatter disease (OS). A complete medical history is important for diagnosis, especially noting a history of RA, gout, DJD in other joints, and any oncologic or infectious disease that could affect the bones around the knee. The history of progression of pain, locking, and/or catching of the joint should be obtained.

Modalities

Radiography is the appropriate initial imaging evaluation. AP, lateral, and Merchant's are good initial views to obtain. Standing AP (or PA) radiographs are important in evaluating DJD of the knee by showing definitively the loss of articular cartilage space in weight-bearing compartments, most often the medial compartment of the knee. The lateral view is important for identifying arthritis, OS disease, loose bodies, and effusions. Merchant views help determine if there is normal alignment of the patella or a patellar tracking disorder.

Patients who have negative radiographs but have pain in the medial or lateral joint lines and complain of locking, clicking, or catching could have meniscal problems. The patients may or may not remember an injury. An MRI is usually indicated for suspected meniscal tear.

COST-EFFECTIVE MEDICINE

If the radiographs of a patient with a clinically suspected meniscal problem show advanced DJD, diagnosis of a meniscal tear does not change treatment; when DJD becomes severe, the definitive treatment is arthroplasty. There is rarely a good indication for MRI when radiographs show moderate to advanced DJD in a patient with chronic knee symptoms.

Patients in whom there is clinical suspicion of meniscal tear and who have a history of prior meniscus surgery may present significant diagnostic difficulty because it can be very difficult on routine MRI to distinguish between post-surgical meniscal changes and a new tear. When evaluating such a patient, it is important that you obtain prior surgical reports as part of the history-taking process. If prior surgery, for example, was on the lateral meniscus and the current symptoms and clinical concern are medial, that information could then be provided to the interpreting radiologist who would then confidently be able to evaluate the medial meniscus. If there is clinical concern about recurrent tear in the previously repaired meniscus, the patient may benefit from MR arthrography of the knee.

Patients who have had prior knee arthroplasty and have recurrent pain are initially evaluated with radiography. If radiographs are negative, CT and/or radionuclide bone scanning is usually obtained.

Patients with osteochondral defects typically have a history of repetitive stress and develop a sudden onset of pain without injury. Radiographs are required for initial evaluation. MRI is valuable, not only in defining the devascularized segment of cortical bone but also in characterizing the lesions as stable or as unstable. Older patients with similar pathology of osteonecrosis (typically middle-aged women) may have sudden sharp pain (usually medial) when they walk or exercise or may have a gradual onset of symptoms and may have locking or catching, especially when the articular cartilage has been disrupted. They are tender over the area and they may have an effusion. These patients may have a history of chronic steroid use, lupus, sickle cell anemia, or renal transplant, conditions that predispose to osteonecrosis.

Patients with pain in the shin, especially after a rapid increase in their activity, may have a stress injury of bone. AP and lateral radiographs should be ordered, but these may not show anything until 3 to 4 weeks after initial onset of symptoms, and by that time the bone may have a frank stress fracture. Bone scans can be used, but sometimes athletes who have repetitive stress on the legs will show areas of increased uptake in asymptomatic locations. MRI will confirm the diagnosis of a stress fracture or stress reaction, although it is not always needed because often diagnosis can be based on history and symptoms.

Interpretation

Patients who have DJD of the knees may report a history of trauma, previous knee surgery (usually meniscectomy), or fractures around the knee. Patients with a history of RA will often have arthritic changes in the knees. With both RA and DJD, patients may develop genu valgus (more common) or genu varus. Pain is most severe when arising in the morning or getting up from a chair. Weight-bearing AP or PA view will show the narrowing of the medial and/or lateral compartments (loss of articular cartilage) and varus or valgus deformity (Fig. 2-61). RA patients will show more symmetric loss of the articular cartilage (medial and lateral compartments) than DJD patients (typically more loss in the medial compartment) and, unless they have developed DJD secondarily, have no osteophytes or sclerosis formation. Patients with chronic patellar tracking disorders often have the most severe changes of DJD in the anterior compartment. Such is likely the case with the patient depicted in Figure 2-62, which shows lateral subluxation of the patella and advanced DJD in the patellofemoral compartment. Note the loss of articular cartilage space in the lateral

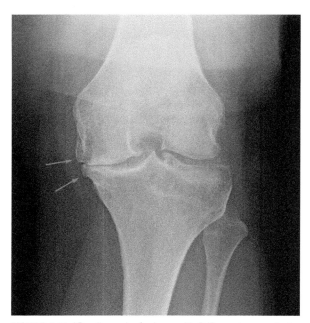

FIGURE 2-61 AP radiograph of a knee with DJD, most severe in the medial compartment. Note loss of medial compartment articular cartilage space and medial osteophytes (arrows).

patellofemoral articulation (arrowheads), and the lateral marginal osteophyte (arrow).

Patients who have a patella tilt seen on Merchant's view radiographs can have patellofemoral syndrome. Sometimes the lateral tilt is an incidental finding and the patient may be asymptomatic. This condition is usually treated nonsurgically. Patients with severe patellar tilt who do not respond to non-surgical treatment can be referred to a surgeon to discuss surgical options such as a lateral retinaculum release.

Patients with OS disease have anterior knee pain and/or pain over their tibial tuberosity. They may even notice a more prominent tibial tuberosity or swelling around that area. They will have pain when compressing the tuberosity. Lateral

radiographs can show fragmentation of the tibial tuberosity or ossification of the distal patellar tendon (Fig. 2-63).

Although radiographs in a young patient with suspected osteochondral lesions or an older patient with osteonecrosis radiographs are often normal, they may reveal a crescent-shaped lucency in the subchondral bone or mixed sclerotic and lucent changes in an articular surface; in advanced cases they may show collapse of the articular surface. This is most commonly seen on the posterolateral side of the medial femoral condyle. Over time the necrotic segment may displace and/or fragment, causing a defect in the articular surface. Displaced fragments become loose joint bodies. MRI is the procedure of choice to further evaluate the osteochondral lesion or osteonecrosis (Fig. 2-64). In young patients with osteochondral lesions, the key finding in MRI is the presence (or absence) of fluid beneath the fragment, indicating that the fragment is unstable. Non-surgical treatment is recommended when the articular cartilage is intact and the fragment is stable.

 Children with osteochondral defect should always be referred to orthopedic consultation.

MRI in patients with osteonecrosis will show a hypointense line beneath the articular cortex that demarcates the necrotic segment, as well as significant bone marrow edema. Patients with osteonecrosis may be candidates for debridement, and in cases in which there is progressive collapse of the articular surface, eventual arthroplasty is likely.

Patients who have persistent knee pain with locking and catching and who have joint line tenderness on examination will likely have a chronic meniscus tear. They may or may

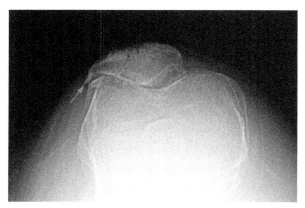

FIGURE 2-62 Merchant view radiograph with lateral subluxation of the patella and advanced DJD in the patellofemoral compartment. Note loss of articular cartilage space in the lateral patellofemoral articulation (arrowheads), and lateral marginal osteophyte (arrow).

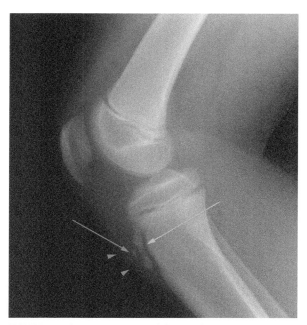

FIGURE 2-63 Lateral radiograph of Osgood-Schlatter's disease (red arrow points to fragmented apophysis). Note overlying soft tissue swelling (arrowheads).

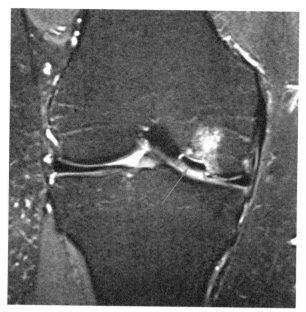

FIGURE 2-64 Coronal T2 MRI of an osteochondral lesion (arrow indicates cortical fragment) of a femoral condyle. Note surrounding bright bone marrow edema.

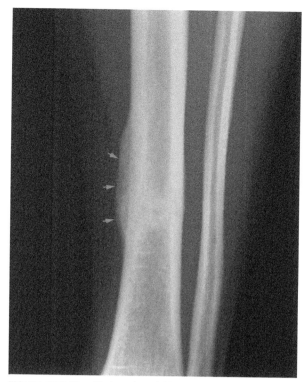

FIGURE 2-65 Magnified section of AP radiograph of the tibia with periosteal new bone formation (arrowheads) consistent with the presence of a healing stress fracture.

not recall an acute injury in the past. MRI should be requested if radiography does not show significant arthritis. Similar to an acute tear, chronic meniscal tears can be treated non-operatively, but when such treatment does not reduce the symptoms, knee arthroscopy with a partial meniscectomy is often done to relieve symptoms.

Typically, tibial stress fractures can be diagnosed by history and physical exam. Radiography of stress fractures may be normal or show very subtle bone lucency and "periosteal reaction," which means that the periosteum of bone is stimulated into producing calcified matrix between elevated periosteum and the bone cortex (Fig. 2-65). In advanced/chronic cases there may be mature periosteal new bone formation along the cortical margin of a stress fracture.

When radiographs of suspected stress fractures are negative and definitive diagnosis is required, a radionuclide bone scan is useful to show the abnormal bone activity that is typical of a stress injury of bone (Fig. 2-66). MRI can also provide a definitive diagnosis of stress injury of bone by various patterns of edema in the marrow space, linear abnormal signal in bone cortex, and edema signal in periosteum and surrounding soft tissue.

ANKLE AND FOOT

Acute Pain and Trauma

Modalities

Initial imaging of the acute ankle should consist of AP, lateral, and mortise views. CT and MRI are rarely used for further evaluation because radiography is usually definitive for the presence or absence of fracture.

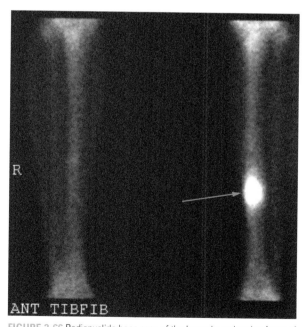

FIGURE 2-66 Radionuclide bone scan of the lower legs showing focus of increased activity (arrow) in the left tibia consistent with the presence of a stress fracture.

COST-EFFECTIVE MEDICINE

Most ligamentous ankle injuries (sprains) are diagnosed clinically and treated appropriately without advanced imaging.

Although a complete tear of the Achilles tendon is a clinical diagnosis that does not require imaging, partial tears that require surgical repair may not be definitively diagnosed clinically. MRI is the procedure of choice in this situation.

Patients who complain of foot pain after an injury or trauma can have swelling, bruising, and/or deformity. Locating the site of maximum tenderness is important for diagnosis. If radiography is requested, that clinical information must be communicated on the imaging order. Initial imaging should consist of AP, lateral, and oblique views. If the patient has significant bruising and swelling around the hindfoot and reports falling from higher than 6 feet or being involved in a motor vehicle accident (MVA), the calcaneus could be fractured. An axial radiographic view of the calcaneus should be done, in addition to routine foot radiographs. For surgical planning of talus and calcaneus fractures, CT is usually done. Complex fractures in the tarsometatarsal regions are often evaluated with CT. Patients who have persistent severe pain and disability that is not explained by ankle and foot radiographs usually are examined with MRI.

If radiographs are negative and there is a high suspicion of a Lisfranc injury, the patient can be immobilized for 2 to 7 days with repeat x-rays with weight bearing. If radiographs are still negative or if weight-bearing views cannot be done due to pain, then an MRI is used to evaluate the midfoot. MRI can also be useful for surgical planning.

Interpretation

Patients with pain and swelling around the ankle who report an inversion, eversion, or twisting injury, and for whom radiographs are negative, likely have an ankle sprain. No other imaging is required. These patients can be treated conservatively. If the patient continues to have instability (recurrent ankle sprains), surgery may be needed for stabilization. MRI to evaluate ankle ligaments may be appropriate for pre-operative planning.

There are several types of ankle fractures, including isolated lateral and medial malleolar fractures, bimalleolar fractures, trimalleolar fractures, fracture-dislocations, and pilon fractures (intra-articular fracture that can be comminuted). In ankle fractures it is important to check for an associated proximal fibular fracture.

For patients who have an isolated lateral malleolus fracture below the ankle mortise (Fig. 2-67) or who show oblique fractures at the level of the mortise and no widening of the mortise, surgery is not needed and the patient can be treated in a cast or boot.

If the syndesmotic ligaments of the distal tibiofibular joint are disrupted and the ankle mortise is widened, the ankle is unstable and surgery is indicated. High lateral malleolar fractures are more likely than low ones to disrupt the

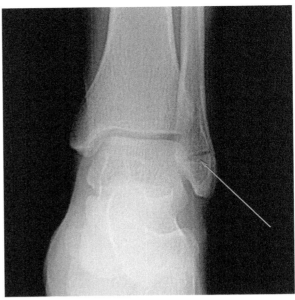

FIGURE 2-67 Mortise view radiograph of a lateral malleolus fracture (arrow) with stable ankle mortise.

distal tibiofibular (syndesmotic) ligaments. Note that a widened mortise secondary to torn syndesmotic ligaments can occur without an ankle fracture. If the tibia and fibula are separated by more than 5 to 6 mm 1 cm superior to the joint line, as in Figure 2-68, the distal tibiofibular syndesmosis is injured. Another radiographic sign of ankle instability that is shown in Figure 2-68 is that the joint space

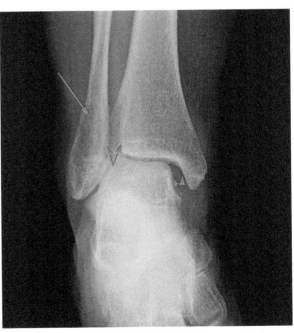

FIGURE 2-68 Mortise view radiograph of a lateral malleolus fracture (long arrow) and an unstable ankle mortise. Short arrows point to the widened tibiofibular space and widened medial joint space. This fracture of the distal fibula was far more evident on other views; mortise view shown to illustrate evidence of disruption of syndesmotic ligaments.

between the medial wall of the talus and medial malleolus is abnormally wide.

Isolated medial malleolus fracture is seen well on the mortise view radiograph shown in Figure 2-69. As long as the fracture is isolated, minimally displaced, and involves the distal portion of the malleolus, it can be treated non-surgically. However, if the fracture is displaced and involves a significant portion of the proximal malleolus, then surgical fixation is needed.

Bimalleolar fractures, as seen in Figure 2-70, involve both the medial and lateral malleoli. Trimalleolar fractures (Fig. 2-71) involve the medial and lateral malleoli and the posterior corner of the distal tibia, which, for clinical purposes, is referred to as a posterior malleolus. With both types of fractures the ankle joint is unstable and surgery is recommended.

Pilon fractures are intra-articular fractures that are comminuted (Fig. 2-72). The fracture can extend in an oblique pattern across the tibia. There can also be an associated distal fibula fracture and a widened ankle mortise. This fracture usually occurs after a high impact injury in which the talar dome impacts the tibia. About 25% of these fractures are open fractures, so wound care is also important in pilon fractures. These fractures are very unstable and need surgical fixation. CT is sometimes done for surgical planning.

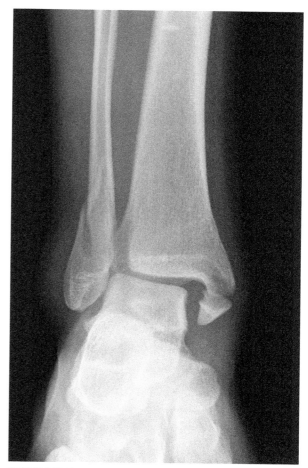

FIGURE 2-70 AP radiograph showing a bimalleolar fracture, with widening of the ankle mortise.

Fracture-dislocation of the ankle show obvious gross disruption of the ankle joint on all radiographic views. The dislocated ankle should be reduced as soon as possible to avoid neurovascular damage. Surgery is always indicated because there will be ankle instability.

Calcaneal fractures from a fall are often bilateral so radiographs from both feet should be examined. Furthermore, these accidents are often also associated with vertebral compression fractures. It would not be uncommon for the severe pain of a calcaneal fracture to "mask" less severe pain in the back. Patients with calcaneal fractures should be carefully evaluated for back pain or tenderness that may require radiologic evaluation of the spine. With calcaneal fracture, a patient will have pain, swelling, and/or deformity of the hind foot. A fracture can typically be seen on the lateral view (Fig. 2-73). An oblique view will show any disruption of the calcaneocuboid joint. An axial view (Fig. 2-74) of the calcaneus will show any displacement of the lateral wall and displacement of the tuberosity. CT scans help with further evaluation of the fracture and surgical planning. Figure 2-75 shows how a CT can also be useful to assess the damage to

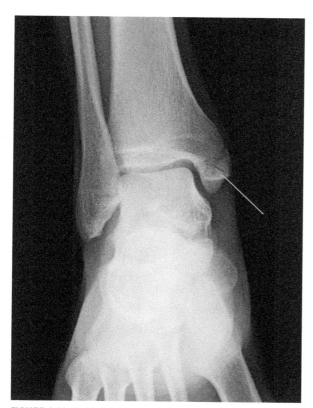

FIGURE 2-69 Mortise view radiograph of a medial malleolus fracture (arrow) with no widening of the ankle mortise.

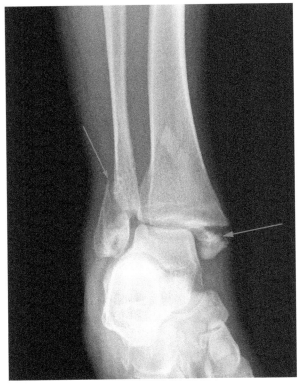

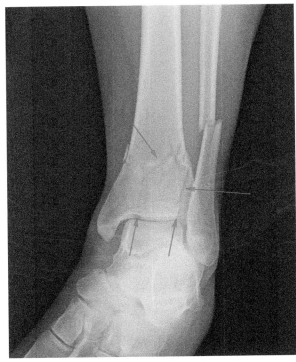

FIGURE 2-72 AP radiograph of a pilon fracture (arrows).

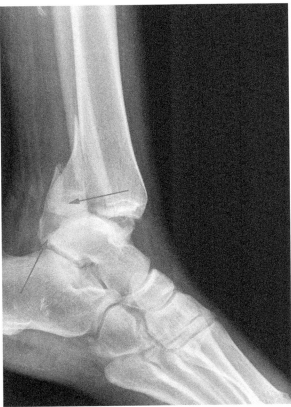

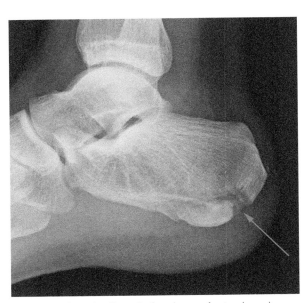

FIGURE 2-73 Lateral radiograph of a calcaneus fracture (arrow).

FIGURE 2-71 AP **(top)** arrows pointing to medial and lateral malleolar fractures) and lateral **(bottom)** radiograph (arrows pointing to displaced fragment of the "posterior malleolus") of a trimalleolar fracture.

the subtalar and calcaneocuboid joints. Non-displaced calcaneal fractures can be treated non-surgically. Displaced and comminuted fractures need surgical fixation.

Talar fractures usually are also the result of high energy trauma. They occur when the foot is forced into severe dorsiflexion. Subluxation or dislocation of the subtalar or ankle joints may accompany this injury. Talar fractures can occur with calcaneal fractures, but this is uncommon. AP and lateral views of the foot help identify the fracture pattern. An

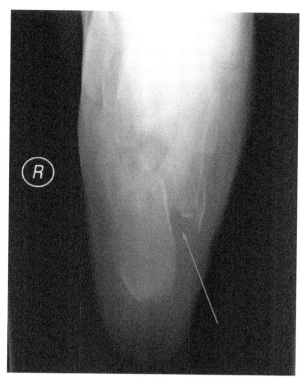

FIGURE 2-74 Axial radiograph of a calcaneus fracture (arrow).

AP or mortise view of the ankle should be obtained to evaluate the tibiotalar joint. CT scans are often used to detect non-displaced fractures, evaluate the fracture patterns, and evaluate for osteochondral injuries. Most often these fractures need internal fixation. The talus' blood supply is limited and if the bone is not repaired there is a high risk of osteonecrosis. Non-displaced fractures may be treated non-operatively.

In a Lisfranc injury there is a lateral dislocation of the second to fifth metatarsals in relation to the distal row of tarsal bones, with or without fractures. More than 2 mm of space between the first and second metatarsal bases is positive for a Lisfranc ligament tear (Fig. 2-76). An avulsion fracture of the second metatarsal base at the insertion of the Lisfranc ligament may be seen. Depending on the severity of the injury, the lateral shift of the second through fifth metatarsal bases may be clearly evident on AP and oblique radiographs. Sometimes there are associated fractures of one or more of the bases of the second to fifth metatarsals. Stable non-displaced injuries can be treated non-operatively, but unstable displaced injuries need surgical fixation. When clinical and radiographic findings for a Lisfranc injury are uncertain, MRI can directly image the Lisfranc ligament and determine if it is intact.

Metatarsal neck and shaft fractures can occur directly with a crush injury. Indirectly, these fractures can occur with twisting forces applied to the foot. There can be bruising and swelling of the foot with or without the ability to bear weight. Metatarsal neck and shaft fractures can be isolated or involve several of the metatarsals. Non-displaced fractures can be treated non-operatively. Multiple metatarsal fractures and fractures with more than 4 mm of displacement may

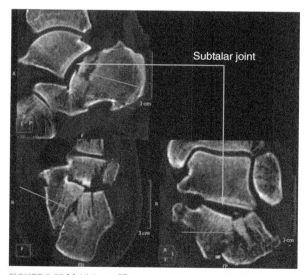

FIGURE 2-75 Multiplanar CT reconstruction images of a highly comminuted fracture (arrows) of the calcaneus.

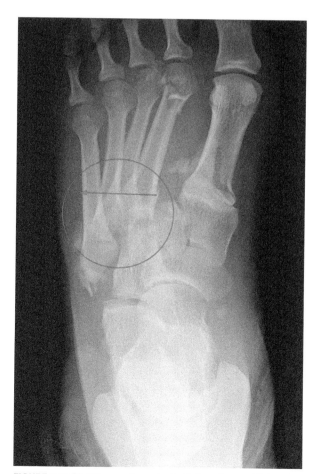

FIGURE 2-76 PA oblique radiograph of a Lisfranc fracture/dislocation. Note lateral shift (arrow) of second through fifth metatarsal bases (within circle).

require surgical treatment. First metatarsal surgery would be considered if there is comminution and displacement of the bone.

Inversion injury or injury that applies an adduction force to the foot can cause fractures of the base of the fifth metatarsal. There may be swelling or bruising and there will be tenderness over the base of the fifth metatarsal. A Jones fracture is a transverse fracture within 15 mm of the base of the fifth metatarsal (Fig. 2-77). Other fractures at the base of the fifth metatarsal are avulsion fractures or fractures of the tuberosity. Usually, these other fractures can be treated non-surgically. Surgical treatment is highly recommended for a Jones fracture to avoid non-union or malunion.

 A common normal finding that may be confused with fracture in this location is the secondary center of ossification along the lateral margin of the base of the fifth metatarsal in the immature skeleton.

Fractures of the phalanges occur usually by dropping objects on the toes or from "jamming" the toe. Patients will have swelling and bruising. A deformity is rarely seen unless the toe is dislocated. Non-operative treatment usually is the best option for these fractures. If fractures are severely angulated and displaced, then closed reduction can be done under a local anesthetic. Markedly displaced and angulated fractures may need open reduction with fixation, especially if they involve the articular surface of the metatarsal or interphalangeal joints of the great toe.

Dislocated toes can be seen on AP, lateral, and oblique views. Dislocated toes can be reduced under a local block.

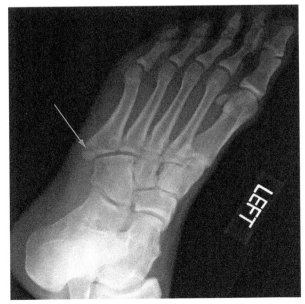

FIGURE 2-77 PA oblique radiograph of a Jones fracture (arrow).

Post-reduction films should be taken to show that the toe has been reduced properly and to evaluate for fractures.

Sesamoid fractures can occur because of direct trauma, dorsiflexion injuries, or repetitive stress. Patient will have pain deep to the sesamoid bones. They may or may not have swelling or bruising. On radiographs, it is important to not mistake a bipartite sesamoid for a fractured sesamoid. Usually a fracture line will look irregular whereas a bipartite sesamoid will have smooth margins. If this differentiation is not clear from the plain films, a bone scan can be done to differentiate between a fractured sesamoid and a bipartite sesamoid. However, a bone scan is sensitive but not specific for fracture. Sesamoiditis or fracture may result in increased activity on a bone scan. High resolution CT scanning may be more specific than a radionuclide study.

Chronic Ankle and Foot Pain

Chronic ankle pain can be the result of arthritis, osteochondral defect of the talar dome, tendonitis, and instability secondary to unresolved severe ankle sprain. Patients with ankle arthritis will complain of chronic pain, swelling, and stiffness of the ankle especially in the anterior aspect. Patients with DJD of the ankle (tibiotalar joint) commonly have a history of trauma to the ankle in the past. A complete medical history is of course important because a history of RA would raise suspicion that ankle pain is arthritic. Patients will complain of pain with flexing and extending the ankle and will have decreased range of motion. Patients with over-pronation of the foot often have chronic ankle pain.

Modalities

Radiography is always the appropriate first imaging procedure. Standard views are AP, lateral, and mortise projections. Weight-bearing images are also helpful to demonstrate joint space narrowing.

 COST-EFFECTIVE MEDICINE
MRI and CT scans are usually not needed for evaluation of ankle arthritis.

Functional imaging, such as weight-bearing ankle and foot radiographs, may have significantly reduced spatial resolution when compared with "table top" images. Subtle bone lesions may be missed. If bone detail is suboptimal on initial functional radiographs, non–weight-bearing tabletop radiographs should be considered

Radiographically visible talar dome osteochondral lesions or suspected osteochondral lesions are evaluated with MRI. In some cases, CT is also needed to best visualize the extent of articular surface damage.

Patients with chronic lateral ankle pain may have tendonitis or a chronic tendon tear. Patients who report lateral ankle pain may have peroneal (fibular) tendonitis, chronic tendon tear, or subluxation of the peroneal (fibular) tendons that can occur with tears of the superior peroneal (fibular) retinaculum. MRI is appropriate to evaluate tendinopathy.

Patients with posterior tibialis tendon dysfunction or tendonitis/tenosynovitis may initially report posteromedial ankle pain and swelling. Over time, dysfunction of this tendon can cause an acquired flatfoot. MRI can be helpful for surgical planning for posterior tibialis tendon abnormalities.

When special expertise is available, ultrasonography may be an ideal imaging procedure for ankle tendons, especially when an experienced examiner can evaluate functional issues such as tendon subluxation.

Patients who complain of pain in the posterior aspect of the ankle and/or heel may have tendonitis of the Achilles tendon. There is usually a gradual onset of pain, which is increased with activity. On examination there may be swelling around the insertion of the Achilles tendon and thickening of the tendon can be palpable. A lateral radiograph of the calcaneus is often sufficient and MRI is not needed unless a diagnosis cannot be made based on radiography, symptoms, and physical exam.

Patients with instability of the ankle may have a history of trauma, such as several ankle sprains. Lateral instability is more common than medial. Ankle instability is appropriately evaluated with MRI.

Chronic foot pain can be from arthritis, tendon dysfunction, pes planus (congenital or acquire flat foot), bunion deformities, toe deformities, stress fractures, and Charcot (neuropathic) foot. AP, lateral, and oblique radiographic views of the foot are the standard for initial evaluation. The standing lateral radiograph is ideal for evaluation of flatfoot. Suspected stress fractures can be evaluated with radionuclide bone scanning or MRI.

Arthritis of the foot typically occurs at the subtalar joint, talonavicular joint, midfoot (tarsometatarsal joints), and first metatarsophalangeal joint (known as Hallux Rigidus). In patients who have pain in the first metatarsophalangeal joint, it is important to rule out gout. Patients with talonavicular arthritis will have pain over the medial aspect of the hind foot. This is a common site for RA. Patients with subtalar arthritis may report pain in their hind foot with walking on uneven surfaces. This type of arthritis may develop after calcaneus fracture. Weight-bearing radiographs should be obtained and, if needed for better bone and joint detail, overhead tabletop radiographs. Radiography is usually sufficient in these cases.

The initial imaging of patients with a clinical presentation of plantar fasciitis should begin with radiography. However, the presence of a plantar calcaneal spur may not always mean that the patient has an active fasciitis that is responsible for pain; MRI is appropriate if diagnosis is uncertain.

COST-EFFECTIVE MEDICINE

Bunion deformities are evaluated radiographically. No further imaging is needed. Patients with toe deformities will have pain in their toes especially when they wear shoes. There are usually clinical findings and radiographs are not needed; weight-bearing films are helpful for further evaluation, especially if surgery is planned.

Patients who present with foot or ankle pain and swelling, especially with increased weight-bearing activity, may have a stress fracture, most commonly in the second metatarsal. Radiographs should be obtained, and high detail is important because the radiographic changes in stress fracture can be quite subtle. When radiographs are normal and stress fracture is suspected, MRI is usually the procedure of choice. When MRI cannot be done, a radionuclide bone scan can be diagnostic.

Diabetic patients with deformity of the foot with or without pain may have Charcot arthropathy. Radiography is usually sufficient, although for treatment planning, MRI or CT is often helpful. It may be difficult to differentiate the neuropathic foot (Charcot foot) from osteomyelitis in the foot, because most commonly both occur in diabetic patients. Contrast-enhanced MRI of the foot, after standard initial radiographic evaluation, has a higher specificity than radionuclide bone scanning in differentiating these cases.

Other conditions causing chronic foot pain, such as Morton's neuroma, Freiberg's disease, and symptomatic accessory ossicles, are evaluated first with radiography and then MRI if needed for more definitive diagnosis.

 Pediatric patients with chronic foot pain may have congenital abnormalities, such as talar coalition, which may be radiographically occult. CT of the foot is often done for further evaluation.

INTERPRETATION

Osteoarthritis in the ankle and foot characteristically shows joint space narrowing, sclerosis, subcortical cysts, and marginal osteophytes (see Table 2-3). Depending on the joint(s) involved, these features may be difficult to completely visualize, especially in the subtalar and mid-foot joints. Be suspicious of any sclerotic changes (Fig. 2-78). RA of the foot usually will have significant bunion deformity at the great toe. The metatarsophalangeal joints of the other toes will

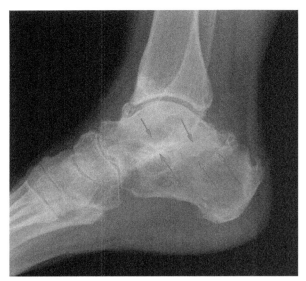

FIGURE 2-78 Lateral radiograph showing signs of subtalar DJD, with sclerotic and irregular cortical bone margins adjacent to the joint, and loss of joint space (arrows).

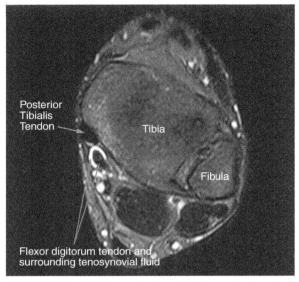

FIGURE 2-80 Axial T2 MRI of ankle. Note fluid-distended tendon sheath (red arrows).

show dorsal joint dislocation. RA is usually bilateral, whereas DJD is often unilateral.

Radiographic findings of talar dome osteochondral lesions can be subtle, often showing only some minimal sclerosis of bone (Fig. 2-79). MRI is done if the lesion cannot be seen on radiographs and can determine the lesion stability of the osteochondral segment of bone by the presence or absence of bright fluid signal along the deep margin of the lesion. Osteochondral lesions of the talar dome can be treated nonsurgically but should always be referred for orthopedic care.

The characteristic MRI (Fig. 2-80) or ultrasound finding for tenosynovitis is fluid distention of the tendon sheath. Tendon tears may be complete transverse tears or may be longitudinal spits of the tendon. Peroneal (fibular) and posterior tibialis tendon dysfunction is usually diagnosed clinically,

with dynamic ultrasound exams providing confirmation when the special expertise for that exam is available.

In patients with the clinical diagnosis of Achilles tendonitis, lateral foot radiographs may show an enthesis (spur) at the insertion of the tendon or Haglund's deformity (Fig. 2-81) of the calcaneus, an osseous prominence that may be resected as part of surgical treatment.

Bunion deformities, as depicted in Figure 2-82, show the characteristic hallux valgus and hypertrophy of the head of the first metatarsal.

Radiographs show sclerosis and fragmentation of bones in a patient with Charcot foot. With advanced osteomyelitis, frank bone destruction may be evident, but usually when osteomyelitis has complicated the diabetic patient's foot,

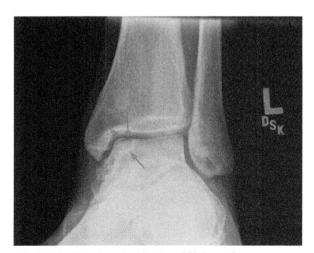

FIGURE 2-79 AP radiograph, talar dome OCD (arrows).

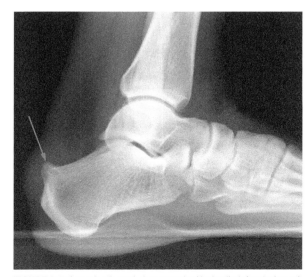

FIGURE 2-81 Lateral radiograph demonstrating Haglund's deformity (arrow).

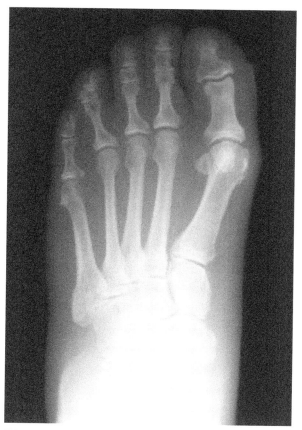

FIGURE 2-82 PA radiograph of bunion deformity.

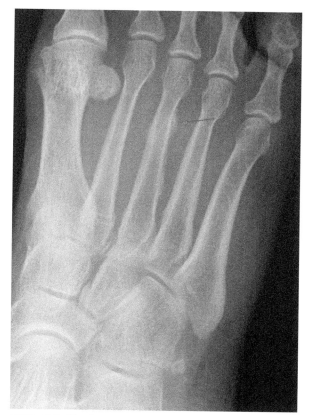

FIGURE 2-83 PA radiograph showing early changes of metatarsal stress fracture (arrow).

findings on radiographs are not specific. MRI will show bone marrow edema, contrast-enhancing marrow space, and sometimes a frank abscess within the marrow compartment of bone.

Radiographs in early stress injury of bone are often normal. Later, subtle periosteal reaction, as in the case shown in Figure 2-83 of the third metatarsal, leads to periosteal new bone formation that forms a subsequent fracture callus, clearly visible on radiographs (Fig. 2-84).

MRI will show bone marrow edema (Fig. 2-85) with stress fracture and may show periosteal high signal. See Patient Communication Box 2-2.

LOWER LIMB VASCULAR DISEASE: PERIPHERAL ARTERIAL INSUFFICIENCY AND VENOUS THROMBOSIS

Arterial insufficiency in the lower extremities leads to the typical symptom of claudication. Clinical examination involves evaluation of arterial pulses and gathering relevant history related to peripheral vascular disease such as smoking or diabetes.

Modalities

The initial procedure used to assess lower extremity arteries consists of **arterial Doppler sonography** that may also be referred to as **lower extremity non-invasive testing.** When Doppler sonography suggests significant stenotic/occlusive disease, then CTA or MRA is usually done for more definitive diagnosis. In cases in which a severe arterial insufficiency may need urgent or semi-urgent intervention, patients may proceed directly to catheter angiography.

Clinical suspicion of deep venous thrombosis (e.g., calf pain and swelling in a post-operative patient) is usually examined with lower extremity **venous Doppler sonography.**

Interpretation

Reduced pulse pressures measured during lower extremity non-invasive arterial testing and dampened pulse waveforms are evidence of arterial occlusive disease. A low ankle-brachial index (ABI) is a basic parameter that indicates possible arterial insufficiency. CTA or MRA demonstrates the location and severity of arterial disease (Fig. 2-86).

Acute deep venous thrombosis (DVT) is revealed on sonography (Fig. 2-87).

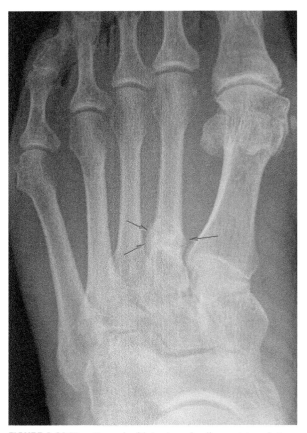

FIGURE 2-84 PA radiograph of late stage, healing metatarsal stress fracture (arrows).

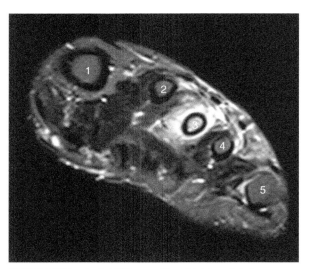

FIGURE 2-85 Short axis MRI image of foot. Metatarsal shafts are numbered. Note the bright T2 hyperintensity of bone marrow in the third metatarsal, as well as of the periosteum and surrounding soft tissues.

Patient understanding and satisfaction with care for many musculoskeletal conditions is often improved when it is explained to them that different abnormalities are visible in different modalities; it is not a simple matter of, for example, MRI being "better" than radiographs.

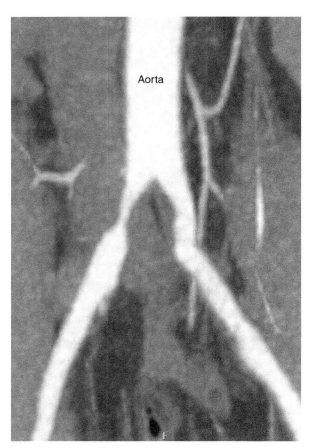

FIGURE 2-86 CTA demonstrating stenosis of the right common iliac artery.

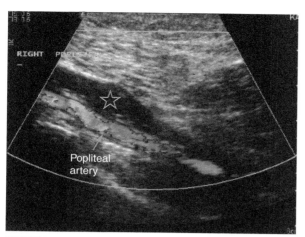

FIGURE 2-87 Lower extremity venous sonography with Doppler Color Flow imaging (Duplex sonography) shows deep venous thrombosis. Note the star within intraluminal thrombus in the popliteal vein.

CASE CONCLUSION

For your 55-year-old patient with shoulder pain, you made a sound clinical decision to not request an MRI of the shoulder just for the sake of "doing something." With physical therapy and nonsteroidal anti-inflammatory medications (NSAIDs), the patient has regained strength and comfort in the shoulder and now has minimal symptoms. In fact, after medical treatment and physical therapy, abduction is quite good and it is doubtful that there could be any significant tear of the supraspinatus tendon.

You outline for your patient some possibilities for the future: Any significant loss of strength of abduction combined with increasing pain would justify getting an MRI to look for a rotator cuff tear. However, gradual progression of joint pain, especially with crepitance, could mean worsening of the glenohumeral joint DJD and repeat shoulder radiographs may be appropriate to follow the arthritis. If that disease becomes severe enough, orthopedic consultation may then be appropriate to consider joint replacement.

Your patient leaves feeling far more satisfied by your explanations and discussions than would have happened with a much shorter interaction accompanied by an order for MRI that did not change the clinical outcome.

Chapter Review

Chapter Review Questions

1. The Salter-Harris classification refers to:
   A. types of comminuted fractures of the humeral head.
   B. types of fractures involving the physis in the immature skeleton.
   C. the degree of pelvis instability following a pubic fracture.
   D. the degree of instability in the ankle joint after fracture.
   E. the different degrees of separation in an AC joint after injury.

2. Articular surface deformities within complex skeletal structures, such as the midfoot, are best seen on:
   A. CT.
   B. MRI.
   C. radiography.
   D. ultrasound.
   E. radionuclide scan.

3. Which of the following is not characteristic of inflammatory (rheumatoid) arthritis?
   A. Joint effusion
   B. Joint deformity
   C. Decreased density in subchondral bone
   D. Loss of articular cartilage
   E. Osteophytes

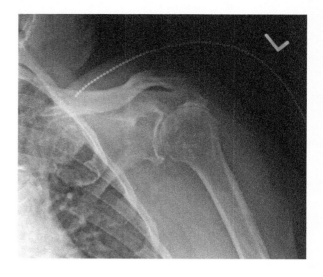

4. Which of the following can be concluded from the above image?
   A. There is a stress fracture in the humeral head
   B. There is a hemarthrosis
   C. There is rotator cuff tear
   D. There is a grade 4 AC separation
   E. There is a posterior humeral dislocation

5. Your patient reports a sudden painful tearing sensation in the cubital fossa and weakness with flexion. There is tenderness and ecchymosis over the cubital fossa and distal upper arm. If physical examination is not definitive, which of the following imaging modalities would be the most likely to confirm the diagnosis of distal biceps tendon tear?
   A. Radiography
   B. CT
   C. MRI
   D. Radionuclide bone scan
   E. Arthrography

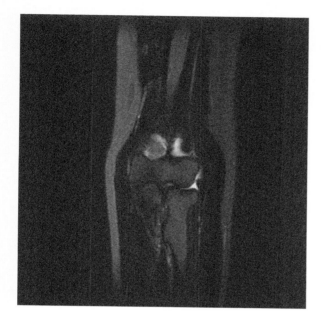

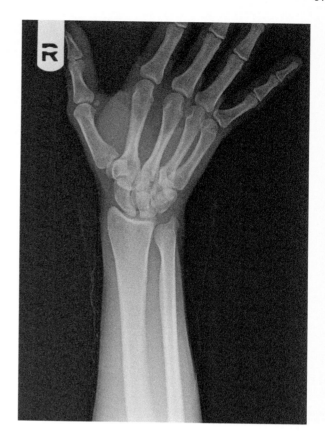

6. The image above shows a:
   A. CT scan of a normal elbow joint.
   B. MRI of a normal elbow.
   C. patient with a torn medial collateral ligament.
   D. patient with a torn lateral collateral ligament.
   E. patient with medial epicondylitis.

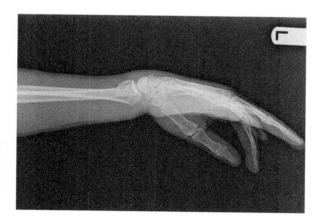

7. The image shown above depicts which of the following fractures?
   A. Colles
   B. Smith
   C. Bankart
   D. Hill-Sachs
   E. Legg-Calve-Perthes

8. Your patient fell on her hand and is now complaining of severe pain and tenderness in the anatomic snuff-box. A radiograph of her wrist is shown above. Which of the following is your likely course of action?
   A. Tell her that her wrist is severely bruised and it may take 6 weeks for the pain and swelling to dissipate
   B. Explain to her that she may have a scaphoid fracture that is not visible on radiographs. Give her the option of repeat radiography after 1 week of immobilization or further examination as soon as possible with MRI
   C. Tell her that she has a fractured scaphoid
   D. Tell her that she has ruptured her triangular fibrocartilage
   E. Send her for an immediate ultrasound exam

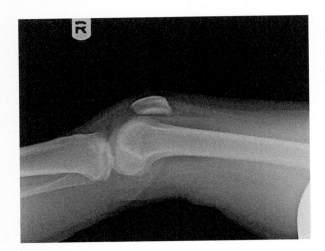

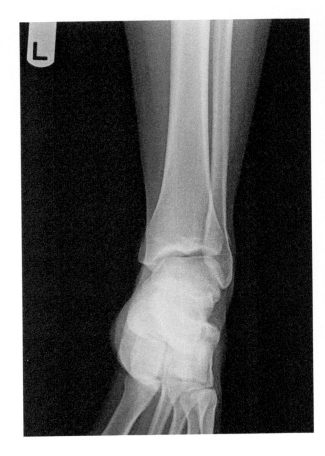

9. The above radiograph, as well as other radiographic projections of the knee, was done after acute trauma. No fracture is visible on any of the radiographic views. Therefore:

   A. patient may be prescribed a knee brace and give a follow-up appointment.

   B. you assure the patient that there is no major injury and recommend physical therapy.

   C. the patient is taught how to use a cane properly and is given a follow-up appointment.

   D. you prescribe nonsteroidal anti-inflammatory medications.

   E. you explain to the patient the likelihood of a fracture that is not visible on radiographs and arrange for urgent CT or MRI of the knee.

10. Your patient has been complaining of severe shin pain, especially during prolonged exercise. Based on the image shown above your likely diagnosis is:

    A. claudication of the lower limb.

    B. pelvic outlet syndrome.

    C. tibial stress fractures.

    D. an osteoblastic tumor.

    E. tetany.

11. A 60-year-old female patient fell off her roof and is now complaining of heel pain. You diagnose a calcaneal fracture on radiographs of the calcaneus. Because of this woman's age and method of injury, you then order:

    A. CT of her pelvis.

    B. MRI of femoral neck.

    C. radiographs of the contralateral foot, if clinical exam reveals any tenderness, and AP and lateral radiographs of her thoracic and lumbar spine if you can elicit any back pain or tenderness.

    D. radionuclide bone scan of tibia.

    E. arterial Doppler sonography of lower limb.

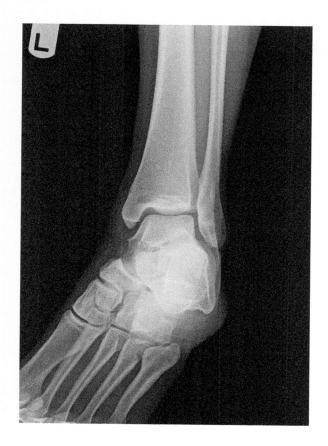

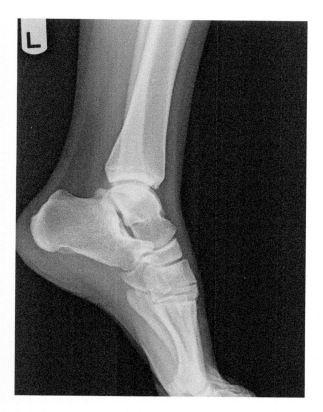

12. Your patient complains of pain on the lateral side of her ankle after "twisting it" yesterday. Her radiographs are shown to the left. Based on these images your likely course of treatment is:

    A. CT scan to look for occult fracture.

    B. referral to a surgeon for internal fixation.

    C. MRI for further evaluation.

    D. conservative treatment—rest, elevation, compression bandaging, and NSAIDs.

    E. casting for 6 weeks.

13. Which of the following is INCORRECT about talar fractures?

    A. Typically associated with Lisfranc fractures

    B. Typically occur with excessive dorsiflexion

    C. Typically need surgery if displaced

    D. Untreated, are often associated with osteonecrosis

    E. May be very subtle or occult on radiographs and may need further study with CT or MRI of the ankle if the patient cannot bear weight on the injured ankle

14. A post-surgical patient is complaining of pain in his calf, which is also swollen. You are most likely to request which of the following imaging modalities to rule out DVT?

    A. Lower extremity non-invasive arterial testing

    B. Venous Doppler sonography

    C. CTA

    D. MRA

    E. Femoral artery angiogram

3 SPINE AND SPINAL CORD

CASE STUDY

On a busy clinic day, you see five patients with back pain:

- Patients A and B are high school football players with progressive low back pain that is limiting their playing. They do not recall any specific severe trauma that precipitated their back pain. You would like to avoid an imaging workup at this time and just see if their symptoms resolve with rest. However, that is unacceptable to these athletes and their parents who are just weeks away from their first competitive events. You order lumbar radiographs.
- Patient C is a 65-year-old female with chronic mild to moderate back pain but no sciatica. Physical examination is normal. You advise her to use over-the-counter NSAIDs judiciously, lose some weight, and join an exercise program at the "YMCA."
- Patients D and E are in their 40's: D has neck pain, numbness, and tingling in the left index finger and thumb, and E has low back pain radiating into the left leg. Physical exam is quite convincing that patient D has a cervical radiculitis and patient E has a lumbar radiculitis. For both of them, you prescribe a short course of steroids.

FUNDAMENTALS OF SPINE AND SPINAL CORD IMAGING

As in any other part of the skeletal system, the spine may suffer from trauma, bone disease, and a variety of arthritic conditions involving the atlantoaxial, facet, costovertebral, and sacroiliac joints.

Unique to the spine is degenerative disc disease (DDD). Intervertebral discs commonly degenerate with age due to dehydration of the nucleus pulposus. As intervertebral discs degenerate, adjacent vertebrae often develop marginal osteophytes. DDD is commonly associated with back and neck pain. However, a major problem with imaging adult patients who have uncomplicated back pain is the finding of pseudo-disease. At least half of adults who have never had back pain can be shown on imaging to have degenerative disc changes. Therefore, when disc abnormalities are found on radiographs, CTs, or MRIs, it

becomes questionable that they are related to a current complaint of back pain, especially the very common finding of small- to moderate-sized anterior vertebral osteophytes.

COST-EFFECTIVE MEDICINE

The documentation of uncomplicated DDD by itself in adults is not likely to change treatment, although the imaging that often shows such disc disease may be useful to rule out other conditions.

Table 3-1 presents examples of the appropriate information that should be part of an imaging request for spine and spinal cord imaging.

SPINAL TRAUMA

Spinal injury that requires medical evaluation and imaging may range from simple twisting or lifting episodes to devastating spinal trauma that results in permanent neurologic deficit. Major spinal trauma, such as that suffered in a severe motor vehicle accident (MVA), is usually managed in the ED. Unless you are working in that environment, your role may be limited to providing follow-up care.

TABLE 3-1 Sample Spine Radiology Requisition Information

Modality	Clinical Data/History
MRI thoracic spine, with contrast if needed	Severe back pain hx: low grade fever, elevated sed rate, hx of active TB, R/O Pott's d.
MRI lumbar spine (w/o contrast)	Back pain, left L3 radiculopathy
MRI cervical spine w contrast	Left cervical radiculopathy, C6? C7?; prior left C5–C6 decompression/ foraminotomy
Radiography lumbar spine	Progressive severe back pain since fall 2 wks ago
Radionuclide bone scan	Progressive generalized back and hip pain; hx of breast cancer, stage 3A in 2006
Lumbar myelogram and CT myelogram	Back pain, bilat leg weakness, DDD, DJD on x-rays; pt. has pacemaker; R/O spinal canal stenosis

Minor spinal trauma may sometimes be accompanied by compression fractures of the vertebrae that occur because the vertebral body was weakened by tumor or osteoporosis (see Chapter 11).

Because cervical spine fractures usually occur from different mechanisms of injury than those in the thoracic and lumbar spine, this region of the spine is discussed separately later in this chapter. Furthermore, you should be aware that because of the increased mobility of the spine below T11 compared with the rib cage–stabilized thoracic region, most non-cervical spine fractures occur near the thoracolumbar junction.

Modalities

For relatively minor to moderate trauma, radiography is an appropriate initial imaging procedure whenever there is reasonable clinical concern about fracture. AP and lateral views are sufficient when the primary concern is that of vertebral body compression fracture of the thoracolumbar spine. In young athletic patients with lumbosacral pain after trauma, in whom you suspect a pars interarticularis fracture, oblique lumbar radiographs should be also be done. In cases in which radiography does not provide definitive diagnosis of a pars interarticularis injury or defect, CT is ideal for further evaluation.

In patients with suspected cervical injury, the "cross-table lateral cervical spine x-ray" is a procedure that has been commonly used to rule out unstable cervical spine injury (i.e., to "clear" the patient). This is now used mainly when CT is not immediately available or when an unstable patient should not be transported to CT.

COST-EFFECTIVE MEDICINE

In patients who meet low-risk clinical criteria for cervical spine trauma, such as the Canadian C-Spine Rule or the NEXUS Low-Risk Criteria, neither this radiograph nor CT is always necessary. However, studies have shown limitations of published decision-making rules; clinical judgment is always required.

In cases of severe trauma transported to the ED that meet high risk clinical criteria for spine fracture, the imaging procedure of choice is CT. When severe spinal trauma is associated with myelopathy, MRI may be preferred because the spinal cord and cauda equina can be evaluated better than with CT. In the severely injured patient, however, patient management issues prevail, and it is far easier to manage patients during a CT exam than during a more confining and lengthy MRI procedure. In complicated cases in which the osseous detail available from CT is needed for operative planning, and neurologic injury requires evaluation with MRI, both procedures may be appropriately performed.

Interpretation

Three conceptual structural "columns" of the spine determine its mechanical stability and are referred to in specific sections of this chapter. The anterior column consists of the anterior longitudinal ligament and the anterior 2/3 of the vertebrae. The middle column includes the posterior 1/3 of the vertebrae and the posterior longitudinal ligament. The posterior column includes the neural arches, ligamentum flava, and interspinous ligaments. Generally, when only the anterior column is injured, stability of the spine is maintained.

When viewing spine radiographs, be certain that fine bone detail can be seen by checking for the sharp appearance of bone trabeculae within the vertebral bodies. This is especially important because any destructive or erosive bone findings, or blastic changes in bone density, raise suspicion of infection or tumor.

Cervical Spine

If a lateral cervical spine radiograph is done (that is, if the patient does not immediately have a CT scan), it should first be inspected for normal alignment of the skull base and all cervical spine segments, as well as the cervicothoracic junction. To check for proper alignment, visualize smooth curved lines along the anterior and posterior margins of the vertebrae and along the posterior margin of the spinal canal as illustrated in Figure 3-1.

After assessing alignment of spinal segments on a lateral radiograph, each level must be carefully inspected for fracture, and you must look for prevertebral soft tissue swelling that could indicate an underlying vertebral fracture. This is most reliable above the level of the glottis where the prevertebral tissues are normally very thin, unlike the case illustrated in Figure 3-2 in which thick soft tissue between the spinal column and the airway could indicate a hematoma from spinal fracture.

Most fatal cervical spine injuries occur at the craniocervical junction, C1, or C2 levels. Fractures that disrupt the C1 ring are called Jefferson fractures and appear on CT as two, three, or four part fractures (Fig. 3-3). When a hyperextension injury, such as in an MVA or hanging, results in a fracture of both C2 pedicles, it is called, surprisingly enough, a Hangman's fracture (Fig. 3-4).

Flexion injuries may cause simple anterior wedge-type compression fractures of cervical vertebrae (Fig. 3-5) without disruption of the middle or posterior columns. These injuries are stable because the middle and posterior columns are intact.

In a flexion "teardrop" fracture such as the one presented as Figure 3-6, anterior displacement of the anteroinferior aspect of the vertebra indicates that the anterior longitudinal ligament (ALL) has been torn. There is also associated widening of the posterior intervertebral space, indicating that the posterior longitudinal ligament (PLL) has been torn, and widening of the space between the posterior elements of affected segments,

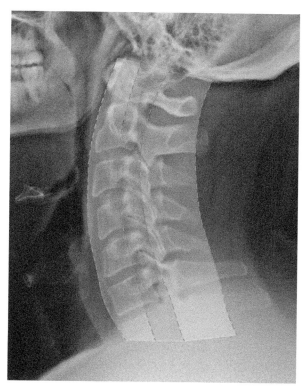

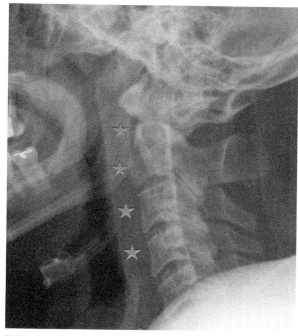

FIGURE 3-2 Lateral radiograph of the cervical spine showing prevertebral soft tissue swelling (stars).

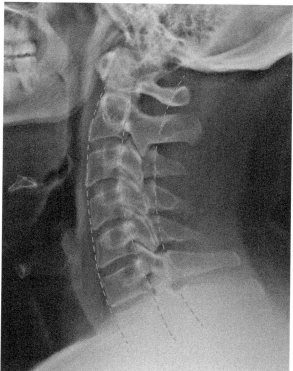

FIGURE 3-1 **Top:** Lateral radiograph of the cervical spine illustrating the concept of the three structural columns. **Bottom:** Lateral radiograph of the cervical spine with dashed lines drawn along the anterior and posterior margins of the vertebral column and the posterior margin of the spinal canal.

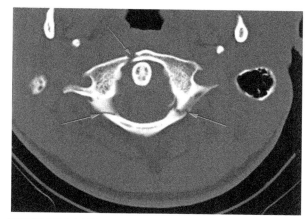

FIGURE 3-3 Axial CT of a Jefferson fracture (arrows indicate multiple fractures of C1).

indicating that the posterior column has been disrupted. Teardrop fractures are unstable and require fixation.

Vertical compression injuries may result in a burst fracture of cervical vertebrae, disrupting the anterior and middle columns. Associated spinal cord injury depends upon the degree of retropulsion of a fractured segment of the posterior wall of the affected vertebral body, which is very well demonstrated on CT, as shown in Figure 3-7, or MRI.

The patient shown in Figure 3-8 has a clay shoveler's fracture, which is an avulsion fracture of the C7 spinous process in which the tip of the spinous process is distracted posteriorly. Note arrow indicating the distracted fracture fragment of the tip of the spinous process. These fractures do not result in any instability and can be treated conservatively.

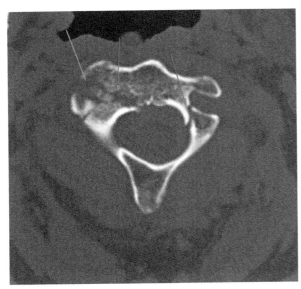

FIGURE 3-4 Axial CT of a Hangman's fracture (arrows indicate fractures involving pedicles of C2).

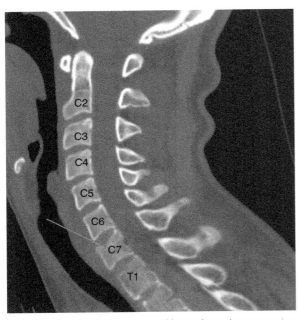

C2
C3
C4
C5
C6
C7
T1

FIGURE 3-5 Sagittal CT with simple, stable anterior wedge compression fracture of C7 (arrow).

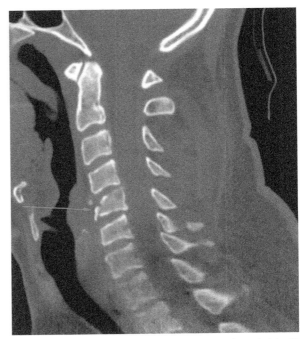

FIGURE 3-6 Sagittal CT with flexion teardrop fracture (arrow) of the C5 vertebral body.

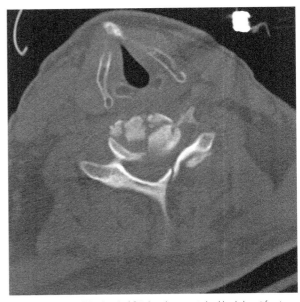

FIGURE 3-7 Axial CT at level of C5 showing a vertebral body burst fracture.

Bilateral cervical facet joint dislocation ("jumped facets") is almost always associated with severe injury to the spinal cord. Unilateral dislocations can occur in which the facets on one side appear to be abnormally overlapping or "perched" as shown in Figure 3-9. These are stable injuries, generally with little associated spinal cord injury.

Thoracolumbar Spine

On a lateral thoracic spine radiograph, you should apply the same principles described in the cervical section above pertaining to checking for normal alignment of the three vertebral columns, and inspect each segment for fracture.

The AP radiograph of the thoracic spine is valuable in trauma for detecting paravertebral soft tissue swelling which, as shown in Figure 3-10, appears as smooth localized soft tissue density along the spine.

In the thoracic spine superior to T11, the middle column may be involved in fracture but the spine remains stable if there are no associated rib and sternal fractures, because an intact rib cage can stabilize the thoracic spine even when the middle column is fractured.

If a lateral radiograph shows an abrupt kyphotic curvature of 20 degrees or more because of an acute

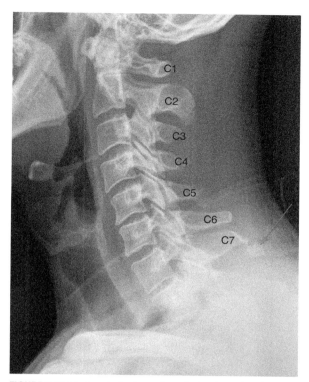

FIGURE 3-8 Lateral cervical spine radiograph showing a clay-shoveler's fracture. Note arrow indicating the distracted fracture fragment of the tip of the C7 spinous process.

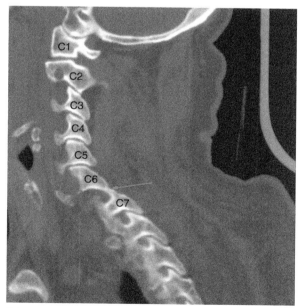

FIGURE 3-9 Sagittal CT of the cervical spine showing dislocated, over-lapping "jumped" facets at C6/7 (arrow). Note the anterior position of the articular column C1-C6 in relation to C7.

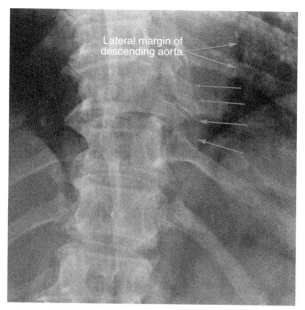

FIGURE 3-10 AP thoracic spine radiograph. Red arrows indicate paravertebral soft tissue swelling, medial to the lateral margin of the descending aorta.

compression fracture, it is assumed that the middle column is involved.

The Chance or seat belt fracture, which is shown in Figure 3-11, is most often seen from T11 to L2 (and mid-lumbar in children) and is a compression fracture of the anterior part of the vertebral body with a transverse fracture through the posterior arch. A large percentage of Chance fractures are associated with pancreatic and duodenal injuries.

Because there is little space within the thoracic spinal canal, injuries that involve the middle column are often associated with cord injury when there is significant retropulsion of a vertebral fracture fragment into the spinal canal as shown in Figure 3-12. These patients usually have clinically evident neurologic injury. Direct visualization of a cord injury is provided by MRI, which shows abnormally high T2 signal (edema or fluid) within the cord or frank disruption of the cord. Such disruption is shown in Figure 3-13, a sagittal MRI after surgical reduction of displaced fractures of T11 and T12.

CASE UPDATE

The radiographs that you ordered on Patient A showed obvious and moderately wide pars interarticularis defects bilaterally at L5 on the oblique radiographs without spondylolisthesis evident on the lateral view. You discuss the case with a radiologist whose opinion is that when pars defects are as wide and as easily seen on radiographs as those of your patient, they are never acute or subacute fractures, but are old defects that will not heal; further imaging will not change this diagnosis. You refer the patient to an orthopedic surgeon who specializes in sports medicine, mainly for counseling about how this diagnosis impacts on participation in contact sports like football.

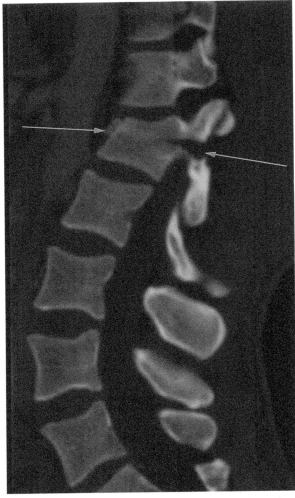

FIGURE 3-11 Sagittal CT of the thoracolumbar spine with a Chance fracture (arrows).

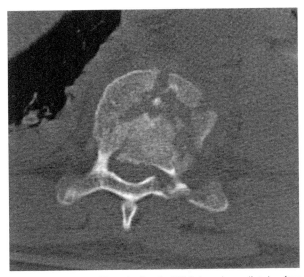

FIGURE 3-12 Axial CT at the level of T10 done immediately after MVA shows a vertebral body burst fracture and markedly narrowed spinal canal.

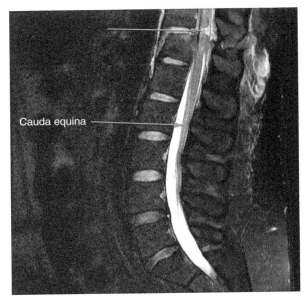

Cauda equina

FIGURE 3-13 Sagittal MRI of the lumbar spine after injury to the lower spinal cord resulting in transection of cord (red arrow).

NECK AND BACK PAIN (No Neurologic Signs or Symptoms)

COST-EFFECTIVE MEDICINE
Acute or short-term neck and back pain is very common and most often unrelated to serious pathology. Treatment decisions do not generally require imaging.

In contrast, the following "red flags" suggest that imaging of the spine may be indicated:

- Persistent spinal pain that does not respond to conservative treatment
- Persistent pain that develops in a patient with a cancer history or who is immunosuppressed
- Severe back pain with unexplained weight loss or fever

Spondyloarthropathies are related arthritic spinal disorders that often cause back pain and that are "seronegative," meaning that patients with these disorders do not test positive for rheumatoid factor. The characteristic radiologic finding is the development of inflammation leading to calcification or ossification of connective tissue that attaches to the vertebrae, an enthesis.

Modalities

Radiography is a useful "baseline" imaging procedure, if any imaging is indicated, in uncomplicated neck and back pain. Often, AP and lateral views are sufficient. Lumbar radiographs are often done with the patient standing, in an effort to acquire functional information about stability and alignment of segments while the patient is weight bearing. Although flexion and extension lateral radiographs may be helpful in evaluating instability, some of the apparent "functional" findings with upright radiography are not perfectly reproducible and may provide pseudo-information that does not explain a patient's symptoms. Especially in a patient who is obese, bone fine detail is often lacking in standing radiographs compared with overhead "table-top" radiography. If standing lumbar radiographs do not provide ideal bone detail, better radiographs should be obtained with overhead "table-top" radiography.

COST-EFFECTIVE MEDICINE

When cervical spine or lumbar pain has a clinical presentation that suggests facet joint arthritis, radiography that includes oblique projections can establish a diagnosis without the need for more expensive CT or MRI.

In addition to AP, lateral, and oblique radiographs, a standard radiographic cervical spine series usually includes an open mouth AP odontoid view, which is valuable in evaluating patients with rotational subluxations at C1–C2 and erosion of the odontoid in patients with RA.

Children with Down's syndrome have atlantoaxial joint instability caused by ligamentous laxity or odontoid hypoplasia, or both. When a child with Down's syndrome is entering athletic competition, screening radiography for atlantoaxial instability is advisable.

When measurement of scoliosis is the essential clinical question, a "scoliosis series" or "scoliosis study" should be ordered rather than radiography of the cervical, thoracic, and lumbar spine.

When MRI is indicated—for example, when pain does not respond to conservative treatment—unenhanced MRI is appropriate if there has been no prior spinal surgery or if previous surgery was from an anterior approach or was a posterior decompression *without* discectomy or foraminotomy. Otherwise, contrast-enhanced MR sequences are needed in the patient with a surgical history to differentiate possible recurrent disc herniations from normal post-operative epidural scar tissue. Also, for suspected infection or tumor in the spine, MRI is usually done with contrast enhancement.

COST-EFFECTIVE MEDICINE

Many health plans and payment systems have created a suboptimal situation in which the physician who is most directly and intimately involved in medical imaging, the radiologist, is prevented from making a clinical judgment about the use of contrast enhancement for the benefit of your patient. However, an imaging order written for "unenhanced

MRI, contrast as needed" may provide some flexibility to the radiologist. For example, if on the routine unenhanced sequences of an MRI done for spinal pain there are unexpected findings that suggest infection, then contrast-enhanced sequences could be done immediately, without the need for a return visit by the patient.

For patients with serious spinal conditions who cannot undergo MRI, CT is the next choice for examining the spine. For patients who are suspected of having skeletal metastatic disease, the radionuclide bone scan may be appropriate. However, you should be aware that multiple myeloma can be associated with severe back pain but often results in false negative bone scans.

PET scanning is becoming more widely used in staging of oncology patients and in the diagnosis of metastatic disease, including metastases to the spine.

In cases of spinal infection or tumor in which the extent of bone destruction may impact treatment decisions or surgical planning, CT is superior to MRI. After a diagnosis of spinal infection had been established by clinical, laboratory, and MRI findings, CT was done in the case shown in Figure 3-14 to visualize the extent of bone erosion.

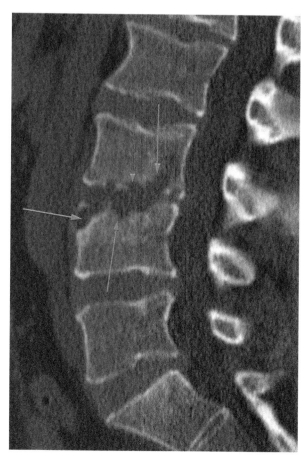

FIGURE 3-14 Sagittal CT of a patient with Pott's disease. Arrows indicate areas of bone erosion in the L3 and L4 vertebrae.

Interpretation

Cervical Spine

The AP open-mouth odontoid radiograph should be inspected for normal contour of the odontoid process and symmetry of the atlanto-axial articulation. Asymmetry may indicate rotational subluxation at C1–C2 as show in Figure 3-15.

As discussed for trauma, alignment of cervical segments should be examined on the lateral radiograph. Straightening or loss of the normal cervical lordotic curvature or a frank cervical kyphosis on the lateral view may be associated with muscle spasm and/or disc disease. Search the radiograph for abnormalities of bone density; look for lytic or blastic bone lesions. Facet joints should be inspected for arthritic changes. Osteoarthritic facet joints show typical changes of joint space narrowing, sclerosis, and marginal osteophytes on oblique views as shown in Figure 3-16. Intervertebral disc height should be evaluated at each level. Vertebral osteophytes associated with chronic degenerative disc disease are often referred to, along with osteophytes of the small synovial uncovertebral joints, as "spondylotic changes" which, as shown on the oblique radiograph in Figure 3-17, can both contribute to narrowing of neuroforamina and impinge on exiting cervical nerves.

On radiographs of patients, such as the one depicted in Figure 3-18, who have had prior anterior cervical discectomy and anterior plate fixation, you must carefully examine the integrity of the hardware and intervertebral fusion. There should be intimate metal to bone contact. When you have a concern about loosening or infection of hardware, or pseudarthrosis of a cervical fusion, CT is ideal after radiography and may show

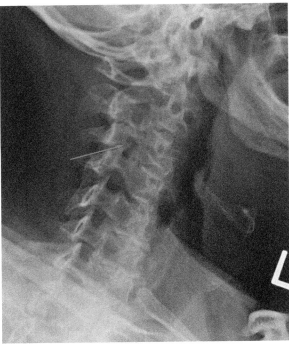

FIGURE 3-16 Oblique radiograph of the cervical spine. Note ventral marginal osteophyte of arthritic right C3–C4 facet joint (arrow) that projects into the neuroforamen.

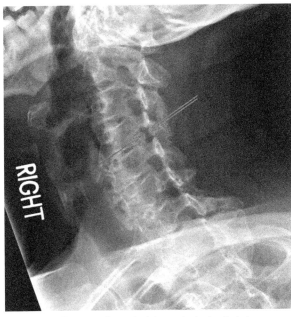

FIGURE 3-17 Oblique radiograph of the cervical spine that shows a narrowed left C4–C5 neuroforamen caused by uncovertebral joint spurring (arrow) and facet joint osteophyte (double arrow).

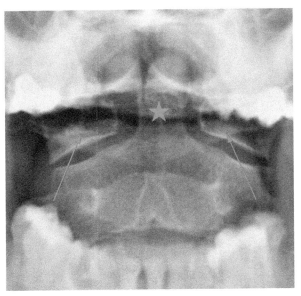

FIGURE 3-15 Open mouth AP odontoid view radiograph. Note asymmetry in the interval between the odontoid process (star) and the articular masses of C1 (arrows). The horizontal dark band crossing the odontoid process is air within a skin fold, probably in the occipital region of the scalp.

radiolucency (bone resorption) adjacent to fixation screws and discontinuities in the intervertebral fusion, as is the case for the patient shown in Figure 3-19.

CT and MRI findings of bone disease such as tumor or infection (bone marrow signal abnormalities on MRI or lytic or blastic bone changes on CT) in the cervical spine are similar to these findings in the rest of the skeletal system. Such disease is more common in the thoracolumbar spine than in the cervical spine and discussed more completely later in this chapter. Arthritic findings on cross-sectional imaging may explain cervical spinal pain, especially if there are secondary signs of an active process. For example, in a patient with arthritic facet joints, the MRI finding of a large joint effusion implies the presence of an active arthritis or joint instability.

Thoracolumbar Spine

Lateral radiographs should be inspected for disc disease, bone disease, and normal contour of the vertebral bodies. AP radiographs are evaluated for scoliosis and evidence of bone and disc disease. Furthermore, unless your "search pattern" of the AP view consistently includes an examination of the pedicles, you may not notice that a lytic metastatic tumor has caused one or more of the pedicles to become radiolucent. An absent pedicle on an AP view of the thoracic spine is known as the **pedicle sign** (Fig. 3-20).

Degenerative disc disease may be related to spinal pain and is evident on radiographs as loss of disc thickness and development of vertebral marginal spurs as shown at L2–L3 and L3–L4 in Figure 3-21.

Vacuum disc phenomenon (gas within the disc space) is commonly seen within degenerated discs as very dark radiographic density within the disc space.

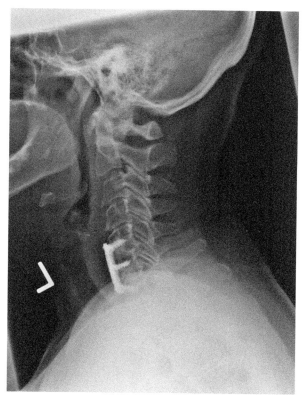

FIGURE 3-18 Lateral cervical spine radiograph of patient who has had anterior cervical discectomy and fusion (ACDF) with anterior plate fixation at C5–C6 and C6–C7.

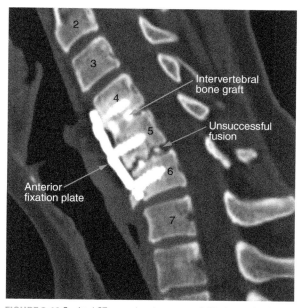

FIGURE 3-19 Sagittal CT scan showing successful fusion at C4–C5 but failure of surgical fusion (pseudarthrosis) at C5–C6 (red arrow). Fixation hardware was not visibly loose in this case.

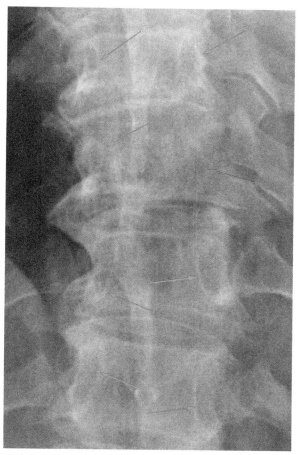

FIGURE 3-20 Pedicle sign. Note the "missing" pedicle (red arrow) compared with normal pedicles (blue arrows).

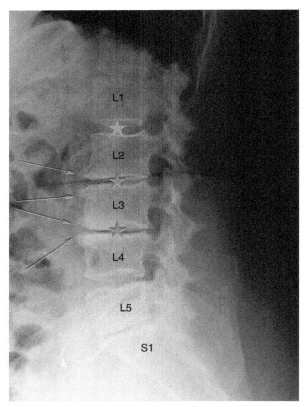

FIGURE 3-21 Lateral spine radiograph of a patient with degenerative disc disease. Compare the well maintained disc space at L1–L2 (blue star) with the flattened degenerated discs at L2–L3 and L3–L4 (red stars). Arrows indicate ventral spondylotic spurs. Note the advanced degenerative flattening of the L5–S1 disc.

When thick, bridging **syndesmophytes** involve four or more contiguous vertebrae, criteria are met for a diagnosis of diffuse idiopathic skeletal hyperostosis (DISH syndrome). This is often seen in the cervicothoracic and thoracolumbar regions of the spine, as shown in Figure 3-22.

Spondylolisthesis, abnormal alignment of vertebrae, is most common in the lumbar spine. Spondylolisthesis of the superior segment anterior to the inferior segment (anterolisthesis) is considered degenerative when secondary to facet joint arthropathy. This is most common at L4–L5 in adults with advanced facet joint DJD at this level. The "slip" is evident on the lateral view (Fig. 3-23) and the facet joint disease is shown on the oblique view (Fig. 3-24).

Spondylolisthesis also results from pars interarticularis defects. Pars defects may represent acute or old non-united fractures or from stress fractures that did not heal and progressed to complete fractures. They may present in the clinical context of subacute or repetitive trauma—for example, in young athletes. The presence of chronic pars interarticularis defects is classically referred to as spondylolysis. The characteristic radiographic finding (Fig. 3-25) on the oblique lumbar radiograph is a linear lucency (arrow) in the "neck" of the "scottie dog" shown in the figure.

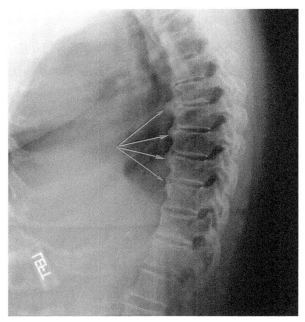

FIGURE 3-22 Lateral radiograph of the thoracic spine. Note the bridging syndesmophytes (arrows) that "flow" continuously along the anterior margin of the thoracic spine.

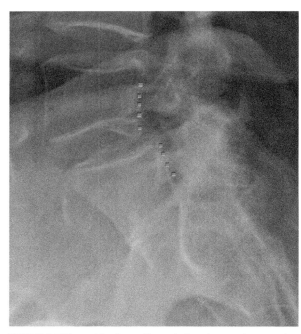

FIGURE 3-23 Lateral lumbar radiograph that shows a degenerative spondylolisthesis at L5–S1, illustrated by the dotted lines. Oblique radiographs (not shown) revealed arthritic facet joints and showed no pars defects.

When radiographs are not diagnostic in a patient suspected of having a pars interarticularis injury, many clinicians get a bone scan to search for abnormal activity as evidence for subacute bone injury. However, CT is ideal for demonstrating fine non-displaced pars defects or fractures or for differentiating incomplete stress injury of a pars interarticularis from a complete fracture or defect (Fig. 3-26).

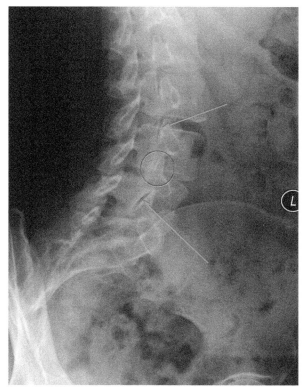

FIGURE 3-24 Oblique lumbar radiograph showing an arthritic left L4–L5 facet joint (circle), with loss of articular cartilage (joint "space") compared with normal facet joints above and below (arrows).

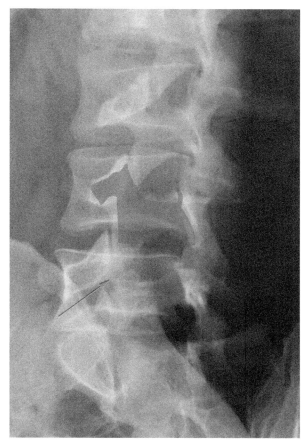

FIGURE 3-25 Oblique lumbar radiograph showing an L5 pars defect (arrow) that is perceived as a break in the neck of the "scottie dog" formed by posterior spinal elements in the oblique projection. Note the shadow of a scottie dog that is superimposed on the posterior elements of the segment above.

In some cases of degenerative disc collapse, the superior vertebral segment is positioned posterior to the inferior segment (Fig. 3-27) and may be referred to as a "retrolisthesis."

The characteristic radiographic finding for the most common of the spondyloarthropathies, ankylosing spondylitis, is the "bamboo spine" shown in Figure 3-28, which results from extensive thin, smooth, bridges syndesmophytes. There is often associated sacroiliitis, which, as shown in Figure 3-29, may be seen in active stages as widening of the joint and loss of cortical margins.

Bamboo spine and sacroiliitis are findings that are usually seen on radiographs long after clinical diagnosis is established based on history (there is a strong genetic link in ankylosing spondylitis) and appropriate laboratory testing, such as elevated sedimentation rate and C-reactive protein (CRP) during acute episodes. In a patient who has the HLA-B27 genotype, there is a high index of suspicion for ankylosing spondylitis as an explanation for back pain.

On MRI both spinal tumor and infection may cause bone marrow signal abnormalities. One differentiating finding is disc involvement, which is common with infection (Fig. 3-30) and unusual with tumor (Fig. 3-31).

MRI and CT may show features of arthritic facet joints or, in the thoracic spine, arthritic costovertebral joints that may explain spinal symptoms. In the lumbar spine in particular,

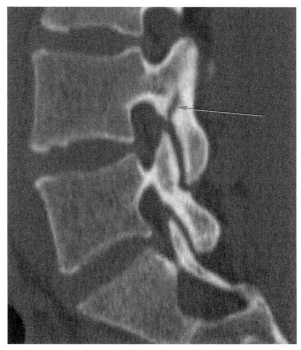

FIGURE 3-26 Sagittal CT demonstrating an incomplete pars interarticularis fracture (arrow) that extends vertically.

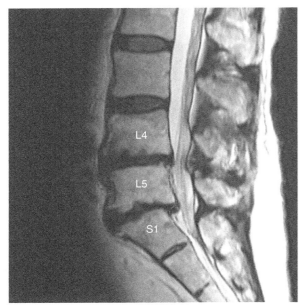

FIGURE 3-27 Sagittal MRI showing retrolisthesis of L5 in relation to the first sacral segment, secondary to collapse of a degenerated L5–S1 disc. Note abnormal alignment of the posterior margins of the L5 and S1 segments indicated by the dashed line.

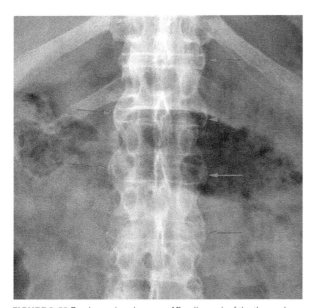

FIGURE 3-28 Bamboo spine shown on AP radiograph of the thoracolumbar spine. Thin, smooth osteophytes or syndesmophytes (arrows) "flow" smoothly from vertebra to vertebra, resulting in a spinal column with a contour resembling a stalk of bamboo.

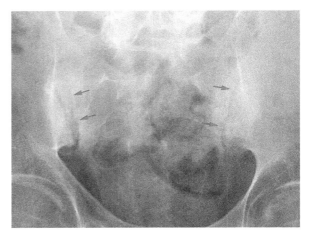

FIGURE 3-29 AP radiograph. Cortical erosions in active sacroiliitis cause irregularity, blurring, and loss of the cortical margins of the SI joints (arrows).

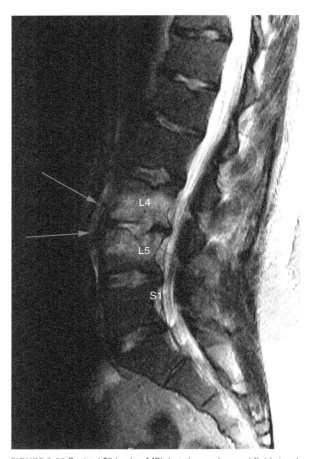

FIGURE 3-30 Sagittal T2 lumbar MRI that shows abnormal fluid signal in the L4–L5 intervertebral disc space and prevertebral fluid signal (arrows) as well as bone marrow edema (stars). These are findings highly suspicious for infectious discitis and vertebral osteomyelitis.

MRI may show disc annulus tears, which are hyperintense on T2 sequences. These may be causally related to back symptoms.

Associated with disc disease are very common reactive marrow signal changes in adjacent vertebra (Modic changes). You will see these findings reported on many radiology reports of spinal MR studies. Modic type 1 changes, indicating bone marrow edema adjacent to a diseased disc, have the highest correlation with acute spinal pain and therefore

increase the likelihood that the disc disease is the cause of back pain. Modic types 2 and 3 are associated with chronic degenerative disc disease.

In patients with active sacroiliitis, bone marrow edema will be shown on MRI adjacent to the SI joints, and as a radionuclide bone scan will show increased activity in bone adjacent to an inflamed joint.

CASE UPDATE

Patient B had normal lumbar radiographs and you ordered a CT scan that showed mild sclerosis of a pars interarticularis at L4 that suggested stress injury of bone. On the other side, there was a partial pars fracture, as shown in Figure 3-26. You referred the patient to a spine surgeon who has a great deal of experience in working with athletes. The surgeon's consultation letter to you indicates that because the fracture of one pars is incomplete and because the contralateral pars at that level in still intact, no surgical fixation was recommended. The surgeon advised the patient to stop playing football now, and there was a reasonable possibility of bone healing. The surgeon prescribed a back brace and recommended a repeat CT scan in several months to see if the fracture was healing.

Patient C has had little relief from over-the-counter NSAIDS and reports that her back is worse, especially in the mornings. There is nothing in the patient history or on your neurologic examination to suggest spinal canal stenosis. You order radiographs that demonstrate moderate to advanced DJD of multiple facet joints. You treat her with a prescription NSAID on a more regular schedule and refer the patient to the back pain clinic at your local hospital. The patient was diagnosed and is being appropriately treated based upon physical examination, thorough history, and supportive radiographs. Cross-sectional imaging such as MRI would not have changed clinical management of the patient.

NECK OR BACK PAIN WITH RADICULOPATHY OR MYELOPATHY

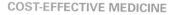

COST-EFFECTIVE MEDICINE

The presence of radiculopathy is not an automatic indication for imaging, but when conservative treatment fails and the patient becomes a candidate for surgery or procedure such as epidural steroid injection, then radiographic study becomes appropriate.

The cause of a specific radiculopathy can be subtle, and it is not uncommon for patients with a radiculopathy to have many pathologic findings, such as several disc abnormalities and arthritic facet joints that are not related to the current clinical concern. Therefore, as exemplified in Table 3-1, it is important, whenever possible, to provide specific clinical information on an imaging order.

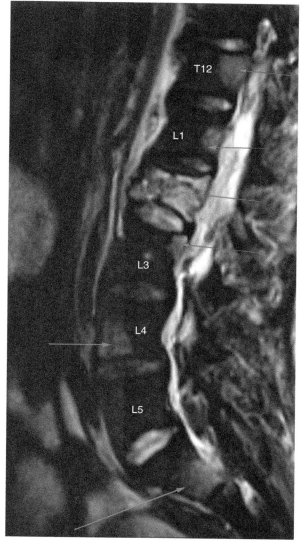

FIGURE 3-31 Sagittal fat suppressed T2 lumbar MRI that shows vertebral metastases (arrows). The L2 vertebra is not only infiltrated by metastatic tumor but also has suffered a pathologic fracture and is edematous. Well hydrated intervertebral discs are moderately intense but not as bright as fluid that might suggest infection. There is no significant disc degeneration to suggest that marrow signal changes are secondary to disc disease.

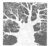 Elderly patients with spinal symptoms are frequently found to have extensive and complex degenerative and arthritic spinal abnormalities, and with advancing age it becomes less likely that there will be an imaging diagnosis that is amenable to a specific treatment other than symptomatic relief. One exception to this is the insufficiency fracture or osteoporotic vertebral fracture, which will be discussed in Chapter 11.

Modalities

Radiography does not typically provide significant diagnostic information in cases of myelopathy/radiculopathy. However, few surgeons would feel comfortable operating without any radiographs for orientation. Radiographs can also be very helpful when there is variant or ambiguous lumbar segmentation, and flexion and extension lateral views may sometimes be helpful in determining spinal stability. Therefore, even when cross-sectional imaging is indicated for definitive spinal diagnosis, radiography usually has clinical value.

Gradually progressive myelopathy may be a benign process in a patient with advanced disc disease and/or facet joint DJD causing spinal canal stenosis. These patients may present with symptoms that somewhat mimic lower extremity arterial insufficiency, referred to as "spinal claudication." Rapid onset myelopathy, especially in an oncologic or infectious disease patient, is a "red flag" indicating the need for urgent imaging.

MRI is the procedure of choice for patients with clinical findings of myelopathy or radiculopathy, often without contrast enhancement. However, when the patient has had prior disc surgery, or if there is suspicion of infection or tumor, MRI without and with enhancement is indicated. For those patients who cannot undergo MRI, CT or CT myelography is recommended.

Interpretation

Medical imaging of any kind is often used to triage patients between surgical and medical management. For the spinal conditions discussed here, the essential imaging feature is whether or not there is significant mechanical impingement of the spinal cord or of spinal nerves. However, even when such impingement is not apparent, imaging can sometimes still explain your patient's pain. For example, an intervertebral disc annulus tear visible as a T2 hyperintensity on MRI, as shown in Figure 3-32, can result in inflammation that irritates a nerve root and causes a radiculopathy without mechanical impingement of a nerve.

The terminology used to describe intervertebral disc herniations found on imaging can be confusing and is not always consistent. Generally, a bulging disc is one in which there is generalized expansion of the annular material beyond the limits of the disc space that encompasses at least 50% (180 degrees) of the disc contour. A disc herniation refers to a localized displacement of disc material that extends beyond the confines of the intervertebral disc space. The disc material may consist of nucleus, cartilage, fragmented bone, annular material, or any combination of these tissues. Both bulging and herniated discs may be further classified based on their form and extent. For example, a disc "protrusion," as shown in the lumbar MRI in Figure 3-33, is a herniated fragment of disc material that shows a maximum displacement less than the diameter of its base at the location of the normal disc margin. The same terminology is used in the cervical spine (Fig. 3-34). When the herniated disc fragment is displaced from the normal position of the disc edge an amount that is greater than the diameter of its base, it is "extruded" (Fig. 3-35). You may also see the phrase "sequestered" disc fragment, which indicates the presence of a disc fragment that has become detached from its parent disc.

The variable language used in reports that describe a disc herniation itself may not matter so much as the clarity of description of the effect of the herniated disc fragment on an adjacent nerve. A report should clearly indicate whether a herniated disc fragment is contacting, displacing (Fig. 3-36), or frankly compressing (Fig. 3-37) a nerve.

Therefore, a small disc herniation in a congenitally small cervical canal could compress the spinal cord, and a large disc fragment may not cause any neural compression in a patient who has a large spinal canal. Furthermore, the location of a disc fragment is very significant; for example, an intraforaminal disc protrusion as shown in Figure 3-38 may cause more neural impingement and clinical symptoms than a posterior midline protrusion of the same size.

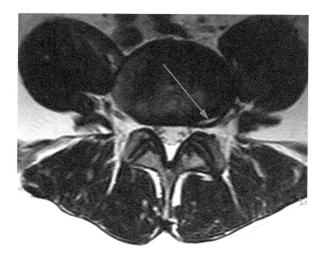

FIGURE 3-32 Axial MRI with conspicuous T2 hyperintense lumbar disc annulus tear (arrow).

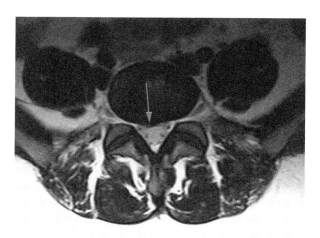

FIGURE 3-33 Axial lumbar MRI showing a small posterior disc protrusion (arrow).

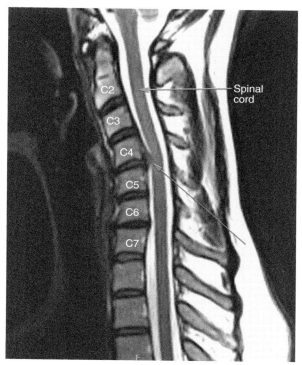

FIGURE 3-34 Sagittal cervical spine MRI with a posterior protruding disc fragment (arrow).

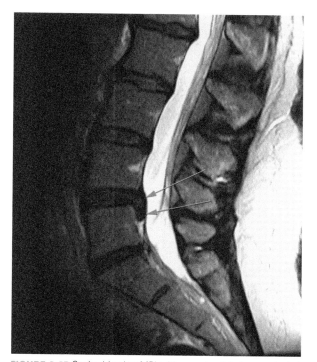

FIGURE 3-35 Sagittal lumbar MRI with a moderately large extruded disc fragment (arrows).

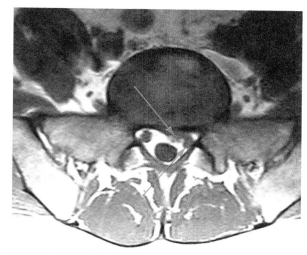

FIGURE 3-36 Axial MRI with a protruding disc fragment (red arrow) that is contacting and mildly displacing the left S1 nerve (blue arrow).

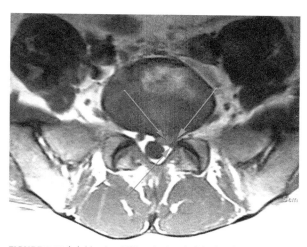

FIGURE 3-37 Axial lumbar MRI at the level of the L5–S1 disc showing a protruding disc fragment (red arrow). The left S1 nerve (blue arrows) is compressed between the disc fragment and the ventral margin of the left L5–S1 facet joint.

Radiology reports may describe disc abnormalities as "soft disc" herniations, implying a disc lesion that is acute or subacute, or as "hard disc" herniations, indicating a chronic disc herniation that is marginated by spondylotic spurs. Figure 3-39 is a sagittal CT myelogram image that shows both an acute "soft disc" herniation and chronic disc herniation with marginal spondylotic spurs.

In unusual cases, multiple sclerosis may present with primarily cord involvement and myelopathy and can be visualized as T2 hyperintense lesions within the cord on MRI. Intramedullary spinal cord tumors usually present with myelopathy and are usually contrast-enhancing lesions on MRI. Intradural tumors, such as spinal meniningioma, may present with pain and/or myelopathy. These enhance on MRI, as shown on the pre- and post-contrast sagittal MRI images shown in Figure 3-40.

Primary or metastatic disease to the vertebral column can cause neural impingement when it causes expansion of bone or penetrates through bone and forms an extradural mass that compresses the cord or nerve roots, as shown by the case of lung cancer metastatic to a lumbar pedicle shown in Figure 3-41. The

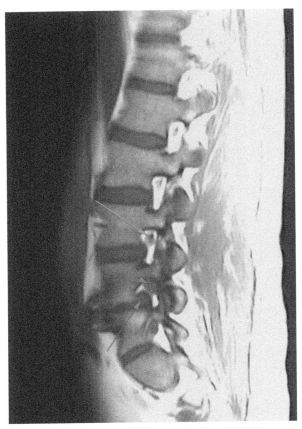

FIGURE 3-38 Sagittal lumbar MRI showing intraforaminal disc fragment (long red arrow). Compare the displaced and edematous nerve (short red arrow) with the nerve in the neuroforamen above (blue arrow).

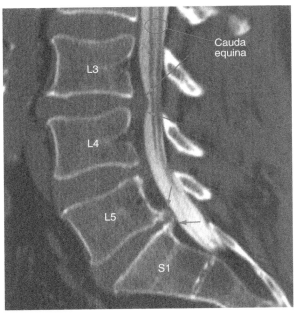

FIGURE 3-39 Sagittal CT myelogram that shows an acute or subacute protruding disc fragment at L3–L4 (long arrows) and spondylotic spurs (short arrows) secondary to chronic disc disease at L5–S1.

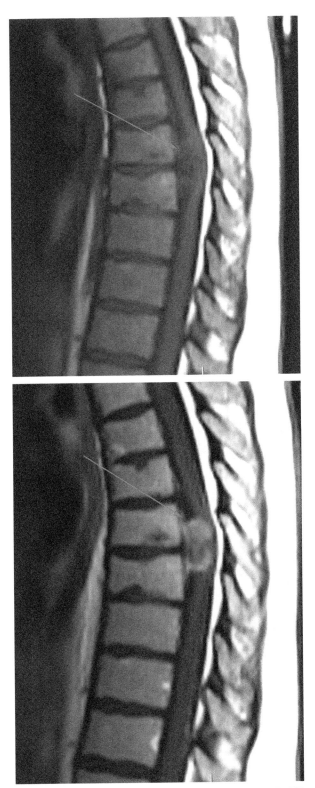

FIGURE 3-40 Pre- (top) and post-contrast (bottom) sagittal T1 MR images show a contrast-enhancing intradural mass (arrows).

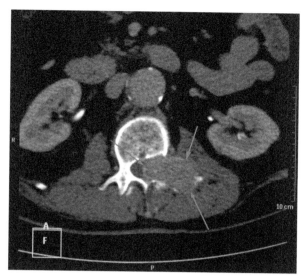

FIGURE 3-41 Axial lumbar CT of a patient with metastatic lung cancer. Spinal metastases frequently go to pedicles and in this case the enlarging tumor (arrows) has destroyed the left pedicle; the patient presented with sciatica because of neural impingement by the tumor.

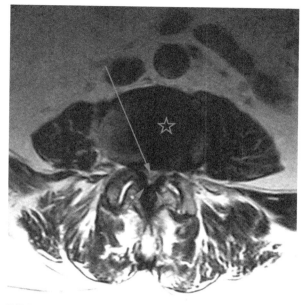

FIGURE 3-42 Axial MRI that shows a degenerated and bulging disc (star) and thickened ligamenta flava (short arrows) adjacent to hypertrophic, arthritic facet joints that severely narrow the spinal canal (long arrow).

metastatic tumor has destroyed the pedicle and severely encroaches on the spinal canal. In the case shown in Figure 3-40, the patient was not known to have lung cancer; after lumbar studies done for sciatica showed the tumor, the patient was asked if he smoked. He did, chest radiographs were done, and the primary lung cancer was found (see Chapter 6).

Symptomatic spinal canal stenosis, especially in the lumbar region, is often caused by a combination of a congenitally small canal, disc disease, hypertrophic (arthritic) facets, and thickened ligamenta flava, all of which are demonstrated in Figure 3-42. Symptomatic degenerative stenosis may not be within the central spinal canal, but rather in the lateral recesses of the canal.

Spondylosis and spurring of facet joints may result in progressive chronic stenosis of the neuroforamen or "nerve root canal" and cause neural impingement. Ventral spurring of arthritic facet joints that encroach upon neural foramina are better appreciated on radiography or CT than on MRI.

CASE CONCLUSION

Patient D initially responded well to a short course of treatment with oral steroids but several months later had recurrent symptoms of cervical radiculopathy. MRI that you ordered showed a left posterior cervical disc herniation at C5–C6 that impinged on the C6 nerve and accounted for the patient's symptoms. A spine surgeon to whom you referred her thought that surgery was not needed, at least for the present, and arranged for an epidural steroid injection by a physiatrist.

Patient E did not respond to steroid therapy; on a follow-up exam you find a dimished Achilles reflex, suggesting signficant neural impingement. You order MRI, which shows a disc herniation at L5–S1 (see Fig. 3-37) that is severely compressing the S1 nerve. Post-operatively the patient was pain-free.

Chapter Review

Chapter Review Questions

1. A 14-year-old male high school football running back is seeing you on a Saturday morning after a game the previous evening in which he was tackled from behind and hit the ground very hard. He is complaining of lumbosacral pain; you suspect a pars interarticularis fracture. Appropriate initial imaging would be:

   A. contrast-enhanced MRI of the lumbar spine.

   B. Radionuclide bone scan.

   C. complete lumbar radiographic series that includes AP, lateral, and oblique views.

   D. AP and lateral lumbar radiographs.

   E. lumbosacral CT.

2. On a lateral cervical radiograph, proper alignment of the cervical vertebrae is determined by visualizing:

   A. two smooth lines, one along the anterior margins of the vertebrae and one along the posterior margin.

   B. three smooth lines, one along anterior margins of the vertebrae, one along the posterior margin of the spinal canal, and one along the posterior margin of the vertebrae.

   C. an unbroken line along the anterior margins of the vertebrae.

   D. a dotted line along the tips of the spinous processes.

   E. the relationship of the foramen magnum to the cervical spine.

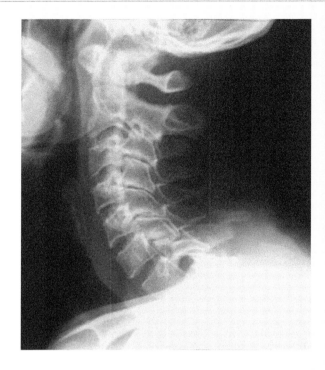

3. Which of the following is correct based on the image above, for a patient who did not have any accompanying neurological signs?

   A. You treat the patient with pain medications as needed and recommend reduced activity levels for 6 weeks

   B. You make an immediate referral to a neurosurgeon or orthopedic surgeon for spinal fixation

   C. You tell the patient that he has a Jefferson burst fracture that has potential instability

   D. You order cervical spine MRI

   E. You order cervical spine CT

4. After a Chance fracture is identified on a lateral spine radiograph, you should:

   A. obtain serum amylase and lipase levels to assess for possible pancreatic injury.

   B. order an immediate thoracolumbar MRI.

   C. order CT myelography.

   D. obtain an upright abdominal radiograph to look for free intra-abdominal air.

   E. no other testing is needed for abdominal imaging if the FAST exam is negative.

5. Which of the following is correct about the radio-
   logic diagnosis of degenerative disk disease in a
   65-year-old patient?
   A. It is consistently well correlated with the patient's
      symptoms
   B. It is associated with the pedicle sign
   C. It is recognizable on radiographs by a loss of disc
      space and presence of marginal osteophytes
   D. It only occurs with DISH syndrome
   E. It requires complete evaluation with MRI

7. The most important information that should be
   provided in a radiology report of a patient with
   lumbar radiculopathy is:
   A. the exact measurement of a herniated disc
      fragment.
   B. the percentage of spinal stenosis at the associ-
      ated level.
   C. the degree of impingement on a spinal nerve.
   D. whether or not there is an annulus tear.
   E. if Modic type 2 marrow changes are seen
      adjacent to a spinal nerve.

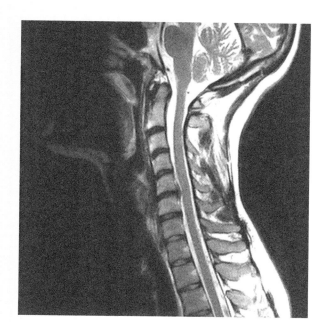

6. Your patient is a 55-year-old woman complaining
   of pain in her neck and shoulder. Which of the fol-
   lowing is correct based on the image shown
   above, which you ordered to be done for this
   patient?
   A. It is a CT myelogram
   B. It shows a sequestered disc at C5–C6
   C. It shows a cervical disk burst fracture
   D. It shows an extradural tumor at C5–C6
   E. It is a sagittal T2 MR image showing a protruding
      cervical disk fragment

4 BRAIN

A 65-year-old woman with no significant medical history other than mild hypertension presents with complaint of progressive headache during the last month. She has no allergies or any symptoms or signs of sinus disease. There is no nuchal rigidity. Although she denies other symptoms, her husband reports that her speech is mildly changed, with slight slurring of speech that is new for her. You order MRI with contrast enhancement.

FUNDAMENTALS OF BRAIN IMAGING

Radiography of the skull has little or no value because it does not directly visualize intracranial contents. For example, a skull fracture can be seen on radiographs but that finding poorly correlates with the degree of intracranial injury.

The ability to directly visualize the central nervous system with CT and MRI in adults, and with ultrasound in infants, has revolutionized the triage of neurologic patients between medical and surgical conditions. The speed of CT imaging and its sensitivity to detection of hemorrhage has great advantages in the setting of an acute emergency. The soft tissue contrast of MRI provides much more information than CT about the brain in subacute and chronic neurologic conditions.

Neuroradiology also includes diseases of the spinal cord, which in this text is covered in Spine Imaging (see Chapter 3), and overlaps with EENT imaging (see Chapter 5).

TRAUMA

The fundamental clinical issues in closed head trauma include level of consciousness and determining whether there was loss of consciousness after trauma. These details of the clinical history are part of well established and widely used clinical criteria for deciding if imaging is indicated after head trauma. For example, patients who suffer an epidural hematoma often have a "lucid interval" after an immediate post-trauma loss of consciousness, but that lucid interval should not distract from the essential historical point of loss of consciousness, which suggests that a serious intracranial injury may have occurred.

Modalities

When imaging is indicated for closed head trauma based on clinical criteria such as the Glasgow Coma Scale, non-contrast (unenhanced) CT is the appropriate imaging procedure.

COST-EFFECTIVE MEDICINE
There is low diagnostic yield from CT when patients have had minor head injury and high Glasgow Coma scores.

Closed head trauma is often associated with cervical spine trauma. In this case, both the cervical spine and head can be immediately studied with CT. In some cases, especially when there is a neurologic deficit not completely explained by the findings on CT, additional examination with MRI is needed. When there is clinical concern that traumatic carotid or vertebral artery dissection has occurred, MR angiography (MRA) or CT angiography (CTA) may be necessary.

When you suspect skull base injury, perhaps along with injuries to the craniocervical junction, thin section helical CT scanning with multiplanar reconstructions should be done, rather than the routine protocol for head CT, usually axial 5 mm slice thickness, which does not provide the imaging dataset needed for viewing complex skeletal structures in multiple planes.

Interpretation

CT images are viewed with a bone window setting (see Chapter 1) to inspect for skull fracture, as well as window settings ideal for the supratentorial brain and the posterior fossa. Very precise windowing may be needed during interpretation to ideally display intracranial blood (dense on CT) just deep to the also radiographically very dense skull.

The classic appearance of an acute epidural hematoma is a biconvex or lentiform high density fluid between the depressed brain surface and the skull, most often deep to a fracture that crosses the groove for the middle meningeal artery, as shown in Figure 4-1.

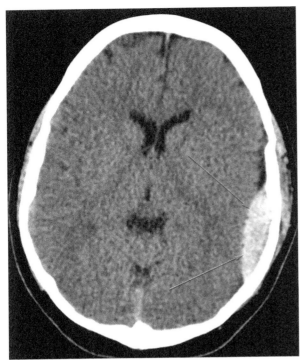

FIGURE 4-1 Axial CT image with brain window setting showing an epidural hematoma (arrows). Images using bone window setting (not shown) revealed a skull fracture.

An acute subdural hematoma has a broader extent of the high density blood than an epidural hematoma and often has a concave inner margin rather than the biconcave shape of an epidural hematoma, as demonstrated in Figure 4-2.

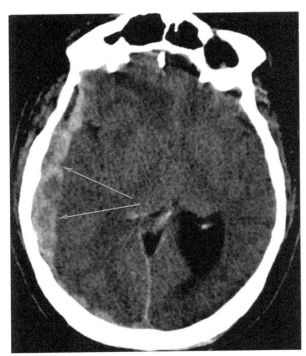

FIGURE 4-2 Axial CT demonstrating an acute subdural hematoma (arrows). Deep to the hematoma there is severe cerebral edema with positive mass effect.

When the otoscopic exam of a trauma patient shows blood in the external auditory canal and/or behind the tympanic membrane, thin section temporal bone CT will show not only the opacification of the middle ear with blood but also a temporal bone fracture, such as the one in Figure 4-3.

 A cephalhematoma (Fig. 4-4), a sequel of childbirth trauma, is a subperiosteal hematoma of the outer surface of the skull that does not have neurologic significance. As the hematoma matures and calcifies it produces a hard lump or "knot" that is often quite persistent, causing alarm in parents, which may lead to imaging that has little diagnostic value.

 In older patients with cerebral cortical atrophy, bridging veins associated with the dura become more susceptible to shearing injuries and episodes of slow

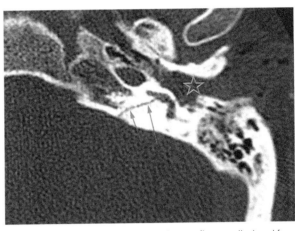

FIGURE 4-3 Thin section axial CT that shows a fine non-displaced fracture of the petrous portion of the temporal bone (arrows) with hematoma (star) in the external auditory canal.

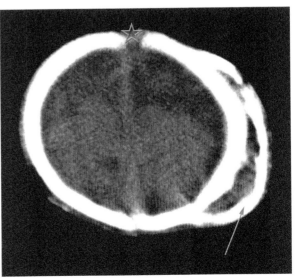

FIGURE 4-4 Axial CT of an infant with a cephalhematoma with a densely calcified rim (arrow). Note the fontanelle (star).

subdural bleeding with relatively minor trauma. The slow development of these subdural fluid collections is often associated with a delayed clinical presentation, unlike the clinical presentation of an acute post-traumatic subdural hematoma. The most common complaint for a chronic subdural hematoma is headache, often with the patient unable to recall an episode of trauma (see Fig. 4-16).

ACUTE NON-TRAUMA NEUROLOGIC EMERGENCY (Stroke and Hemorrhage)

A stroke is defined as a cerebrovascular event (or "accident" [CVA]) that results in a neurologic deficit that persists for more than 24 hours. An acute cerebrovascular event with neurologic deficit that resolves within 24 hours is called a transient ischemic attack (TIA). Strokes are divided into ischemic strokes (with no intracranial bleeding) and hemorrhagic strokes. Acute subarachnoid hemorrhage (SAH) is a separate category from strokes because it has a different clinical presentation. Stroke and SAH are common medical emergencies for which successful treatment is critically time-dependent and requires immediate and appropriate medical imaging.

It is critically important that those stroke patients with intracerebral hemorrhage be identified (by imaging) because the thrombolytic treatments used for ischemic stroke increase bleeding, perhaps fatally, if used on a patient with a hemorrhagic stroke.

The characteristic history for a patient with an acute SAH (usually caused by a ruptured aneurysm) is the acute or hyperacute onset of "the worst headache of my life," often associated with decreased level of consciousness, photophobia and other visual problems, and neck stiffness. Symptoms of acute ischemic stroke include dizziness, slurred speech, ataxia, double vision, unilateral motor deficits, unilateral paresthesias, paralysis, and decreased cognition.

Modalities

Although acute hemorrhage can be detected with MRI, it is more common to perform an urgent CT scan to differentiate ischemic from hemorrhagic stroke because unenhanced CT is a readily accessible and rapid procedure for imaging stroke victims during the time-critical hyperacute phase, the very few hours of the *therapeutic window* in which cerebral damage can be minimized by the use of thrombolytic treatment. When no hemorrhage is found on CT, intravenous thrombolytic therapy can be administered even while further imaging is done. CTA and a CT brain perfusion study may be done to identify an obstructed artery and assess the territory of the brain deprived of blood flow.

 COST-EFFECTIVE MEDICINE
As an alternate to CTA and CT brain perfusion, many patients with stroke undergo multimodality evaluation with both CT and MRI. Although it may seem costly for a patient to undergo multiple expensive procedures, quality care sometimes requires an aggressive approach in order to minimize complications and achieve the best possible outcome.

In the patient with (non-hemorrhagic) ischemic stroke, the **diffusion weighted MRI sequence** (DWI) can detect an ischemic stroke as early as 30 minutes after an arterial occlusion, prior to any other positive imaging finding on CT or other MRI sequences. Almost immediately after the onset of stroke, there is increased intracellular water content within ischemic brain parenchyma. Those water molecules now in the intracellular compartment are less free to move than interstitial water molecules, and it is this *restricted diffusion* that is demonstrated with DWI. During the acute and subacute phases, DWI has an extremely high sensitivity and a high specificity (few false positives). MRA and MR brain perfusion studies are used in stroke patients as well.

Perfusion studies, whether CT or MRI, are used in ischemic stroke to map the extent of infarcted brain tissue and borderline ischemic tissue, *the ischemic penumbra*, which is at risk for infarction.

Stroke protocols for imaging vary among institutions but have in common the goal of a rapid assessment of stroke when brain parenchyma is at risk of infarction, adhering to the principle that "time is brain."

Causes of intracerebral hemorrhage include tumors, hypertension, amyloid angiopathy, and vascular malformations. Additionally, thromboembolic (ischemic) strokes may cause infarction that is not initially hemorrhagic, but later hemorrhages as infarcted parenchyma breaks down. For these patients, MRI is needed for complete evaluation, even when a diagnosis has been initially established with CT.

SAH is usually caused by rupture of an aneurysm of the circle of Willis. When an SAH is found on CT or MRI, an immediate CTA or MRA can be performed to identify the bleeding vessel. (In patients with a family history of intracranial aneurysm, MRA is recommended for non-invasive screening for asymptomatic intracranial aneurysms.)

In the appropriate setting where aggressive intervention is available, invasive catheter angiography may be used in hemorrhagic stroke and SAH to stop bleeding. In ischemic stroke this intervention can be used for lysis and the physical removal of intraluminal thrombus from an obstructed vessel.

Unfortunately, not every patient who suffers a stroke seeks immediate medical attention. Subacute ischemic strokes/cerebral infarctions and subacute intracranial hemorrhage are much better seen on MRI than CT.

Interpretation

Acute intracerebral hemorrhage is seen as a hyperintensity on CT within brain parenchyma, as shown in Figure 4-5, which is associated with **positive mass effect** that describes how the space occupied by a hematoma (or tumor, focal brain edema, abscess, cyst, etc.) displaces adjacent tissue. Within the confines of the skull, positive mass effect is a more critical issue than in other parts of the body. As a neurologic emergency, the complication of positive mass effect of an intracranial lesion (e.g., uncal herniation, subfalcine herniation) can be more immediately significant than the lesion itself (Fig. 4-6).

SAH, which is associated with a high mortality rate, is seen on unenhanced CT as localized or diffuse increased CT density within the subarachnoid space in sulci, fissures, or basal cisterns. An example of an acute SAH is shown in Figure 4-7.

The imaging appearance of any intracerebral hemorrhage or hematoma varies over time due to the changes in characteristics of blood products over time on both CT and MR. In MRI, T1 and T2 signal intensity varies as a hematoma ages. You may likely see the phrase *magnetic susceptibility* in MRI reports that refer to the paramagnetic effect of the iron content in hemoglobin on an MR image, specifically in **gradient echo sequences**. Hemosiderin within macrophages that linger at the site of even a very old hemorrhage can be detected on these sequences. For example, the MRI of a patient seen for an acutely bleeding arteriovenous malformation (AVM) may not only have a new

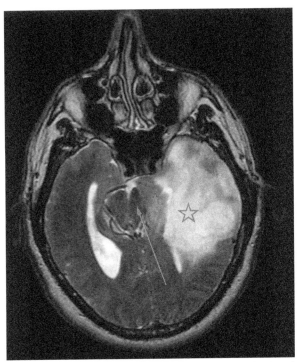

FIGURE 4-6 Axial T2 MRI of the brain with uncal herniation (solid star) impinging on the pons (arrow). There is a large area of vasogenic edema (open star) in the temporal lobe.

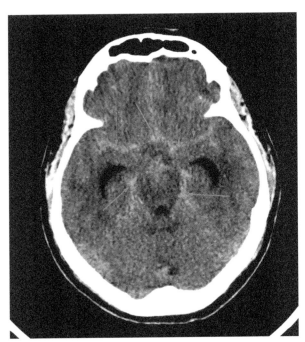

FIGURE 4-7 Axial CT that shows hemorrhage (arrows) in the subarachnoid space.

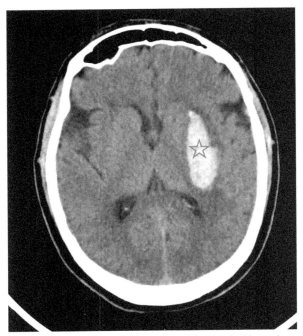

FIGURE 4-5 Axial CT demonstrating an acute intracerebral hemorrhage (star).

hematoma but also a focus of magnetic susceptibility at the site of an old hemorrhage from another AVM (they are often multiple), as shown in Figure 4-8. Another example of the imaging of blood changing over time is that immediately after SAH, CT has extremely high sensitivity, but in the absence of continued

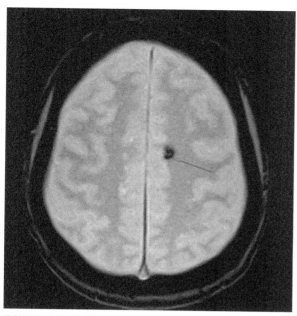

FIGURE 4-8 Axial MRI, gradient echo sequence image on a patient with multiple AVMs. The focus of magnetic susceptibility (arrow) is at the site of an old hemorrhage. The acute hemorrhage (not shown) was at a different location.

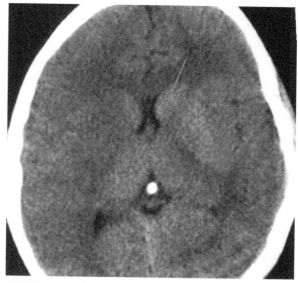

FIGURE 4-9 Axial CT of acute stroke patient in which there is visibility of the head of the caudate and lentiform nuclei on the normal left side (arrows). An acute right MCA infarction has caused vasogenic edema that obscures the basal ganglia on the affected side.

bleeding, blood in the subarachnoid space becomes diluted with CSF, so there is progressive decrease in CT sensitivity in the hours and days after a hemorrhage. Therefore, CT can become significantly less sensitive for detecting SAH in the subacute phase than it is in the acute phase.

When a patient has suffered a TIA, imaging is focused on finding an underlying cause, such as an ulcerated plaque in the carotid artery that may be responsible for microemboli to the intracranial circulation. Similarly, when a patient presents with amaurosis fugax, a search is made for a cause of microemboli to the ophthalmic artery.

The CT findings of acute cerebral infarction in unenhanced CT may be very subtle, especially within the first few hours after ictus. A finding that suggests cerebral infarction is a decrease ("blurring") of the visible difference between gray and white matter, such as the **insular ribbon sign**, in which the insular cortex is no longer visible as slightly hyperdense to the underlying subcortical white matter, and *obscuration* of the normal CT visibility of the basal ganglia (Fig. 4-9). Another significant CT finding that you may see in radiology reports of CT done on stroke patients is the presence of the **hyperdense vessel sign**, in which a thrombosed artery (most commonly the proximal middle cerebral artery [MCA]) is visible because intraluminal thrombus is denser than blood, as shown in Figure 4-10.

Large cerebral infarctions, usually in the distribution of the MCA, can cause cerebral edema of the infarcted tissue that can be appreciated as effacement of sulci and narrowing

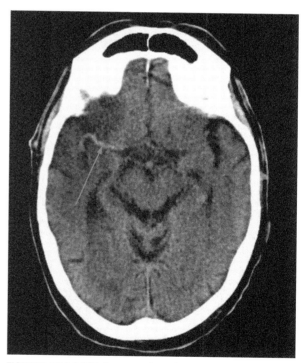

FIGURE 4-10 Axial CT of acute stroke patient that shows a hyperdense MCA (arrow).

of the Sylvian fissure. These findings are usually seen in the more extensive and severe cerebral infarctions. Acute cytotoxic edema may result in conspicuous decrease in density of affected parenchyma.

When acute ischemic stroke is diagnosed after unenhanced CT or MRI, treatment commonly involves the use of intravenous tissue plasminogen activator (tPA). However, advanced imaging procedures such as CT or MR perfusion studies, CTA, or MRA may rapidly be done in many hospital settings when more aggressive treatment such as intra-arterial tPA or transcatheter clot retrieval are being considered. As an example, Figure 4-11 is a volume rendered display from a CTA on an acute stroke patient in whom the right MCA is occluded.

Patients with mild strokes often present to the practitioner in the subacute phase (days to several weeks), when CT may have a low sensitivity. In MRI, the DWI sequence is nearly 100% sensitive in detecting early subacute cerebral infarction, as shown in Figure 4-12.

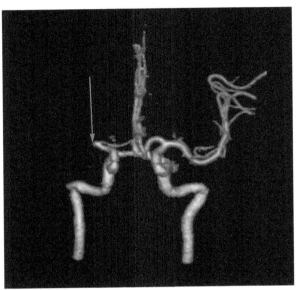

FIGURE 4-11 The truncation of the right MCA caused by an acute thrombus (arrow) is shown on a volume rendered (3D) display of an intracranial CTA.

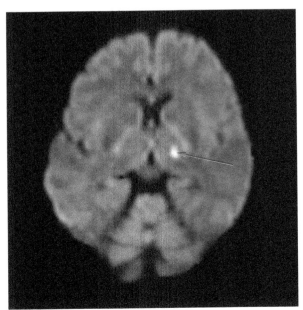

FIGURE 4-12 DWI revealed a focus of restricted diffusion (arrow) indicating an acute (or early subacute) infarction in the left thalamus.

HEADACHE

Although most headaches are idiopathic, headache may be a presenting symptom of serious pathology, such as brain tumor or abscess. Clinical judgment is essential in the very difficult task of separating the typical headaches, likely to have very low diagnostic yield with imaging from those headaches that might be associated with serious pathology.

When headache is frontal, clinical evaluation may suggest that sinusitis is present (see Chapter 5). Some headaches, such as migraine and cluster headaches, have characteristic clinical histories.

The following Modalities section applies to patients with generalized headache; a separate Modalities section is presented for unilateral headache.

Modalities

Unenhanced CT may be useful when there is a limited goal for imaging of ruling out large lesions or hydrocephalus. For chronic clinical problems, CT without and with contrast enhancement is better than unenhanced CT alone but is not as sensitive or specific as unenhanced MRI of the brain. The most thorough and accurate examination can be expected from MRI without and with contrast enhancement. Unenhanced MRI has a very low false negative rate and is usually sufficient to rule out significant pathology. But when pathology becomes evident on unenhanced images, further refinement of imaging diagnosis with contrast-enhanced image sequences may be critical. It can be very efficient to order "brain MRI, contrast enhancement if needed," as shown in Table 4-1.

When brain imaging is ordered for an oncology patient for suspected intracranial metastases, it should always be done without and with contrast enhancement. Remember that for older and diabetic patients and those with known renal insufficiency, serum creatinine level and creatinine clearance should be obtained prior to MRI if the use of a gadolinium-based contrast agent might be needed.

TABLE 4-1 **Sample Neuroradiology Requisition Information**

Modality	Clinical Data/History
MRI brain, with contrast if needed	Progressive h/a, confusion, no focal findings
MRI brain wo/w Gd, attn. pituitary	Hyperprolactinemia
CT head w/o (pacemaker pt.)	Dementia—R/O hydrocephalus
MRI brain, wo/w contrast	h/a, weakness left side, stage 4 breast ca
Intracranial MRA	Intermittent h/a; fam hx intracranial aneurysm
MRI brain and orbits wo/w Gd	Visual disturbance, bilat arm and leg paresthesias—R/O optic neuritis, MS

Chronic Headache

There is a very low yield in neuroimaging on patients who have a history of headaches for many months or years. Chronic migraine patients do, however, have positive MR findings that reflect the micro-ischemic effects of the vasospasm that occurs with this disorder. Although MRI may have a low yield for detecting pathology that changes clinical management in these patients, a negative imaging study can have psychosocial value in providing needed reassurance to the patient.

Although most imaging studies that are done for chronic headache show no significant pathology or result in change in clinical management, there can be an association between the chronic headache found with pseudotumor cerebri and the finding on MRI of an *empty sella* (in which the pituitary is flattened along the inferior aspect of a CSF-filled sella turcica).

Recent Onset or Change in Character of Headache

Unlike chronic headache with no new neurologic problems, imaging is often appropriate, even mandatory, when headache in the adult is new, progressive, different than previous "routine" headache, and associated with neurologic complaints.

With Other Neurologic Symptoms and Signs

With major intracranial pathology, such as hydrocephalus, tumor, or abscess, the patient may present with a combination of complaints (e.g., nausea, visual problems, slurred speech, behavioral changes, and ataxia or dizziness) but also a new onset, change in the pattern of, or progression of headache. Additionally, seizure in an adult with no previous history of seizure and no history of brain trauma that could have caused an epileptogenic lesion is a very clear sign that the associated headache is not benign.

 Elderly patients with chronic subdural hematomas may present with chronic headache, often with slowly progressive neurologic dysfunction such as difficulty with speech, memory, and ambulation.

INTERPRETATION

In children, adolescents, and younger adults, hydrocephalus is likely to be secondary to a tumor causing an obstructive (non-communicating) hydrocephalus, such as a mass in the fourth ventricle, as shown in Figure 4-13, or an extraventricular mass impinging on the cerebral aqueduct (of Sylvius). A third ventricle lesion may cause the lateral ventricles to dilate; the fourth ventricle is normal in these cases. See Box 4-1 for specific information regarding hydrocephalus in the pediatric and geriatric patient. This condition is discussed later in this chapter under Movement Disorders.

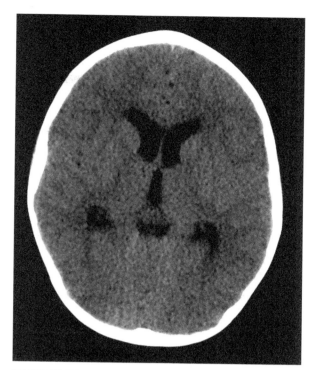

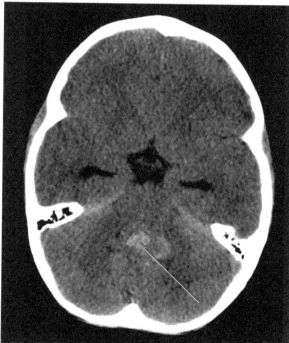

FIGURE 4-13 CT section **(top)** of a pediatric patient shows hydrocephalus (this section shows dilated third and lateral ventricles). CT section of the same study **(bottom)** at a lower level demonstrates the cause of this obstructive hydrocephalus, a mass in the fourth ventricle (arrow).

A common, usually benign intracranial tumor, the meningioma, is characteristically a sharply marginated, homogeneously enhancing dural-based mass. A finding that is highly associated with the origin of this lesion from the dura, not the underlying brain, is that of a "dural tail," as

Box 4-1 **Hydrocephalus**

● **Pediatric**

Hydrocephalus in infants is typically manifest as an enlarged head, usually detected during neonatal exams.

● **Geriatric**

In elderly patients, hydrocephalus is more commonly a normal pressure hydrocephalus (NPH) and symptoms other than headache predominate.

shown in Figure 4-14. Although these are usually benign histologically, the pressure they exert upon adjacent intracranial structures (mass effect) can lead to a wide variety of symptoms, including headache.

Intracerebral abscesses and malignant brain tumors are typically contrast-enhancing masses. Depending upon the histologic type, these may be centrally cystic or necrotic and be accompanied by varied degrees of edema in adjacent brain tissue. When brain edema is caused by pathology such as trauma, infection, or tumor, there is increased water content in the interstitial space (unlike the intracellular edema that is found in an ischemic stroke) and is described as vasogenic edema. It is shown in MRI as decreased T1 signal and increased T2 signal. The vasogenic edema surrounding a brain lesion may also have significant positive mass effect that may be more profound than the mass itself. The vasogenic edema that is adjacent to tumor may obscure its margins; therefore, gadolinium-enhanced images are needed to

provide precise delineation of its margins, an important issue for treatment (Fig. 4-15).

As stated earlier, acute subdural hematomas are usually conspicuously dense in CT, whereas subacute subdural hematomas may be isodense to brain on CT and may therefore be difficult to perceive.

 In the elderly patient, as subdural hematomas evolve from subacute to chronic, the resorption of blood products in the hematoma may be so complete that the subdural fluid is low density on CT and easily seen. These are sometimes referred to as a subdural *hygroma*, common in

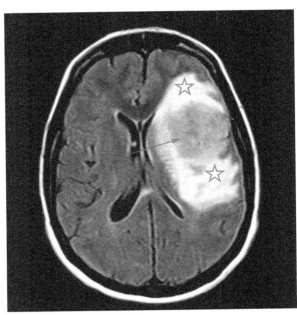

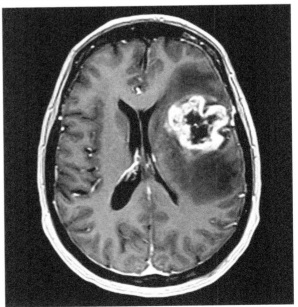

FIGURE 4-15 Axial T2 MRI **(top)** that shows a glioma (arrow) surrounded by broad areas of vasogenic edema (stars). On the subsequent contrast-enhanced axial T1 sequence **(bottom)**, the enhancing tumor is clearly demarcated from the surrounding edema.

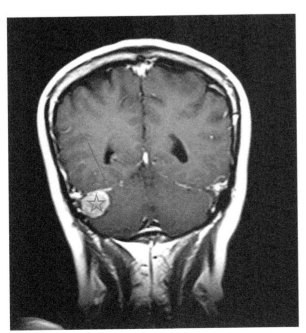

FIGURE 4-14 Coronal contrast-enhanced T1 MRI. The contrast-enhancing mass (star) that arises from the tentorium has a dural tail (arrow), characteristic of a meningioma.

the elderly, who may develop a subdural fluid collection slowly after relatively minor trauma. A chronic subdural hematoma (hygroma) is shown in Figure 4-16.

The radiologist interpreting the MRI on your 65-year-old female patient with dysarthria calls you with the unfortunate finding (which you suspected) of a left posterior frontal lobe enhancing mass (probable glioma). There is mild to moderate vasogenic edema. You arrange for the patient an immediate consultation with a neurosurgeon. She is prescribed steroids to reduce the vasogenic edema and arrangements are made for surgery the following week.

With Signs of Meningeal Irritation

When nuchal rigidity suggests meningeal irritation and is associated with extremely severe headache and decreased cognition, imaging is immediately done to rule out intracranial hemorrhage. However, when signs of meningeal disease are associated with fever and slow onset of headache, clinical concern may be directed toward meningitis. In this situation, a lumbar puncture (*spinal tap*) becomes an important diagnostic procedure but must be done after a CT scan. The CT scan is used to rule out the presence of major intracranial pathology that may result in brain herniation through the foramen magnum when fluid is removed from the spinal canal during lumbar puncture. During the course of

meningitis, additional imaging may be needed to identify intracranial meningeal inflammation, development of intracranial abscess, or the development of communicating hydrocephalus, which may be a complication of meningeal disease.

INTERPRETATION

For the complete intracranial evaluation of leptomeningeal disease, MRI done without and with contrast can directly visualize thickened and inflamed meninges, as shown by the red arrow in Figure 4-17.

In the Pregnant Patient

Headaches are common in pregnancy, mostly tension and migraine, but when there is a new onset of headache or very severe headache, the clinician should be alert to the possibility of serious neurologic conditions. The hormonal changes in pregnancy may cause rapid growth in a preexisting intracranial lesion, such as meningioma or pituitary adenoma. Because pregnancy is a hypercoagulable state, intracranial vascular events such as intracranial venous thrombosis and pituitary apoplexy sometimes occur in the pregnant patient. Immediate and appropriate imaging is needed for prompt diagnosis and specific treatment of these conditions.

When the clinical presentation in the pregnant patient suggests acute intracranial hemorrhage such as with a ruptured intracranial aneurysm, unenhanced CT is indicated. The tight **collimation** (restricting and shaping by shielding) of the x-ray beam in a CT scan of the head and the simple application of a lead drape ensures that the fetus will not be exposed to a significant dose of radiation.

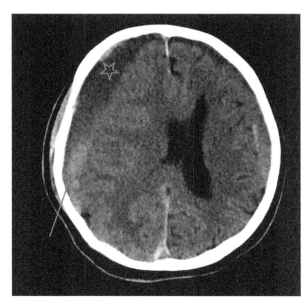

FIGURE 4-16 Axial CT of a patient with a chronic subdural hematoma (star) that is hypodense to brain (because of resorption of blood products over time). In this case, the patient has just suffered some rebleeding into the old subdural collection, and the fresh blood is visible as a higher density (arrow).

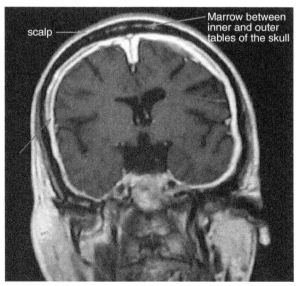

FIGURE 4-17 Coronal contrast-enhanced T1 MRI that shows thickened and brightly enhancing meninges (red arrow).

94

Chapter 4

Pituitary apoplexy usually develops over days, not hours as in a more typical intracranial hemorrhage, and, because of mass effect on the optic chiasm, frequently is associated with visual disturbances. Unenhanced MRI provides a more comprehensive exam than CT, and enhanced MRI is usually not needed for this diagnosis. As noted earlier, there is a relative contraindication to the use of gadolinium-based contrast agents for MRI in pregnant patients because these agents pass through the placenta into fetal circulation.

INTERPRETATION

Using special *flow-sensitive MR pulse sequences* in which blood flow determines signal intensity, an unenhanced MR venogram (MRV) can be done when there is clinical suspicion of intracranial venous thrombosis (Fig. 4-18).

Pituitary apoplexy results in an enlarged pituitary that often has mixed signal characteristics of venous hemorrhage and thrombosis on MRI, as shown in Figure 4-19.

Unilateral Headache

Most unilateral headaches fall within the clinical patterns of those chronic headaches, such as migraine and cluster headaches, for which imaging is not generally needed. Temporal arteritis (giant cell arteritis) is most definitively diagnosed by temporal artery biopsy, although imaging is sometimes used during the workup and can be helpful. Acute unilateral headache with pain radiation and neurologic signs and symptoms that suggest arterial dissection requires urgent imaging.

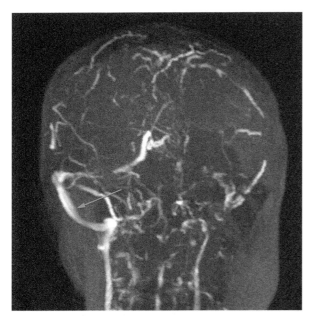

FIGURE 4-18 MR venogram in which there is good flow in the right sigmoid sinus (arrow), but the contralateral sigmoid sinus is thrombosed. In addition, the expected bright signal from the superior sagittal sinus is absent because of extensive venous thrombosis.

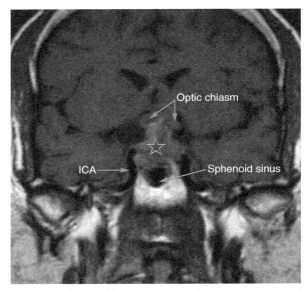

FIGURE 4-19 Coronal MRI without contrast enhancement on a pregnant patient with headache and visual field defect. The T1 hyperintensity within the greatly enlarged pituitary (star) indicates subacute hemorrhage (ICA, internal carotid artery).

MODALITIES

Imaging is often not needed for evaluation of temporal arteritis. When clinical management may be altered by imaging, the superficial temporal artery can be evaluated with ultrasonography, but this modality is less sensitive in detecting mild vascular changes than CTA, MRA, or invasive catheter angiography. Because non-invasive vascular imaging techniques have progressively improved, there is declining use of invasive catheter angiography for such a vascular diagnosis.

For imaging of suspected carotid or vertebral artery dissection, CTA or MRA is done, usually along with unenhanced brain CT to rule out hemorrhage, or along with brain MRI without and with contrast enhancement. When non-invasive imaging is not definitive or when transcatheter intervention is planned, invasive catheter angiography is appropriate.

INTERPRETATION

In temporal arteritis, ultrasonography and high resolution MRI demonstrate evidence of arterial wall edema. In ultrasonography, the edema surrounding the artery results in a hypoechoic halo around the vessel.

Carotid or vertebral artery dissections are revealed by the presence of a dark line within the vessel that is the elevated flap of intima, as shown in the CTA presented in Figure 4-20.

MOVEMENT DISORDERS

Movement disorders are degenerative diseases that are primarily diagnosed clinically. They include ataxia, dystonia, Huntington's disease, Parkinson's disease (PD), motor neuron diseases, and spasticity. In patients with movement

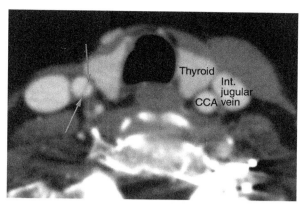

FIGURE 4-20 Axial image, carotid CTA. The dark line (arrows) within the right common carotid artery (CCA) is a raised flap of intima that indicates carotid artery dissection.

disorders, imaging is done mainly for exclusion of treatable structural abnormalities, such as tumor, and as a research tool. However, there is one treatable condition that may present with a gait disturbance as a major symptom, along with some degree of dementia and often urinary incontinence, and that is normal pressure hydrocephalus (NPH). Patients with NPH in whom the gait disturbance predominates show favorable response rates to shunting. Therefore, NPH is presented here rather than in the section on dementia.

Ataxia may sometimes present acutely, and in those cases patients should be treated as in any potential neurologic emergency.

Modalities

MRI is preferred for any patients with chronic movement disorders. This is often done with contrast enhancement. However, many of these patients do not tolerate lengthy scans and there may be contraindications to the use of gadolinium-based contrast agents, in which case unenhanced MRI is considered appropriate. CT is used for patients who have a contraindication to MRI (e.g., pacemaker).

Advanced imaging in patients with movement disorders in major centers may involve **functional MRI, MRI brain spectroscopy,** FDG-PET scanning, and SPECT scanning.

Patients suspected of having NPH clinically and on MRI may undergo a special nuclear medicine procedure called **cisternography** to study the flow of CSF in the brain to determine the likelihood of response to shunting. Flow-sensitive MR sequences (similar to those used in MRA) may be used to assess flow dynamics of CSF in the cerebral aqueduct.

Interpretation

NPH is characterized as a communicating hydrocephalus without significant cerebral cortical atrophy; characteristically it is seen as a dilation of the lateral ventricles that is

disproportionate to any cortical atrophy, as shown in Figure 4-21. Transependymal flow of CSF may results in diffuse periventricular white matter hyperintensity on T2 weighted sequences, most pronounced on **T2 FLAIR** sequence images. Even without special flow-sensitive sequences, the hyperdynamic flow of CSF within the cerebral aqueduct may cause a flow void (as seen often in arteries) on T2 images, resulting in dark fluid within the cerebral aqueduct.

Neurodegenerative movement disorders usually have either unremarkable or non-specific findings on CT and MRI. In Parkinson's disease, MRI may show decreased width of the pars compacta of the substantia nigra, but this is not reliable and many patients with this condition do not show this morphologic change. A common motor neuron disease, amyotrophic lateral sclerosis, may show corticospinal tract atrophy and T2 hyperintensity that can be traced from the motor cortex to the spinal cord. For both these diseases, MRI is used for exclusion of other pathology, not for establishing a diagnosis.

When chronic ataxia is unexplained by imaging study of the brain, pathology may be spinal; imaging of the spine should be considered.

FOCAL NEUROLOGIC DYSFUNCTION

A wide clinical spectrum of clinical presentations with neurologic disease, including disordered thought and altered level of consciousness exists in which neuroimaging has little or no indication. However, imaging is indicated for diagnosis

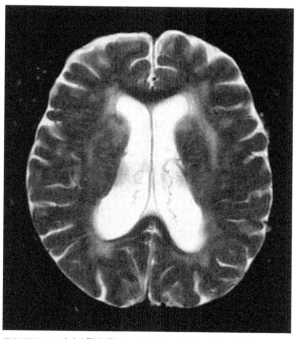

FIGURE 4-21 Axial T2 MRI showing dilated lateral ventricles with no cortical atrophy. There was no mass that would cause an obstructive hydrocephalus. NPH was later proven with radionuclide cisternography.

for many specific neurologic symptoms, including aphasia, sensory and motor deficits, cranial nerve deficits, and suspected white matter disease such as multiple sclerosis (MS).

Many white matter diseases are the result of small vessel disease and are referred to as *microangiopathic white matter changes*. These are discussed in the section on dementia later in this chapter. Multiple sclerosis, the most common demyelinating white matter disease, is diagnosed through a combination of clinical findings with confirmatory findings on MRI. Because this is a disease characterized by a course that progresses in patterns over time (e.g. progressive or relapsing-remitting MS), the diagnosis may depend upon visible progressive changes seen on repeated MR scans.

The results of a thorough neurologic examination direct imaging decisions—both the need for imaging and the specific imaging procedure that is needed. The visual disturbance that may accompany MS may call for a different MRI protocol than the visual disturbance caused by an enlarged pituitary that is compressing the optic chiasm, a lesion in the occipital lobe, or one that originates within the orbit itself.

Modalities

MRI is the procedure of choice for structural brain abnormalities and white matter diseases. In many cases, contrast-enhanced scanning is not needed and unenhanced MRI may be sufficient. However, when a mass or potentially active inflammatory or demyelinating disease is found, contrast-enhanced sequences become important.

Although the use of contrast enhancement in the neuroimaging in many "routine" clinical situations may be optional, when there is a high index of suspicion for structural pathology, as in an oncology patient, the yield from contrast-enhanced imaging requires brain MRI without and with contrast enhancement.

When a brainstem lesion is suspected, such as in a patient with ophthalmoplegia and no orbital findings, a very small brainstem lesion may be responsible and contrast-enhanced MRI is recommended.

When a visual disturbance suggests involvement of the optic chiasm, a pituitary protocol MRI without and with contrast enhancement should be requested for best visualization of a suprasellar mass impinging on the optic chiasm. If MS is a suspected or known diagnosis in a patient with visual disturbance, MRI of the brain and orbits should be requested; this will include special sequences of the orbit that will improve detection of optic neuritis. When MRI is done for MS, contrast enhancement is important to distinguish chronic from active white matter lesions.

For cranial nerve deficits with symptoms that suggest disease at the skull base, it is helpful if that concern is specified on the imaging requisition because special sequences with fat suppression may be used that are not usually part of routine brain imaging protocols. CT is useful mainly for cases in which MRI is contraindicated, such as a patient with a pacemaker, and for disease at the skull base that requires ideal depiction of a bone abnormality—for example, in a patient with a cranial nerve deficit caused by tumor eroding bone at the skull base.

Interpretation

Intracranial tumors, either metastatic or primary, are generally contrast-enhancing masses, with a range of enhancement patterns, cystic components, central tumor necrosis, and widely varied degrees of associated vasogenic edema and positive mass effect. An example of a mass found in a patient who presented with mild headache and disorientation, and a motor deficit because of the location of the tumor affecting the motor cortex, is shown in Figure 4-22.

Because metastatic disease to the brain often results in multiple lesions in different parts of the brain, as shown in Figure 4-23, there is a very wide range of possible symptoms, including multiple motor and sensory deficits. The presence of many small metastatic lesions involving numerous parts of the brain explains the protean nature of this patient's neurologic symptoms.

Pituitary and other sellar and suprasellar lesions may impinge on the optic chiasm, resulting in the characteristic visual field deficit of homonymous hemianopsia if the impingement is midline. Pathology responsible for this includes pituitary tumor, craniopharyngioma, and Rathke's cleft cyst, as shown in Figure 4-24 of a patient referred for

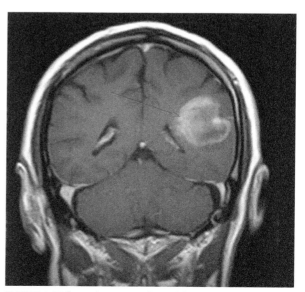

FIGURE 4-22 Coronal contrast-enhanced MRI of a patient who presented with a right motor deficit shows a contrast-enhancing primary brain tumor (arrow) with no surrounding vasogenic edema.

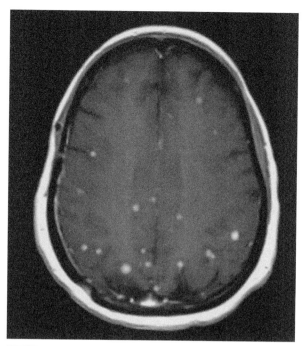

FIGURE 4-23 Axial contrast-enhanced MRI of a patient with stage 4 breast cancer shows many small enhancing (hyperintense) metastatic brain lesions.

matter signal changes in MRI provides diagnostic information that helps establish the diagnosis for a large number of white matter diseases.

The white matter imaging findings in MS include a variety of peripheral (subcortical, less common) and deep (periventricular, more common) white matter lesions. Focal T2 hyperintense lesions that are most characteristic are those periventricular lesions oriented perpendicular to the adjacent lateral ventricle (*Dawson's fingers*), as shown in Figure 4-25. These white matter lesions, however, are non-specific with respect to the pathologic changes and may represent acute, evolving, or chronic foci of cellular damage. Non-focal white matter changes are those of atrophy from chronic disease. In the course of MS, there are *normal appearing white matter changes* that are not yet visible on conventional MR sequences but that can be detected using research tools such as *magnetization transfer MR sequences.*

MS lesions are usually T1 isointense to adjacent white matter. Lesions with more advanced cellular damage may be T1 hypointense. An important feature in imaging of MS patients is the presence of MS plaque enhancement, as shown in Figure 4-26, indicating the presence of active inflammation.

MRI by an ophthalmologist who found that the patient had a bitemporal hemianopsia.

A common finding in all white matter disease is T2 hyperintensity, seen well on all T2 sequences but most conspicuous on the T2 FLAIR sequence. The pattern of white

COST-EFFECTIVE MEDICINE

If the clinical situation does not call for a specific protocol, ordering "Brain MRI, with contrast as needed" may provide the flexibility needed for a radiologist to review an initial set of unenhanced sequence images and proceed appropriately (see Table 4-1).

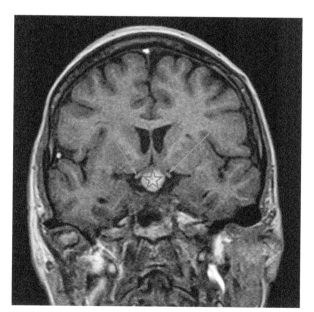

FIGURE 4-24 Coronal thin section pre-contrast T1 MRI image just posterior to the optic chiasm from pituitary protocol MRI. Blue arrows indicate the optic tracts. A Rathke's cleft cyst filled with simple serous fluid would be T1 hypointense, but in this case the cyst (star) has fluid that is T1 hyperintense because there has been hemorrhage into the cyst.

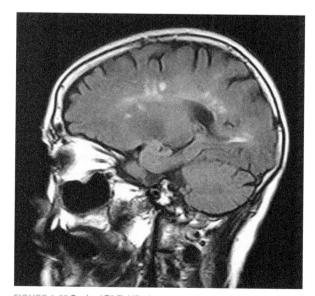

FIGURE 4-25 Sagittal T2 FLAIR of a patient that reveals the presence of periventricular T2 hyperintense white matter lesions, several of which are oriented perpendicular to the adjacent lateral ventricle (two of these indicated with arrows).

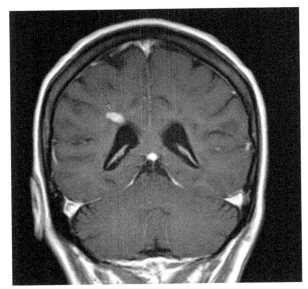

FIGURE 4-26 Coronal contrast-enhanced T1 MRI. The contrast enhancement of a periventricular white matter lesion (arrow) indicates that this is an active MS plaque. Other (older) plaques in this case that were T2 hyperintense showed no enhancement.

NEUROENDOCRINE DYSFUNCTION

Endocrine diseases for which CNS imaging is appropriate include hypopituitarism, hyperthyroidism secondary to high thyroid-stimulating hormone (TSH) levels, Cushing's syndrome, hyperprolactinemia, and acromegaly. For other disorders, such as diabetes insipidus, growth hormone deficiency, and precocious puberty, the need for imaging as part of the routine medical workup is less clear.

Obesity, anorexia, sleep disorders, and hypo- or hyperthermia may be related to the neuroendocrine axis, for which the diagnostic yield of imaging is low.

Empty sella syndrome may be associated with hypopituitarism and with pseudotumor cerebri, in which the finding of papilledema often leads to neuroimaging to rule out an intracranial mass.

Modalities

"Pituitary protocol" or "MRI special attention to the pituitary" of the brain without and with contrast enhancement should be requested for neuroendocrine patients, not a routine MRI of the brain. If the use of gadolinium-based contrast material is contraindicated, then unenhanced MRI with thin section imaging of the sella is superior to CT scanning with contrast enhancement.

Interpretation

Hypopituitarism can be caused by suprasellar lesions that disrupt the neuroendocrine axis, such as a CNS lymphoma or brain malignancy that involves the hypothalamus. However,

more commonly the cause is a non-functioning pituitary tumor that compresses or invades normal pituitary tissue. Endocrine dysfunction caused by elevated levels of TSH, adrenocorticotropic hormone (ACTH), prolactin, growth hormone, and gonadotropins are the result of functioning pituitary adenomas. Because normal pituitary tissue enhances intensely after the administration of a contrast material, a microadenoma (<1 cm) can be seen as a hypo-enhancing focus with the pituitary, as shown in Figure 4-27.

The MRI finding in which the pituitary fossa (the sella turcica) is mostly filled with CSF and the pituitary is found to be flattened along the inferior margin of the sella (Fig. 4-28) is called empty sella syndrome. This syndrome may be found in patients with hypopituitarism, although it is commonly observed on MRI as an incidental finding, or may be associated with chronic headache, often in obese young women.

EPILEPSY AND SEIZURES

Seizures are either focal or generalized; a patient with chronic seizures is diagnosed with epilepsy. As discussed earlier, the new onset of seizure in the adult may be associated with a mass lesion, such as tumor, abscess, traumatic brain injury, or vascular malformation such as AVM.

 Children between the age of 6 months and 6 years may have febrile seizures. When there is a normal neurologic examination and normal developmental history, neuroimaging is usually not needed.

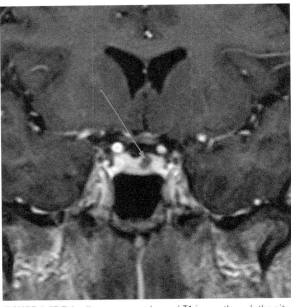

FIGURE 4-27 Thin slice contrast-enhanced T1 image through the pituitary that shows a hypo-enhancing pituitary microadenoma (arrow), surrounded by brightly enhancing normal pituitary tissue, in a patient with hyperprolactinemia.

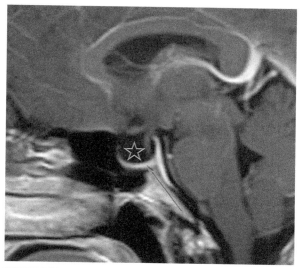

FIGURE 4-28 Midline sagittal contrast-enhanced T1 image of the brain in which the sella was noted to be filled with CSF, referred to as an empty sella (star). Note the compressed pituitary gland (arrow) along the floor of the sella. This is presumed to be caused by a deficiency of the diaphragma sella.

Modalities

Seizure may result acutely with trauma; unenhanced CT should be done immediately as discussed in the trauma Modalities section earlier. New onset seizure that is not likely to be explained by drug or alcohol use, and with no history of trauma, should be investigated with MRI of the head without and with contrast enhancement. The yield from the additional contrast-enhanced sequences is typically not high and seizure patients can be examined satisfactorily with unenhanced MRI. CT without and with contrast enhancement is a secondary alternative.

During the neurology/neurosurgical evaluation of epilepsy, special procedures used for diagnosis and surgical planning include FDG-PET, functional MRI, MR spectroscopy, SPECT, and EEG and **magnetoencephalography.**

Interpretation

In the adult with new onset seizure, vascular malformations, tumors, and other mass lesions that may precipitate seizure have no distinguishing features.

Congenital brain malformations may be associated with seizures, along with other neurologic abnormalities; the spectrum of imaging findings in these cases is beyond the scope of this text.

Most seizure activity arises in the temporal lobe. The most common epileptogenic focus is in the hippocampus and is associated with the imaging finding of mesial temporal sclerosis. This may be visible as increased T2 signal and decreased volume of the hippocampus, as shown in Figure 4-29. More advanced MRI analysis in epilepsy uses software programs

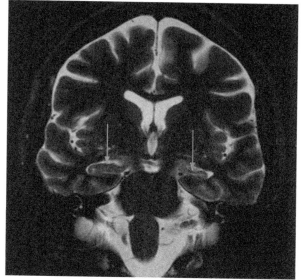

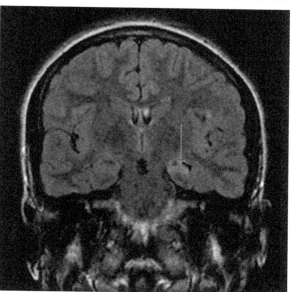

FIGURE 4-29 Left mesial temporal sclerosis. **Top:** The hippocampal atrophy is best appreciated on a coronal T2 fast spin echo sequence (red arrow). Compare to normal contralateral side (blue arrow). **Bottom:** The T2 hyperintensity (red arrow) of the abnormal left hippocampus is best shown on the coronal FLAIR sequence

that can accurately measure the volume of the hippocampus from the MR images.

 COST-EFFECTIVE MEDICINE

The structural abnormalities associated with epilepsy can be very subtle; therefore imaging for epilepsy is one area in which the scanner used is a fundamental issue; the use of low field strength "open" magnets is discouraged; patients should be scanned in a high field strength 1.5 T scanner or in the newest generation of 3.0 T scanners.

DEMENTIA

Just as dementia is the loss of cognitive abilities beyond that expected of normal aging, the imaging findings in dementia may be significantly different quantitatively and qualitatively from the common (and expected) imaging changes of the aging brain. The diagnosis of dementias, including Alzheimer's disease (AD), is primarily clinical. Imaging is ancillary in the diagnostic workup of dementia; however, it has been shown to increase diagnostic accuracy.

Vascular dementias are very common, either from small vessel disease causing white matter changes or multi-infarct dementia.

Modalities

MRI is the procedure of choice for identifying the white matter changes and cortical atrophy associated with dementia and the hydrocephalus associated with dementia in NPH. For these goals, unenhanced MRI is usually sufficient, with relatively little increased diagnostic yield from contrast-enhanced MR sequences; therefore, contrast-enhanced MRI is considered optional. In patients who cannot undergo MRI, unenhanced CT can reveal severe degrees of cerebral cortical atrophy and hydrocephalus. There is now also growing use of PET scanning in the diagnosis of dementia, because the information gained from PET scanning can be applied to newer specific treatment options.

Beyond routine MRI, advanced volumetric analysis of the hippocampus from MRI data is used in evaluation of AD. Emerging imaging techniques for evaluating patients with dementia include functional MRI and SPECT scanning.

Interpretation

The normal aging brain commonly shows white matter changes that are progressive. The most common of these findings are so widely seen that they have been given the dismissive moniker of the "UBO," the unidentified bright object. These small foci of high T2 signal are commonly multiple, and widely distributed in the major white matter tracts of both cerebral hemispheres, as shown in Figure 4-30. UBOs should not be misinterpreted as evidence of specific disease in patients older than 65.

More advanced and confluent white matter hyperintensity is often the result of widespread microangiopathic (small vessel) white matter changes, as shown in Figure 4-31.

Multi-infarct dementia is evident on imaging by the finding of multiple foci of gliosis and cystic encephalomalacia at the sites of numerous cerebral infarctions, as seen in Figure 4-32.

In addition to UBOs and more extensive white hyperintensity of chronic ischemic white matter changes, diffuse

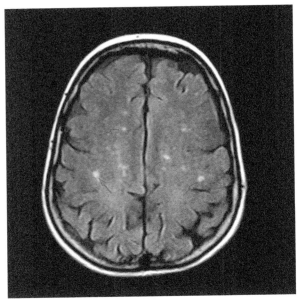

FIGURE 4-30 Axial T2 FLAIR sequence. The foci of T2 hyperintensity in the centrum semiovale (several indicated with arrows) are characteristic of UBOs (see text) that are common in the normal aging brain.

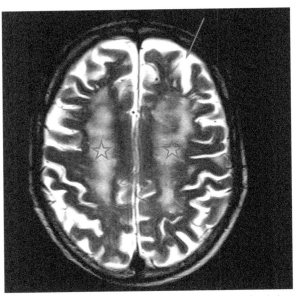

FIGURE 4-31 Axial T2 MRI at the level of the centrum semiovale in a patient with advanced microangiopathic white matter changes (stars) and widened sulci (arrow) secondary to cortical atrophy.

cerebral cortical atrophy is often seen in the aging brain. When there is disproportionate hippocampal cortical atrophy, a diagnosis of AD is considered (Fig. 4-33).

The frontotemporal dementias, of which Pick's disease is best known, are difficult to differentiate from AD. The imaging findings reflect the description of these disorders by showing disproportionate cortical atrophy in the frontal and temporal lobes (Fig. 4-34).

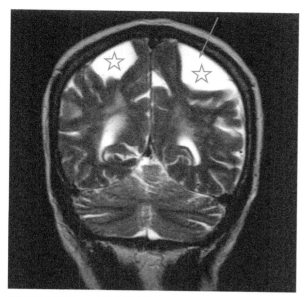

FIGURE 4-32 Coronal T2 MRI. Widened subarachnoid spaces (stars) result from loss of gyri secondary to multiple old cortical infarctions.

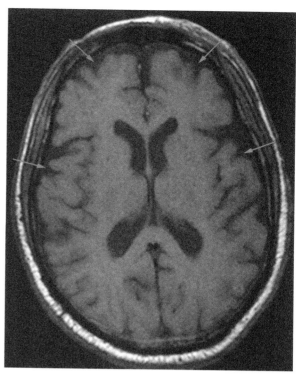

FIGURE 4-34 Axial MRI of a patient with frontotemporal cortical atrophy. Note widened subarachnoid space in frontal and temporal regions (arrows) but normal sulci and gyri in the occipital lobes.

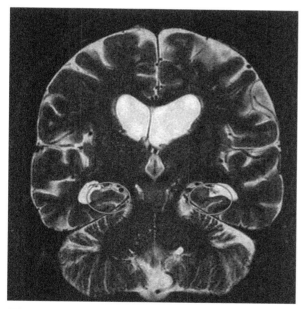

FIGURE 4-33 Coronal MRI that shows hippocampal atrophy (circled). The adjacent temporal horns of the lateral ventricles are dilated ex vacuo secondary to the hippocampal atrophy.

CASE CONCLUSION

Your 65-year-old female patient, who was given steroids for the vasogenic edema around her brain tumor, had been feeling better, but the weekend before her planned surgery she experienced an explosive onset of headache, which she called "the worst headache of her life." She is rushed to the emergency department, where an immediate unenhanced CT is performed, revealing an intracerebral hemorrhage in the left frontal lobe, a positive mass effect, and signs of uncal herniation. She undergoes urgent neurosurgery to evacuate the hematoma and to biopsy the mass that pathology revealed to be a glioblastoma multiforme.

She has done well since surgery and is now enrolled in a clinical trial of new treatment for this usually fatal cancer.

Chapter Review

Chapter Review Questions

1. Which of the following associations is not correct?

    A. Epidural hematoma: skull fracture across groove for middle meningeal artery

    B. Chronic subdural hematoma: shearing of dural bridging veins

    C. Cephalhematoma: immediate CT and MRI needed

    D. Otoscopic exam showing blood behind tympanic membrane in a trauma patient: thin section CT temporal bone

    E. Head trauma: unenhanced CT

2. DWI MRI sequences are most important for the diagnosis of:

    A. chronic subdural hematoma.

    B. acute ischemic stroke.

    C. hemosiderin.

    D. pituitary apoplexy.

    E. empty sella syndrome.

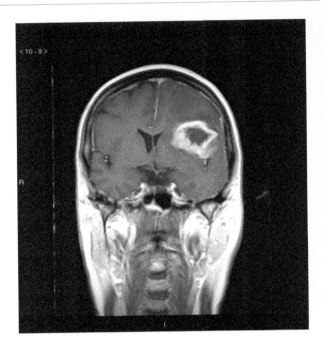

3. The contrast-enhanced coronal T1 image shown above is important:

    A. to determine if this is a tumor that is malignant.

    B. to definitively differentiate tumor from abscess.

    C. to define margins of the tumor for treatment planning.

    D. to determine if there is mass effect.

    E. to determine if there is bleeding.

4. Which of the following is TRUE pertaining to the appearance of blood in neuroimaging?

    A. Acute and chronic hematomas have the same density on CT images

    B. Acute and chronic hematomas have the same intensity on MR images

    C. On CT, an acute hematoma appears less dense than a chronic hematoma

    D. Magnetic susceptibility is associated with residual hemosiderin from an old hemorrhage on MR

    E. MRI is not useful in cases of intracranial hemorrhage

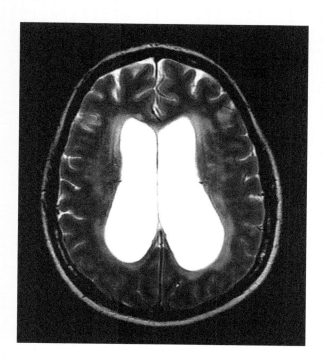

5. What is your diagnosis based on the MRI image above?

   A. Hydrocephalus

   B. Epidural hematoma

   C. Subdural hematoma

   D. SAH

   E. Meningitis

6. T2 hyperintensity is consistently associated with which of the following?

   A. Parkinson's disease

   B. White matter diseases

   C. Alzheimer's disease

   D. Frontotemporal dementia

   E. Pituitary apoplexy

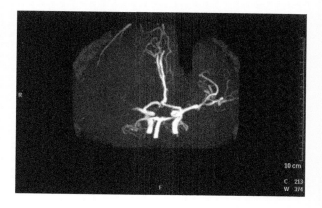

7. What is your diagnosis based on the image above?

   A. Ischemic stroke in the territory of the right MCA

   B. Hemorrhagic stroke in the territory of the right of the ICA

   C. Empty sella syndrome

   D. Sigmoid sinus venous thrombosis

   E. SAH

8. Which of the following is incorrect pertaining to the images of patients with seizures?

   A. Children younger than 6 with febrile seizures need immediate imaging

   B. Chronic seizure patients can usually be satisfactorily evaluated with unenhanced MRI

   C. Seizure activity is often associated with mesial temporal sclerosis

   D. Seizure activity may be associated with MRI showing increased T2 signal in the hippocampus

9. UBOs are:

   A. diagnostic for MS.

   B. diagnostic for AD.

   C. associated with venous thrombosis in pregnancy.

   D. associated with empty sella syndrome.

   E. normally found in the aging brain.

10. Neuroimaging should routinely be ordered for patients with any of the following except:

   A. progressive headache.

   B. chronic headache.

   C. headache with focal neurologic signs.

   D. acute, severe headache described as the worst headache of the patient's life.

5 EENT IMAGING

CASE STUDY

Two patients have appointments with you on the same day for routine physical exams. Patient A is 55 years old and is found to have an enlarged left thyroid lobe and a right carotid bruit. You order thyroid and carotid ultrasonography and thyroid lab studies. Patient B is 57 years old and found to also have a right carotid bruit. You order a carotid ultrasound. Family history includes vascular disease in both parents and a brother (perhaps related to the history of smoking in all family members), and there is a maternal history of goiter.

FUNDAMENTALS OF EYES, EAR, NOSE, AND THROAT IMAGING

Some radiologists in large practices or at universities specialize in Eyes, Ear, Nose, and Throat (EENT) radiology (head and neck radiology), which partially overlaps neuroradiology. Similarly, here we differentiate EENT and neuroradiology (see Chapter 4), but the reader should realize that the two are often closely related. Imaging procedures for diseases in the region may be very highly specific, such as the nearly universal use of sonography to evaluate the morphology of thyroid disease and the ubiquitous use of CT for paranasal sinus inflammatory disease, or the dynamic (barium) swallowing study done to visualize pharyngeal swallowing dysfunction.

NASAL CONGESTION AND SINUSITIS

Appropriate evaluation and treatment of nasal congestion due to allergies usually requires no imaging. Similarly, most cases of acute rhinosinusitis, whether viral or bacterial in origin, do not require imaging.

The American Academy of Pediatrics does not recommend radiologic study of children younger than age 6 who meet clinical criteria for uncomplicated bacterial sinusitis, because of concern about radiation exposure in children and the infrequency of a misleading clinical presentation in this situation.

The role of imaging when sinusitis is suspected clinically is to establish the presence or absence of paranasal sinus inflammatory disease (especially purulent sinusitis), to evaluate any impairment to sinus drainage, and to evaluate complications of sinusitis.

Modalities

Unenhanced CT scanning of the paranasal sinuses is indicated in the following two situations:

- When sinusitis persists for longer than 4 weeks
- When several episodes of infectious sinusitis occur per year with at least 8 weeks free of disease between episodes (recurrent sinusitis)

If orbital or intracranial spread of a sinus infection is suspected (or routine unenhanced sinus CT show evidence of such complication), CT or MRI of the brain and orbits, without and with contrast enhancement, is indicated. The choice between these two modalities typically depends on patient factors and available expertise and specialty preferences.

 COST-EFFECTIVE MEDICINE

When the clinical diagnosis of acute infectious sinusitis is certain, or if clinical evaluation determines that sinusitis is very unlikely, no imaging is needed.

In patients who have been diagnosed with purulent sinusitis on CT, an upright occipitomental (Waters) view radiograph to evaluate response to treatment may be useful as a low-cost follow-up imaging procedure rather than repeat CT.

Interpretation

Sinusitis is diagnosed on CT by the finding of inflammatory hyperplastic mucoperiosteal thickening. This thickening, along with secretions, may opacify (replace air) in portions of the sinuses, such as a frontal recess or an air cell of the ethmoid or sphenoid sinuses, or may opacify an entire sinus. When the process is extensive, it may be reported as *pansinusitis*, which is evident on the several selected coronal sections through the paranasal sinuses shown in Figure 5-1.

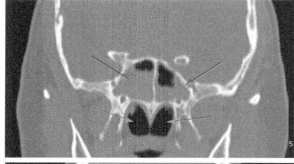

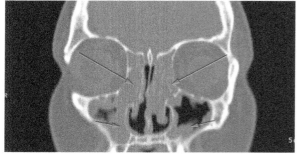

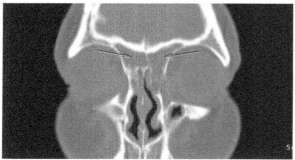

FIGURE 5-1 CT of paranasal sinuses from posterior to anterior. The most posterior **(top)** of the selected "slices" shows mucoperiosteal thickening in the sphenoid sinus (red arrows). Note air in the posterior nasopharynx (blue arrows). The **middle** coronal section shows complete opacification of the ethmoid sinus (long red arrows) and nodular circumferential mucoperiosteal thickening of the maxillary sinuses (short red arrows). The **bottom** image shows complete opacification of the frontal sinus (red arrows).

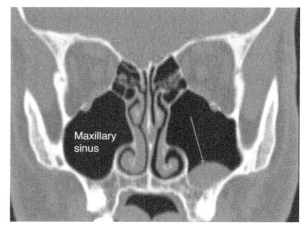

FIGURE 5-2 Coronal CT. Characteristic mucous retention cyst (arrow) but no other mucosal thickening that would suggest the presence of an active sinusitis.

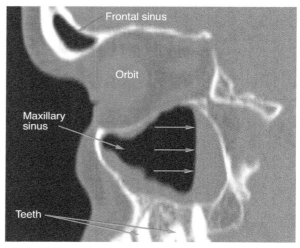

FIGURE 5-3 Sagittal CT of the paranasal sinuses showing an air–fluid level in a maxillary sinus. The patient was scanned supine, so the straight edge (arrows) that represents the air–fluid level was horizontal in the patient.

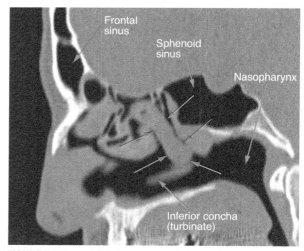

FIGURE 5-4 Sagittal CT of the paranasal sinuses that shows a nasal polyp (red arrows).

The mucoperiosteum of the nasal sinuses may also be focally thickened due to post-inflammatory mucous retention cysts. These are very common and, as shown in Figure 5-2, are typically rounded lesions that have relatively abrupt margins with normal mucosa, which is normally so thin that no soft tissue should be seen adjacent to the cortical bone of the paranasal sinuses.

The presence of air fluid levels within a sinus results from purulent sinusitis and provides reliable evidence of a bacterial infection (Fig. 5-3).

Nasal polyps, which may impair sinus drainage, may be very difficult to identify on CT because they are the same density as the soft tissues of the nasal turbinates (concha). In Figure 5-4, the imaging order included relevant clinical data, including the finding of a nasal polyp on physical exam. This information resulted in the radiologist evaluating the patient using a sagittally reconstructed image (not usually done on paranasal sinus CT studies), which clearly showed the polyp that may be obstructing drainage of the right maxillary sinus.

When opacification of paranasal sinuses is associated with bone erosion of the skull base or orbit, or when orbital fat is replaced with abnormal soft tissue density, an unusual aggressive infection, such as fungal sinusitis is suspected, especially in immunocompromised patients. In a patient with no immunologic compromise and no clinical findings that suggest infection, erosive bone changes raise suspicion of tumor, as shown in Figure 5-5.

When sinus tumors or complications of sinusitis are found, contrast-enhanced CT or MRI will demonstrate enhancement of tumor, inflammatory tissue, or abscess wall. For example, see the pre-contrast (Fig. 5-6, top) and post-contrast (Fig. 5-6, bottom) axial T1 MR images of a sinus malignancy that has invaded the left orbit.

NECK LUMPS

Palpable masses in the neck are most often in the thyroid or salivary glands, or represent adenopathy, and imaging is fundamental to the diagnostic workup. Palpable thyroid nodules, for which thyroid ultrasound exams are commonly done, are most often benign.

Up to half of all patients with papillary thyroid cancer present initially with enlarged metastatic lymph nodes, rather than presenting with a thyroid nodule, and imaging is initially directed toward evaluating cervical adenopathy.

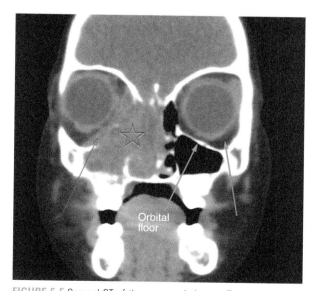

FIGURE 5-5 Coronal CT of the paranasal sinuses. Tumor in the right maxillary sinus (star) has destroyed the osseous floor of the right orbit (note contralateral normal orbital floor). Sinus tumor has invaded the right orbit (red arrow) and infiltrates intraorbital fat (note normal hypodense left intraorbital fat indicated by the blue arrow).

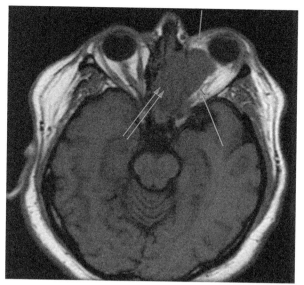

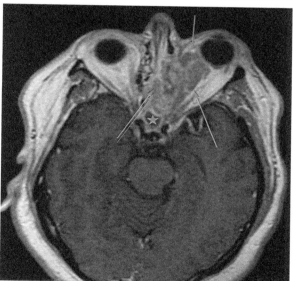

FIGURE 5-6 Pre- (top) and post-contrast (bottom) axial T1 MR images demonstrate the irregular enhancement of ethmoid sinus tumor (double arrow) invading the orbit (single arrows) and expanding posteriorly into the sphenoid sinus. This kind of heterogeneous enhancement is often seen in rapidly growing malignancies, with areas of tumor that are highly vascularized and some areas that have become necrotic (star) because they have outgrown their blood supply and therefore do not enhance.

Nasopharyngeal, oropharyngeal, and laryngeal cancers do not present with a palpable mass unless there is already metastatic disease to regional nodes. The diagnosis of such tumors is usually done by direct inspection and biopsy, with imaging then important for staging and treatment planning.

The most common salivary gland mass that is evaluated with imaging is a benign pleomorphic adenoma of the parotid gland, but malignant masses of the salivary glands also occur. Not all salivary gland enlargement that is evaluated with imaging is the result of a mass. For example, Sjögren's syndrome, an autoimmune disease, may present with generalized parotid gland swelling, in addition to the complaint of decreased salivation.

Non-thyroid cystic masses in the neck are typically congenital lesions such as a thyroglossal duct cyst.

Modalities

Determining which CT and MRI procedural designation to use for head and neck imaging can be confusing because of existing procedure codes for both maxillofacial and soft tissue neck imaging studies. An example would be a mass in or near the parotid gland that would be within the field of view of either study (Table 5-1). As always, in such situations, talk with your consulting radiologist.

Ultrasonography of the thyroid is performed:

• To evaluate thyroid enlargement
• To evaluate palpable thyroid nodules
• To screen for thyroid nodules in patients at risk for thyroid cancer because of prior neck irradiation
• To confirm clinical suspicion that the cause of neck pain is thyroiditis

CT or MRI of the soft tissues of the neck may be required for thyroid disease when:

• Thyroid masses are larger than 3 cm
• The clinical presentation of thyroid masses is highly suspicious for aggressive malignancy
• There is clinical concern about mediastinal extension of a goiter

When a patient presents with a large thyroid mass that is highly suspicious for cancer based on sonography, or has positive fine needle aspiration (FNA) results for thyroid cancer, CT or MRI of the neck can reveal extracapsular invasion or spread of the tumor and regional adenopathy. CT is advantageous for large thyroid masses because calcifications can be seen on CT that are not apparent on MRI.

Radionuclide (usually I^{123}) thyroid scanning is useful in assessing types of hyperthyroidism and in determining the functional status of thyroid nodules. However, iodine administered during any contrast-enhanced CT scan will suppress subsequent uptake of iodine by the thyroid for 4 to 8 weeks. Therefore, radionuclide thyroid exams should not be done within 8 weeks of a prior enhanced CT study.

Patients with salivary calculi often present with a history of intermittent post-prandial pain and swelling of the associated salivary gland. The ideal procedure for demonstrating suspected calculi is CT without contrast enhancement. For evaluation of tumors of the salivary glands, CT scanning is done with contrast enhancement. MRI is also rated very highly for this imaging indication when CT might be contraindicated (e.g., pregnancy) and should be done without and with contrast enhancement.

Enlargement of lymph nodes in the neck may be due to lymphoma or regional or distant metastatic disease, or may commonly occur in response to infection (usually viral), in which case the nodes are termed "reactive nodes."

COST-EFFECTIVE MEDICINE
When the clinical presentation is highly consistent with reactive nodes secondary to infection, no imaging may be needed.

For adults, contrast-enhanced CT of the soft tissue of the neck is usually done. For patients with severe renal disease or other factors that contraindicate the use of contrast agents, unenhanced MRI would be the procedure of choice.

In children, imaging of the soft tissues of the neck for adenopathy is usually done with ultrasonography. A common clinical concern related to neck soft tissues in children with recurrent otitis media and those with chronic nasal obstruction ("mouth breathers") is enlarged adenoids. The best imaging procedure in this situation is a lateral soft tissue radiograph of the neck.

When there is clinical suspicion of a cystic neck lesion such as thyroglossal duct cyst or branchial cleft cyst, ultrasonography is an ideal initial procedure.

In patients with known malignancy who present with neck masses or adenopathy, PET and CT scanning are both indicated, usually now done simultaneously as a PET-CT scan. Depending upon a patient's individual situation, an oncologist may use MRI without and with contrast enhancement as an alternative.

Interpretation

Goiter often has a nodular appearance on ultrasound. Graves disease and the early stage of Hashimoto's thyroiditis are

TABLE 5-1 Sample EENT Radiology Requisition Information

Modality	Body Region	Clinical Data/History
MRI, with contrast	Soft tissue neck	Squamous cancer—base of tongue on left
CT with contrast	Soft tissue neck	Possible left parotid mass
Ultrasound	Thyroid	2 cm palp. nodule L upper, hypothyroid (faxing lab data)
Radiography	Lateral soft tissue neck	R/O enlarged adenoids
CT	Paranasal sinuses	Nasal polyposis, h/a, fever leukocytosis; R/O sinusitis
Radiography	Swallowing study	Dysphagia, chronic sx. of GERD, regurgitation of undigested food; R/O Zenker's
CT	Maxillofacial	Facial trauma—loss of upward gaze L eye

associated with moderate diffuse thyromegaly. Chronic thyroiditis is usually associated with a small hyperechoic thyroid. Doppler sonography may reveal diffuse thyroid hyperemia in both Graves disease and in subacute viral thyroiditis.

Multinodular thyroid enlargement often results from the presence of multiple thyroid nodules that may have varied histology and appearance on sonography, as shown in Figure 5-7.

Criteria for biopsy of either a single thyroid mass or of one or more nodules in multinodular thyroid enlargement are determined by imaging-based morphology and/or nuclear medicine scans. For example, a uniformly hyperechoic thyroid nodule is so consistently benign that it has been called a "white knight" (Fig. 5-8). A nodule that takes up iodine on a radionuclide scan similar to normal thyroid tissue is very unlikely to be malignant and biopsy can be avoided or

deferred. A hyperfunctioning nodule that avidly takes up iodine to the extent that uptake in the rest of the thyroid is suppressed is called a "hot nodule," and these are also rarely malignant. Such a hyperfunctioning nodule is often referred to as an "autonomous nodule" on a radiology report.

Sonographic findings that are suspicious for thyroid malignancy include poor transmission of the ultrasound beam, irregular shape and indistinct margins, and multiple small central calcifications.

When a thyroid nodule meets criteria for biopsy, FNA under ultrasound guidance is indicated (Fig. 5-9).

Sialolithiasis (calculi in salivary ductal system) is clearly shown on unenhanced CT as calcific density structures in the expected location of a salivary duct (Fig. 5-10).

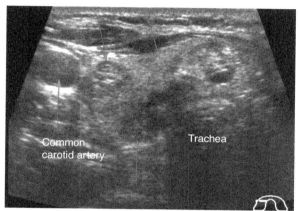

FIGURE 5-7 Transverse thyroid ultrasound image. Red arrows indicate several thyroid nodules with varied levels of echogenicity and tissue texture.

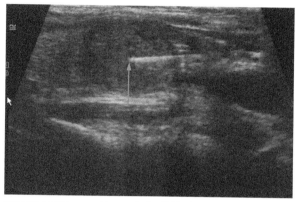

FIGURE 5-9 Ultrasound image during FNA of a thyroid nodule. Image provides documentation of position of needle tip (arrow) within the nodule during tissue sampling.

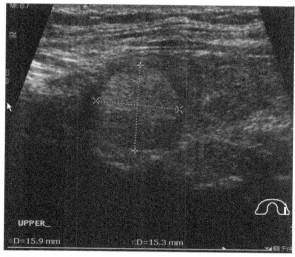

FIGURE 5-8 Thyroid ultrasound. The hyperechoic nodule that was measured by the technologist (note electronic calipers and the measurements of 15.9 mm and 15.3 mm at the bottom of the image) can be considered benign with a high degree of certainty because of its sonographic appearance (see further explanation in text).

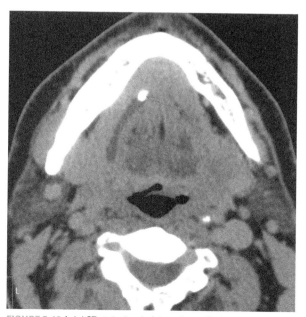

FIGURE 5-10 Axial CT at the level of the submandibular gland and duct. The arrow indicates an obstructing calculus in the distal submandibular duct that causes dilatation of the duct (double arrow).

In Sjögren's syndrome the enlarged parotid gland typically has a CT appearance that is isodense with muscle, rather than the usual CT appearance of the parotid that is intermediate in density between soft tissue and fat.

Pleomorphic adenomas are usually seen as smoothly and sharply marginated masses within a salivary gland (most often the parotid) on CT (Fig. 5-11) or MRI. Because the facial nerve lies close to the retromandibular vein within the parotid gland, the relationship between a parotid tumor and that vein is an important aspect of pre-operative CT or MRI interpretation.

Salivary gland malignancies often have less distinct margins and more variable appearance than pleomorphic adenomas. Histology of salivary gland tumors can be established with ultrasound-guided FNA or core needle biopsy.

You will receive many radiology reports on maxillofacial and soft tissue neck studies in which lymph nodes are described as marginal, borderline, or prominent in size, or as being definitely enlarged but without other significant radiologic findings. This occurs because normal-sized lymph nodes may harbor disease and large nodes may not contain significant pathology. A cervical node is within normal limits in size if its short axis diameter is less than 1 cm, with the exception of the jugulodigastric and jugulo-omohyoid nodes, both of which may normally have a short axis measurement of 1.5 cm.

 Children tend to have larger (absolute) neck nodes than adults.

Enlarged nodes that are round are more suspicious than elongated ovoid nodes. A "necrotic" cervical node (hypodense center on CT or hyperintense center on MRI) of any size is highly suspicious for cancer (especially metastatic squamous cell cancer) or intranodal abscess secondary to neck infection. In Figure 5-12, an enhancing squamous cell carcinoma of the base of the tongue was metastatic to a right cervical node.

Aside from massive adenopathy that is obviously pathologic, the overall accuracy rate for the diagnosis of lymph node disease in the neck, based only upon appearance of nodes on imaging, is about 80%. Thus, PET-CT scanning is an important tool in head and neck oncology. Figure 5-13 is a PET scan that reveals the abnormal activity in cervical nodes caused by metastatic disease.

Massive bilateral cervical adenopathy is most often lymphoma (Fig. 5-14).

Cystic lesions in the neck appear on ultrasound as fluid-filled anechoic lesions that transmit sound well if filled with simple serous fluid, or may show echogenic debris. Figure 5-15 shows an ultrasound image that confirmed the clinical impression that a soft midline anterior neck mass was a thyroglossal duct cyst, and also shows a CT scan that revealed the presence of a small thyroglossal duct cyst, which was an incidental finding.

 The interpretation of a lateral soft tissue radiograph of the neck for adenoid size requires experience with viewing many such images; there are no firm criteria or reference measurements. However, when adenoids are greatly enlarged, as may occur in children, the experienced professional has little difficulty recognizing the markedly thickened

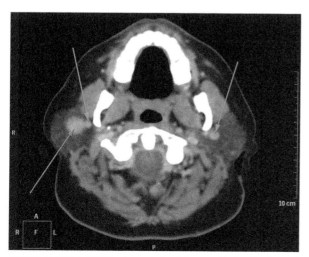

FIGURE 5-11 Axial CT. The tumor in the right parotid gland (red arrow) is well marginated and shows homogenous enhancement, most consistent with pleomorphic adenoma. It is superficial to the retromandibular vein, indicated on both sides by the blue arrows (see text).

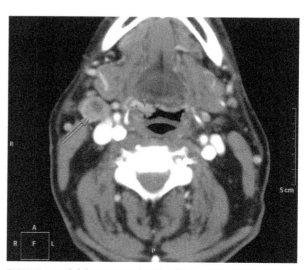

FIGURE 5-12 Axial contrast-enhancing CT. The enhancing squamous cell carcinoma of the right tongue base (arrow) is metastatic to a right cervical node (double arrow).

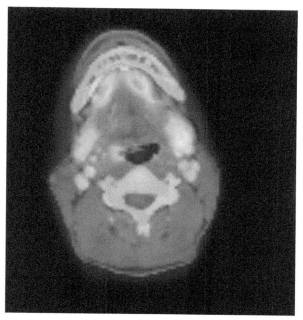

FIGURE 5-13 Axial CT-PET scan image of the neck. Foci of increased glycolytic activity (typical of malignant tissues) are represented by colors toward the red end of the color spectrum and normal glycolytic activity toward the blue end of the spectrum.

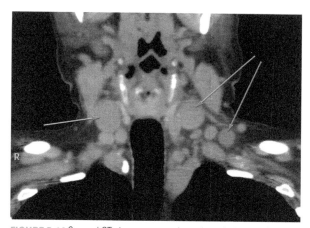

FIGURE 5-14 Coronal CT shows many enlarged cervical nodes (three of them indicated by arrows) in the base of the neck.

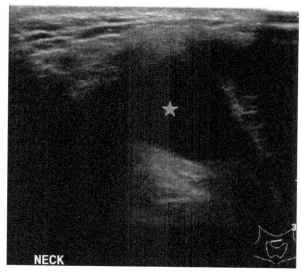

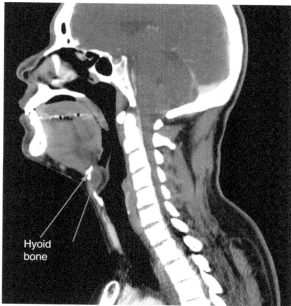

FIGURE 5-15 Transverse ultrasound image **(top)** shows a midline cystic structure (star) just above the thyroid gland, confirming the clinical impression of a thyroglossal duct cyst. Midline sagittal CT **(bottom)** shows a small thyroglossal duct cyst (red arrow) deep to the hyoid bone.

posterior pharyngeal tissues that narrow the nasopharynx (Fig. 5-16), resulting in the mouth breathing typical in patients with this condition.

FACIAL DROOP (Bell's Palsy)

Bell's palsy, the most common cranial neuropathy, is an in-flammation of nerve VII that is now known to be related to infection with herpes simplex virus in many cases. Most cases resolve spontaneously or with medical therapy and do not require any imaging. However, when the clinical course is atypical or surgery is being considered to decompress cranial nerve VII, imaging is appropriate.

Modalities

The procedure of choice for evaluation of cranial nerve VII is MRI of the brain without and with contrast enhancement, with special attention to the internal auditory canals (IACs). If the administration of gadolinium-based contrast material is contraindicated, unenhanced MRI can identify a mass along the course of cranial nerve VII, but only if special thin

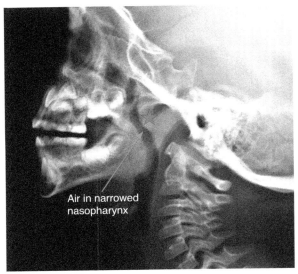

Air in narrowed nasopharynx

FIGURE 5-16 Lateral soft tissue neck radiograph that shows greatly en-larged adenoids (star).

sections through the IACs are requested. The scan will ideally also cover the course of cranial nerve VII within the parotid gland so that a separate MRI of the soft tissues of the neck will not be needed. If MRI is contraindicated, thin section contrast-enhanced CT scanning of the temporal bones may be diagnostic.

Inconsistencies in Terminology

Words or phrases that describe a particular condition or procedure in a textbook often differ from the words or phrases used in actual practice, and that may be the case for terms used in this book.

A "Schwannoma of the vestibulocochlear nerve (cranial nerve VIII)" is commonly called an "acoustic neuroma," even though the nerve involved is no longer officially called the acoustic nerve and the tumor is not really a neuroma. Medical publications describing Bell's palsy usually refer to the "seventh cranial nerve," though an anatomist would prefer the official term, "cranial nerve VII," the terminology used in this chapter.

When you have a patient with degenerative spinal canal stenosis and want to brush up on the anatomy, you may not be able to find spinal canal in an anatomy textbook or atlas. That anatomic feature is more likely to be labeled as vertebral canal in anatomy publications, even though it is labeled spinal canal in surgery and radiology texts and journals.

Don't be surprised by such apparent inconsistencies. Just be aware that you may hear and use slightly different terms as you move from the classroom to the clinic.

Interpretation

The hallmark MRI finding in Bell's palsy is abnormal enhancement of cranial nerve VII, as shown in Figure 5-17, and/or the geniculate ganglion. In unusual cases, an infiltrating malignancy of the parotid gland may involve cranial nerve VII and invade the mastoid portion of the temporal bone.

DYSPHAGIA AND SORE THROAT

Swallowing dysfunction is classically divided into pharyngeal and retrosternal (thoracic esophagus) clinical presentations. Within the pharyngeal presentation, difficulty in initiating a swallow indicates oropharyngeal dysfunction while aspiration with swallowing indicates hypopharyngeal mobility abnormalities, both of which often have a neurologic basis.

When the patient does not have difficulty with initiating swallowing and does not aspirate, but "food gets stuck on the way down," then there is more likely to be thoracic esophageal disease. However, localization of the anatomic derangement based upon symptoms is problematic. The sensation of dysphagia that occurs from lower esophageal disease or even from disorders of the esophagogastric junction is often referred to the upper chest or neck.

With modern antibiotic treatment, complications of sore throat are rare, and therefore imaging to evaluate such complications is often not needed. However, when the clinical evaluation raises concern about peritonsillar or retropharyngeal abscess, then imaging becomes important.

Modalities

A **dynamic swallowing study** is a radiologic exam that involves videography and/or rapid sequence radiographs

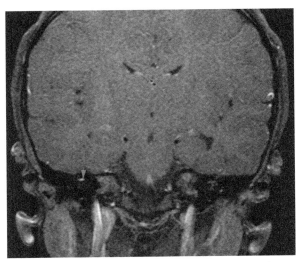

FIGURE 5-17 Coronal contrast-enhanced T1 MRI that shows enhancement of a segment of nerve VII (arrow) in a patient with Bell's palsy.

made during the fluoroscopic observation of a patient drinking barium. You should order such an exam when your patient has difficulty initiating swallowing or you suspect a Zenker's diverticulum, which is a pulsion type of diverticulum of the posterior wall of the junction of the pharynx and cervical esophagus. An upper GI series, which includes an esophagram, should be ordered when dysphagia is likely to be related to thoracic or lower esophageal disease, such as sliding hiatus hernia, Schatzke ring, esophagitis, or esophageal tumor. When the clinical presentation does not provide a clear differentiation between pharyngeal and esophageal disease, it may be appropriate to order both a dynamic swallowing study and an upper GI series. The term "barium swallow" should be avoided because it could refer to either a dynamic swallowing study or an upper GI exam.

For the patient who may have a peritonsillar or retropharyngeal abscess, MRI can clearly demonstrate the abnormalities, but MRI is a lengthy examination that may be difficult to tolerate for these patients. Contrast-enhanced CT of the neck, which may be done with just a few seconds of scanning, is typically recommended for these patients.

Dysphagia associated with retrosternal pain may be part of the clinical presentation of gastroesophageal reflux disease (GERD). When GERD does not respond readily to routine medical therapy, and especially if GERD is complicated by dysphagia, endoscopy or radiographic upper GI series may be indicated.

Interpretation

When a dynamic swallowing study demonstrates abnormalities, these findings are more often related to neurologic disease than to abnormal morphology of the pharynx. An important functional disorder is abnormal movement of the epiglottis that allows aspiration during swallowing. The documentation of such aspiration, as shown in Figure 5-18, may explain why a patient has had repeated episodes of pneumonia.

A common cause of hypopharyngeal or cervical esophageal dysphagia is spasm of the cricopharyngeus muscle, which often has a neurologic basis but may also be a response to GERD. The chronic hypertonicity of this muscle may lead to muscular hypertrophy (Fig. 5-19) that causes a large, smooth indentation of the posterior wall of the junction of the pharynx with the cervical esophagus.

The Zenker diverticulum arises from the posterior wall of the hypopharynx as shown in Figure 5-20.

Dysphagia can result from large masses that deviate or compress the pharynx or esophagus. Cross-sectional studies are often done in these patients because of symptoms unrelated

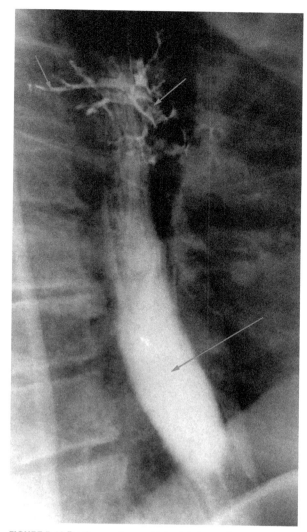

FIGURE 5-18 Esophagram image obtained during performance of a radiographic upper GI exam. Aspirated barium (short arrows) is visible in bronchi. Swallowed barium (long arrow) fills the distal esophagus.

to swallowing. Benign and malignant strictures of the esophagus are seen on an esophagram as persistent or fixed contour deformities such as those shown in Figure 5-21.

Contrast-enhanced CT shows a peritonsillar abscess as an enhancing mass with a low density center as shown in Figure 5-22, often with effacement of the parapharyngeal space.

VISUAL PROBLEMS

Visual problems may arise from disease within the orbits or the optic nerve or from intracranial pathology affecting the visual pathway. Orbital disease and disease of the optic nerve are discussed in this chapter. Visual problems that arise from intracranial disease, including visual field defects, are discussed in Chapter 4.

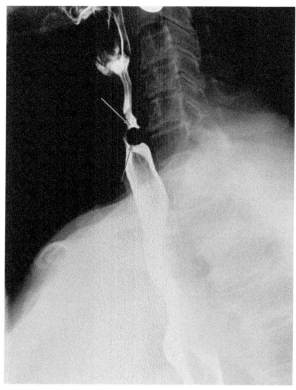

FIGURE 5-19 Dynamic swallowing study. An enlarged cricopharyngeus muscle causes the pronounced indentation (arrows) of the barium-filled (white liquid) esophagus.

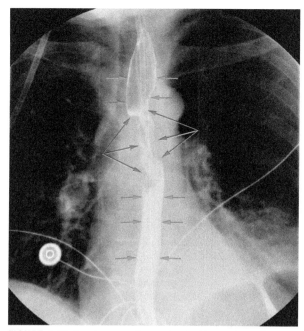

FIGURE 5-21 Esophagram of a patient with esophageal cancer shown as an irregular constriction of the barium-filled esophagus (red arrows). Note the smooth normal esophageal contours above and below the cancer (blue arrows). Fine vertically oriented parallel lines within the esophagus are the walls of a nasogastric tube.

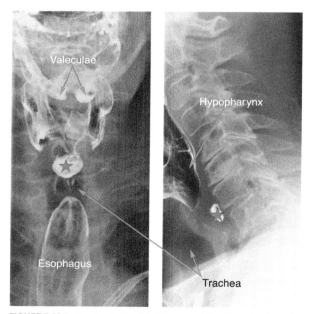

FIGURE 5-20 Zenker diverticulum (star) shown on AP and lateral radiographs acquired by the radiologist while performing a dynamic swallowing study.

Modalities

The best imaging procedure for most visual/orbital conditions, such as sudden vision loss, mass, or exophthalmos, is MRI of the brain and orbits without and with contrast enhancement (this is a more elaborate study than MRI of the

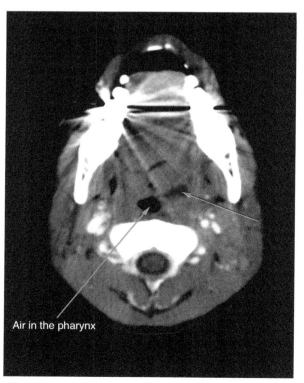

FIGURE 5-22 Axial CT that shows the low density within a peritonsillar abscess (red arrow). Note the streak artifact from metallic dental fillings, a common problem with CT imaging at the level of the teeth.

brain alone). If there is an absolute or relative contraindication to the use of gadolinium-based contrast material, unenhanced MRI of the brain and orbits is often a sufficient examination.

CT scanning is useful for patients who cannot undergo MRI. If available, ophthalmic ultrasonography can provide sufficient diagnostic evaluation for many specific ophthalmic conditions such as drusen.

Interpretation

Exophthalmos (also referred to proptosis), when associated with thyroid disease, is typically caused by enlargement of the extraocular muscles. This can be shown on ultrasonography. However, if the clinical differential diagnosis includes orbital mass, MRI or CT is preferred. Figure 5-23 demonstrates thickening of the left medial rectus muscle in a patient who presented with exophthalmos that led to a diagnosis of Graves disease.

Intraorbital cancers are demonstrated on CT and MRI as contrast-enhancing tumors. These lesions may originate within the orbit, may be metastatic lesions from a distant site (such as breast cancer), or may be a direct spread of malignancy arising in a paranasal sinus (see Figure 5-6). Melanin-containing melanomas of the retina are hyperintense on unenhanced T1 sequences, as in the case shown in Figure 5-24.

Among the contrast-enhancing masses within the orbit, leukemic infiltration may be the first finding leading to a diagnosis of acute myelogenous leukemia. Non-Hodgkin's

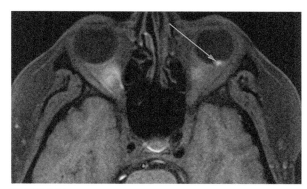

FIGURE 5-24 Axial unenhanced fat-suppressed T1 MRI of the orbits in a patient with a retinal melanoma (arrow), in this case a nearly pathognomonic imaging diagnosis because melanin is T1 hyperintense.

lymphoma, also a contrast-enhancing mass within the orbit, may be the diagnosis in about 10% of all intraorbital masses.

A variety of infectious and non-specific inflammatory conditions that can be seen as enhancing and swollen tissues within the orbit may be diagnosed as a pseudotumor of the orbit, after other more specific diagnoses, such as lymphoma, are excluded by biopsy or laboratory testing. An example is the inflammatory enlargement of a lateral rectus muscle shown in Figure 5-25.

HEARING PROBLEMS

Decreased or lost hearing is classically divided into conductive (middle ear) and sensorineural hearing loss. Conductive

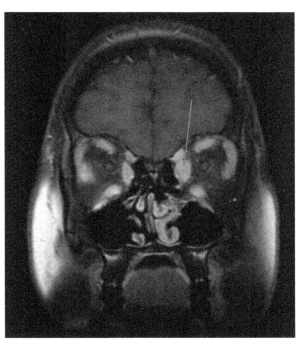

FIGURE 5-23 Coronal MRI of the orbits in a patient with thyroid ophthalmopathy due to Graves disease. Note the enlarged left medial rectus muscle (arrow).

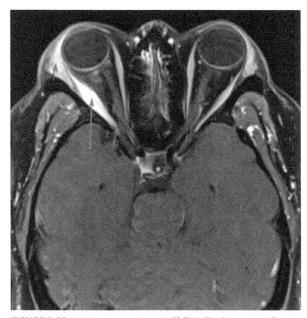

FIGURE 5-25 Axial contrast-enhanced FS T1 MRI of the orbits. The hyperenhancement and thickening of the right lateral rectus muscle (long arrow) extends to the muscle insertion, a feature not seen with thyroid ophthalmopathy (also ruled out by normal thyroid studies in this case). The lacrimal gland (short arrow) is also enlarged and probably inflamed.

hearing loss may be due to congenital abnormalities. It may also be due to inflammatory disease of the middle ear and temporal bone, which is usually successfully treated medically, and no imaging is needed. However, when medical treatment fails and there is progressive conductive hearing loss, imaging becomes appropriate.

Sensorineural hearing loss is divided into cochlear and retrocochlear (neural) diseases, both of which are commonly evaluated with imaging. The most common cause of neural hearing loss is a schwannoma of cranial nerve VIII, commonly called an acoustic neuroma.

Modalities

Because of the need to clearly visualize compact bone, thin section CT scanning of the temporal bones is the preferred imaging modality for disease of the middle ear and cochlea.

For evaluation of a suspected acoustic neuroma, MRI of the brain *and* IACs with and without contrast enhancement should be done.

Interpretation

CT will show opacification caused by fluid and abnormal tissues filling normal air-containing spaces of the temporal bone (such as the mastoid sinuses) and middle ear. When inflammatory disease has progressed beyond the acute stage, granulation tissue within the middle ear and temporal bone shows enhancement on both CT and MRI.

Some cholesteatomas are considered congenital, but most are acquired. The key finding for diagnosis of acquired cholesteatoma on CT is a mass that causes bone erosion in the middle ear (Fig. 5-26).

In a patient with sensorineural hearing loss, a mass (Fig. 5-27) in the IAC is usually a schwannoma of cranial

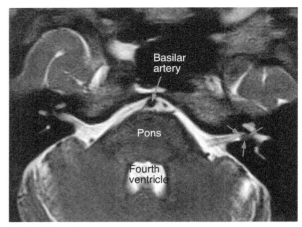

FIGURE 5-27 Axial T2 MRI. At the lateral end of the left IAC, the small mass (red arrows) is a schwannoma of the cranial nerve VIII in a patient who presented with progressive left-sided hearing loss and tinnitus.

nerve VIII. Hearing loss may occur when the tumor is very small and may only be visible as abnormal enhancement of the nerve as in Figure 5-28.

VERTIGO AND TINNITUS

Vertigo is when dizziness is associated with an exaggerated perception of movement or an illusory sensation of movement. Tinnitus may be pulsatile, which may be caused by a vascular lesion, or it may be non-pulsatile, possibly caused by an IAC or cerebellopontine angle mass. Imaging typically does not reveal an etiology for most patients with tinnitus or vertigo.

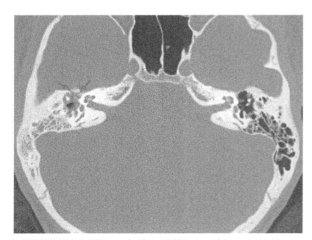

FIGURE 5-26 Axial thin section (1 mm) CT image of the temporal bones. The soft tissue mass (arrows) in the middle ear associated with bone erosion was found at surgery to be a cholesteatoma.

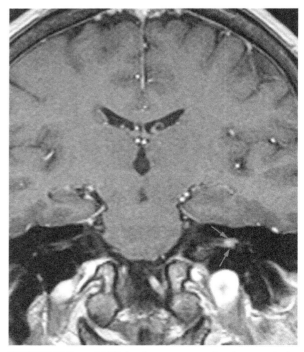

FIGURE 5-28 Coronal MRI showing a contrast-enhancing mass in the left IAC (arrows).

Modalities

The most common imaging procedure done for vertigo and tinnitus is MRI of the brain and IACs without and with contrast enhancement to rule out a correctable cause such as a mass. With pulsatile tinnitus, MRA or CTA is sometimes done to evaluate a suspected vascular lesion such as aneurysms and arterial dissections. In evaluating patients for unusual vascular tumors, such as glomus tympanicum causing pulsatile tinnitus, contrast-enhanced high resolution CT is sometimes indicated.

Interpretation

Schwannomas, similar to the one shown in the MRI in Figure 5-28, may cause tinnitus and vertigo in varied degrees of severity, along with deafness.

Malformations of the temporal bone that cause tinnitus by bringing large vessels into close proximity to the middle ear include dehiscence of the carotid artery canal and jugular bulb, as shown in Figure 5-29.

FACIAL TRAUMA AND TEMPOROMANDIBULAR JOINT (TMJ)

Trauma to facial structures means injury to structures below the skull base. Clinical evaluation often can distinguish whether a facial injury has occurred with or without closed or open brain injury. This affects whether brain, facial, or both brain and facial imaging studies are done. The following discussion addresses facial, not head (brain), injuries. Potential brain injury is discussed in Chapter 4.

Although TMJ dysfunction is considered to be a chronic condition, there is often a history of whiplash-type injury preceding the development of TMJ symptoms.

Modalities

Many special radiograph projections have been developed to display the complicated osseous anatomy of the face for the evaluation of suspected trauma. However, with the superior accuracy of CT, radiographic studies are now limited to a few basic views when CT is not immediately available, the most important of which is the Waters view, an occipitomental projection in which a PA view of the skull and facial bones is typically done with the patient's nose and chin lightly touching the x-ray cassette.

 COST-EFFECTIVE MEDICINE
Trauma that is limited to the nasal bones may be thoroughly examined with lateral nasal and Waters view radiographs.

If CT is not immediately available for evaluation of a patient who has suffered facial trauma, upright radiography of the facial bones may be used to triage patients; a negative radiographic study can suggest that CT can be deferred or may not be necessary. When there is suspected mandibular fracture, a **panorex** is done when the appropriate equipment is available. Panoramic radiographic images are also used to evaluate the mandible for dental disease and for chronic mandibular pain.

TMJ dysfunction is usually evaluated with MRI.

Interpretation

The classic pitfall in the interpretation of the lateral nasal bone radiograph is the nasomaxillary suture, which can be misinterpreted as a fracture. Acute nasal bone fractures usually cause a distinct step-off of the nasal bone surface on the lateral view with a discontinuity of the bone cortex (Fig. 5-30). On the Waters view, mediolateral displacement of nasal fracture fragments is evident.

When a Waters view shows an air–fluid level in a maxillary sinus after facial trauma, as in Figure 5-31, the fluid is presumed to be blood and a CT scan is indicated for definitive facial bone evaluation, even if fractures are not radiographically visible.

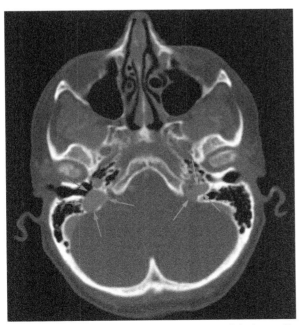

FIGURE 5-29 Unusually high and large right jugular bulb (red arrows) in a patient who presented with right-sided tinnitus. Compare with the normal left jugular bulb (blue arrows).

reconstruction (MPR) in coronal, sagittal, and oblique planes. In addition, as part of pre-operative planning, a volume-rendered (3D) display from maxillofacial CT, as shown in Figure 5-32, may also be provided to the reconstructive surgeon.

Fractures of the floor of the orbit may occur with NOE, ZMC, and **Le Fort** II (see below) fractures, or may be isolated such as in **blowout fracture**. These can be appreciated on a Waters view but typically are now diagnosed on CT, as shown in Figure 5-33. They key finding in these studies is whether or not an extraocular muscle is entrapped in the fracture.

A fracture involving the apex of the obit may require emergency surgical decompression of the optic nerve.

Le Fort fractures were named more than a century ago and consist of a group of fracture patterns. The key feature of these fractures is separation of the maxilla from the skull base after fracture of the junction of the posterior maxillary

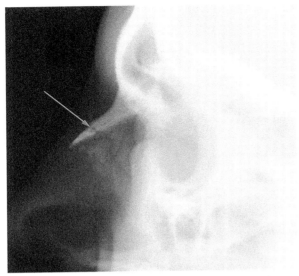

FIGURE 5-30 Lateral nasal bone radiograph that shows an acute fracture (arrow).

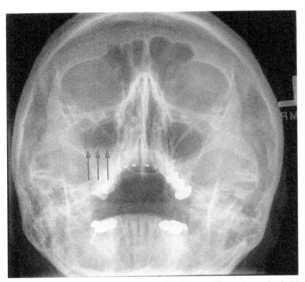

FIGURE 5-31 Waters view radiograph with maxillary sinus air–fluid level (arrows).

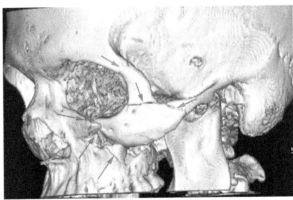

FIGURE 5-32 Volume-rendered (3D) display from a maxillofacial CT scan on a patient with a ZMC fracture (red arrows). Compare the appearance of these fractures with normal sutures (blue arrows).

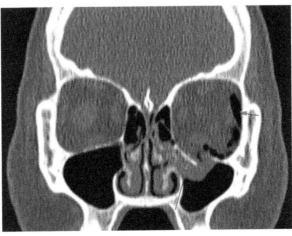

FIGURE 5-33 Coronal facial CT after blowout fracture shows depression of the medial portion of the left orbital floor (long arrow) and intraorbital air (short arrow) that escaped from the maxillary sinus to the orbit.

Naso-orbitoethmoid (NOE) fractures are complex fractures that may disrupt the nasofrontal duct, causing the complication of a frontal mucocele. Disruption of the medial orbital walls by these fractures may impinge on extraocular muscles and cause abnormal positioning of the eyeball. The finding of an NOE fracture is an indication for surgical referral.

Zygomaticomaxillary complex (ZMC) fractures involve the lateral wall of the orbit and possibly the inferior orbital rim and zygomatic arch. When these fractures are displaced, surgery is needed to prevent cosmetic deformity and enophthalmos. The imaging evaluation of complex fractures such as NOE and ZMC benefits greatly from CT multiplanar sinus walls and pterygoid plates. The Le Fort I, II, and III fracture patterns describe how much of the face is moveable in relation to the skull.

A panorex radiograph of the mandible clearly demonstrates the geometry and position of a fracture within the mandible, as shown in Figure 5-34.

When patients have difficulty with jaw opening, pain, and a sensation of popping or clicking in the TMJ, MRI may show displacement of the articular disc ("meniscus") of the joint in relation to the mandibular condyle. These are dynamic studies that include multiple views with varied degrees of mouth opening. In Figure 5-35, an anteriorly displaced TMJ articular disc is shown. This can be surgically corrected.

CAROTID ARTERY DISEASE

Extracranial atherosclerotic carotid artery disease is a major cause of stroke. The steady decline in the incidence of stroke due to carotid artery disease over the last two decades has

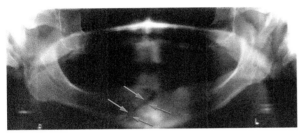

FIGURE 5-34 Panorex radiograph of a mandible after acute fracture (arrows).

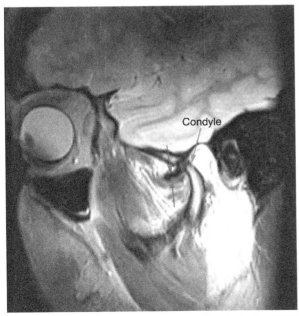

Condyle

FIGURE 5-35 Sagittal MRI demonstrating an anteriorly displaced TMJ meniscus (red arrows).

been attributed to improved diet, decline in smoking, improved and more widespread treatment of hypertension, and the detection of carotid artery disease prior to disease causing a stroke. However, this disease is still quite prevalent in our society, and it is an important clinical responsibility to detect this disease before it can cause devastating neurologic damage.

Modalities

Patients at high risk for carotid atherosclerotic disease because of personal or family medical history frequently have carotid screening exams with either limited or complete carotid Doppler sonography. When patients are found to have a carotid bruit on physical exam, sonography is indicated. A complete carotid duplex carotid sonogram consists of high resolution ultrasound images of the common carotid arteries, the carotid bifurcations, and the proximal segments of the internal and external carotid arteries. Color Doppler flow analysis includes velocity and direction of flow in the carotid and vertebral arteries.

When further diagnostic visualization of these neck vessels is needed for more precise pre-operative triage and planning, CTA or MRA is done. Invasive catheter angiography is sometimes needed, especially if the patient is a candidate for stenting, rather than surgical carotid endarterectomy.

In those rare cases in which there is a pulsatile mass associated with the carotid artery, contrast-enhanced CT of the neck or MRI of the neck without and with contrast enhancement is recommended.

Interpretation

The main goal of carotid imaging is to determine the degree of stenosis of the cervical internal carotid artery (ICA), with additional goals of identifying ulcerated atherosclerotic plaque and evaluating vertebral artery flow. There is now emerging evidence that the risks of surgery and stenting are lower than the stroke risk for patients with stenoses of between 60% and 70%. It has been well established that when an ICA stenosis of 70% or greater is found, the surgical risk and the risk of stroke after endarterectomy are lower than the stroke risk if endarterctomy is not done. In high-risk patients with high-grade stenosis, stenting is a viable alternative to surgery, although stenting may not be possible when the diseased vessel segment is very heavily calcified.

Determination of stenosis on ultrasound is partially based on measurement of the area of remaining patent lumen on cross-sectional images. However, the measurements have significant limitations, and most determinations of stenosis are based upon flow velocities determined by Doppler sonography. Several parameters are examined, such as peak systolic and diastolic velocity at the stenosis. A key measurement is the ratio between the peak systolic velocity at or just beyond the stenosis of the ICA to the peak systolic velocity in the common carotid artery (CCA). An example of a carotid sonogram showing ICA stenosis is shown in Figure 5-36.

The choice between MRA and CTA for further evaluation of a carotid stenosis depends upon patient factors, particulars of equipment used in different imaging facilities, local expertise, and treatment intent (endarterectomy vs. stenting), and may even vary with the appearance of carotid disease on

ultrasonography. As always, good communication between the professionals caring for patients is important, and in this case a discussion with a radiologists may be very helpful in selecting the ideal exam. An example of a carotid CTA is shown in Figure 5-37.

When the unusual clinical presentation of pulsatile mass at the angle of the mandble is examined with imaging, the most common lesion found is the carotid body paraganglioma (also called carotid body tumor or chemodectoma). These masses are characteristically found at the bifurcation of the common carotid artery, as shown in Figure 5-38. Angiographic studies demonstrate the mass to splay the proximal internal and external carotid arteries because they sit in the crotch of the carotid bifurcation.

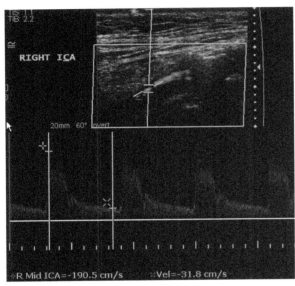

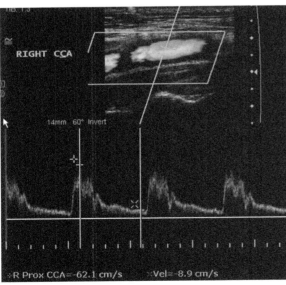

FIGURE 5-36 Carotid ultrasound showing stenosis of the proximal right ICA. The evidence for the presence of a hemodynamically significant stenosis is the high (3.06) ratio between the peak systolic ICA velocity of 190 cm/sec **(top)** and the peak systolic CCA velocity of 62 cm/sec **(bottom)**.

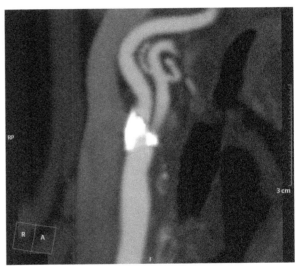

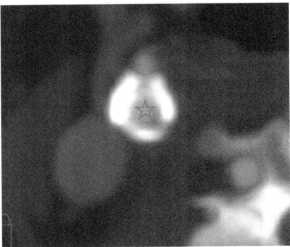

FIGURE 5-37 Maximum intensity projection (MIP) from carotid CTA with densely calcified atherosclerotic plaque at the carotid bifurcation **(top)**. An axial CT image **(bottom)** of the proximal ICA from the same study shows the small residual lumen (star) in this significant stenosis.

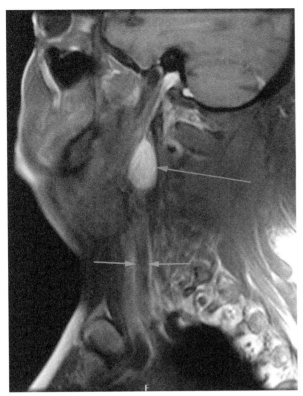

FIGURE 5-38 Sagittal MRI of carotid body tumor (red arrow). The blue arrows indicate the common carotid artery.

CASE UPDATE

The carotid Doppler sonogram of Patient A found very high velocity turbulent flow in her right external carotid artery (ECA) that explains the audible bruit. No significant atherosclerotic disease involving either ICA is found, so no further carotid studies are needed. Her thyroid ultrasound exam is reported to show multiple thyroid nodules, the largest of which is a 1.2 cm hyperechoic mass in the left thyroid lobe. This is the palpable lesion that you found on physical examination. Her thyroid lab studies are all normal. The radiologist has recommended an ultrasound follow-up exam in 6 to 12 months. It is explained to the patient that if the nodule remains perfectly unchanged on follow-up sonography, biopsy could be avoided. The patient, however, is uncomfortable with waiting up to a year before a decision is made to biopsy but is quite fearful of having a thyroid biopsy, even after you explain to her that a thyroid FNA is done with a very thin needle and the risk of complication is extremely low. You order a radionuclide thyroid scan, hoping that it will be normal; a "functioning" nodule would have a very low likelihood of malignancy and this would provide reassurance to the patient.

Patient B had a carotid ultrasound exam that showed irregular atherosclerotic plaque in the right carotid bulb and origin of the right ICA. Velocities were measured for the ICA and the common carotid artery (CCA). The right ICA to CCA systolic velocity ratio was approximately 4:1, consistent with a very high grade stenosis. Incidentally, thyroid nodules were noted during the carotid sonogram. You order a carotid CTA to further evaluate the stenosis and thyroid sonography to evaluate the nodules. Patient A has a normal thyroid radionuclide scan. She will have a follow-up thyroid sonogram in 1 year.

Thyroid sonography on Patient B showed multiple nodules, most of which were small and had a variety of benign imaging features. One nodule, however, was hypoechoic, poorly marginated, and showed numerous tiny bright echoes caused by calcifications throughout the lesion. Her carotid CTA showed a heavily calcified critical stenosis of the origin of her right ICA. She underwent uneventful carotid endarterectomy. Several weeks after this surgery, she had thyroid FNA because of the incidentally found suspicious nodule. The pathology report from the FNA was suspicious for papillary neoplasm. Subtotal thyroidectomy confirmed the presence of a thyroid papillary carcinoma; cervical lymph nodes were positive for metastatic disease. The patient had post-operative treatment with I[131] and was reassured that her prognosis was excellent: 90% long-term survival rate for patients with this disease.

Chapter Review

Chapter Review Questions

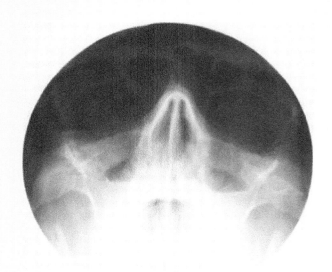

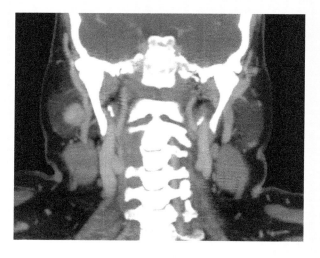

1. Based on the Waters view above, you diagnose the patient as having:
   A. mucous retention cyst.
   B. purulent sinusitis.
   C. nasal polyps.
   D. contrast-enhancing maxillary sinus tumors.
   E. Le Fort fractures.

2. The presence of erosive bone changes on a CT of the paranasal sinuses in a patient with HIV suggests:
   A. mucous retention cyst.
   B. purulent sinusitis.
   C. nasal polyps.
   D. fungal infection.
   E. Le Fort fracture.

3. Your physical examination reveals a large (>3 cm), very firm thyroid mass and possible adenopathy. Instead of thyroid sonography you might order:
   A. fine needle thyroid biopsy.
   B. thyroid MRI.
   C. contrast-enhanced soft tissue neck CT.
   D. radionuclide thyroid scanning.
   E. Waters view thyroid radiograph.

4. A PET-CT would most likely be ordered for:
   A. a child with enlarged cervical nodes.
   B. an adult with enlarged cervical nodes accompanying a viral infection of his oropharynx.
   C. salivary duct calculi.
   D. fungal-caused sinusitis.
   E. adenopathy in a patient with a known malignancy.

5. Which of the following is the most likely diagnosis based on the image above of a contrast-enhanced CT done because of swelling in the patient's right parotid region?
   A. Pleomorphic adenoma
   B. Sjögren's syndrome
   C. Invasive mucoepidermoid cancer
   D. Cyst
   E. Adenopathy

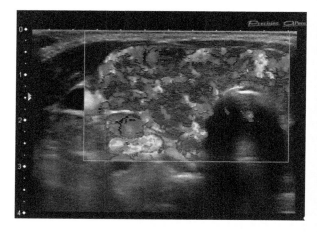

6. The thyroid Doppler flow ultrasound shown above would be most consistent with which of the following?
   A. Graves disease
   B. Multinodular thyroid disease
   C. Thyroid cancer
   D. Goiter
   E. Thyroglossal duct cyst

7. Which of the following sonographic characteristics would NOT be consistent with thyroid nodule malignancy?

    A. Multiple small calcifications

    B. Homogeneously hyperechoic nodules

    C. Irregular shape

    D. Poor transmission of the ultrasound beam

8. Which of the following is not correct for a dynamic swallowing study?

    A. It should be ordered when a patient has difficulty initiating swallowing

    B. It should be ordered when you suspect the patient has a Zenker diverticulum

    C. It involves the patient receiving ionizing radiation

    D. It is a term that may be used interchangeably with "barium swallow"

    E. It is sometimes appropriate to order this exam with an "upper GI"

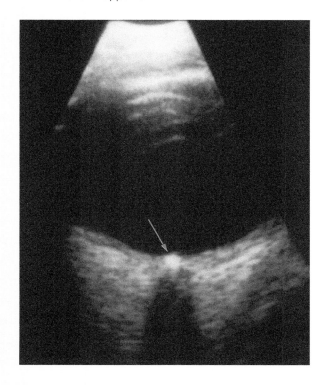

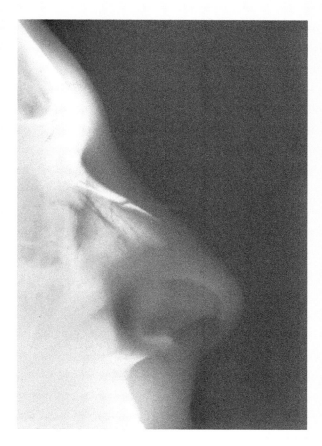

10. The image above shows:

    A. frontal sinusitis.

    B. fractured nasal bones.

    C. Zenker diverticulum.

    D. pansinusitius.

    E. blowout fracture.

11. Which of the following is not true about internal carotid artery stenosis?

    A. The degree of stenosis can be established by Doppler sonography

    B. A stenosis greater than 70% is considered to be hemodynamically significant

    C. Both MRA and CTA may be useful for surgical planning

    D. It is typically associated with a carotid body tumor

9. The above image is an ultrasound of the eye that is clinically diagnostic (note arrow). What is the patient's diagnosis?

    A. Drusen

    B. Graves disease

    C. Non-Hodgkin's lymphoma

    D. Pseudotumor of the orbit

    E. Cancer of the optic nerve

6 CHEST

A 52-year-old male nicotine user whose history includes smoking one pack of cigarettes daily for 30 years complains that he is experiencing more frequent and severe episodes of "breathlessness" during routine chores. A chest x-ray shows "mild diffuse interstitial prominence" that was not evident on radiographs completed 5 years earlier. The current study does not show cardiomegaly or pulmonary venous congestion. You would like to get a more definitive imaging study before referring the patient to a pulmonologist.

FUNDAMENTALS OF CHEST RADIOGRAPHY

The initial workup of many clinical presentations includes chest radiography to evaluate possible cardiac or pulmonary causes for a patient's symptoms. Chest CT is frequently used for a wide variety of symptoms that may have a cardiac or pulmonary origin. Recent progress in technology and techniques has led to more widespread use of MRI for imaging cardiac and thoracic vascular problems (Table 6-1). Also, ultrasound exams of the heart, called **echocardiography,** have been a staple of the cardiac workup for many years. It is widely available and often may be the most readily accessible procedure to examine fundamental issues such as left ventricular contraction, valve function, and presence or absence of pericardial effusion. Nuclear medicine procedures are generally used to provide functional information about the heart.

However, none of these cross-sectional procedures supplants the chest radiograph as a baseline imaging study.

COST-EFFECTIVE MEDICINE
As the lowest cost imaging procedure, chest radiography provides the most imaging information at the least expense and can then direct you to the most efficient use of other imaging modalities.

Selecting the "procedure of choice" for advanced imaging in the chest may not always be straightforward, and the ideal procedure may greatly depend upon available resources. As clinical studies are done, and as imaging equipment continues to evolve and improve, what is considered the "ideal" procedure for a given situation or condition will change. It is important that you realize that the quality of the care you provide may depend on remaining up-to-date on medical publications and in communication with radiologists, cardiologists, and pulmonologists about current recommended imaging procedures.

ROUTINE CHEST RADIOGRAPHY

Routine chest radiography is the most widely performed radiologic imaging study and has been basic to the initial evaluation of patients throughout the world for many decades. It is performed on patients with new symptoms that may be cardiac or pulmonary and as a follow-up exam on known cardiac and pulmonary patients to evaluate response to treatment. Chest radiographs are obtained as a screening exam for public health concerns like communicable diseases, as part of routine general health assessment, and as preoperative evaluation of many patients who will undergo general anesthesia.

Technique

When used as a screening tool for various diseases and cardiac, pulmonary, and chest wall disorders, PA and lateral chest radiography is standard. However, in some situations, a single standing PA view may be all that is needed for a specific evaluation. For example, various health agencies may screen certain populations for active tuberculosis (TB) with only a PA

TABLE 6-1 Sample Chest Radiology Requisition Information

Modality	Body Region	Clinical Data/History
Radiography—PA and lateral	Chest	Cough, fever, left pleuritic pain, leukocytosis, rales left base
CT, unenhanced HRCT	Chest	Progressive dyspnea, scleroderma, +/- interstitial changes on chest x-ray
CT with contrast	Chest	Nicotine addict with hemoptysis and enlarged right hilum on CXR, suspected lung ca

radiograph. A single PA projection is reasonable for TB because TB most commonly involves the pulmonary apices, which are well seen in the PA chest radiograph. Also, TB is rarely at the lung bases that may be below the diaphragm and more difficult to see in the PA projection.

 Single-view, rather than two-view, chest radiography is often preferable in children because of concern for radiation exposure.

High quality chest radiography should not be taken for granted and should never be considered a "simple procedure" that can easily be done well. The wide range of radiographic densities in the chest may be difficult to capture and display without excellent radiographic equipment and proper technique. If you are performing chest radiography in an office setting (not unusual), standards of image quality must be maintained or patient care suffers.

If you do not have radiography equipment in your office and you are referring your patient for chest radiography, the process begins with your order. It is imperative that your order provide sufficient information to clearly demonstrate the medical necessity of the imaging examination and allow for its most effective implementation and interpretation. Radiographic findings may be subtle, and few patients are likely to provide all their pertinent medical information to the personnel at a radiology facility or radiology department.

The PA chest radiograph must show all of both pulmonary apices. This can be ascertained by ensuring that the entire first ribs are visible, including the costovertebral junctions. Both costophrenic sulci should be seen. The patient should not be rotated at all; the thoracic spinous processes should be equidistant from the medial ends of the clavicles. The mediastinum should be "penetrated" sufficiently so that you can see the thoracic spine. The exposure must never render any portions of the lungs black; mid-lung zones should be an intermediate level of gray (Fig. 6-1). You should expect that any medical image that is substandard will be repeated unless the condition of the patient precludes it. It is sometimes difficult to obtain an ideal radiograph. It is not difficult to decide to make the effort to obtain a good imaging study on every patient, even if that requires extra time for repeat radiography.

On the lateral view, the posterior costophrenic sulci must be included. Exposure must be sufficient for good detail of mediastinal structures but also should not render any portion of the lungs black (Fig. 6-2).

Interpretation

The search pattern used to look *for* normal anatomy and *for* radiographic findings of disease in a chest x-ray is a different mental process than just looking *at* a chest x-ray, which is our

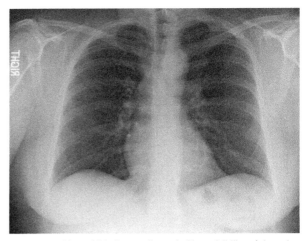

FIGURE 6-1 Normal PA chest radiograph. Note visibility of the spine and the medial aspect of the left hemidiaphragm posterior to the heart. When viewed on a high resolution monitor that meets current standards for radiologic diagnosis, there is clear visibility of normal lung markings (vessels and bronchi) almost to the periphery of the lungs.

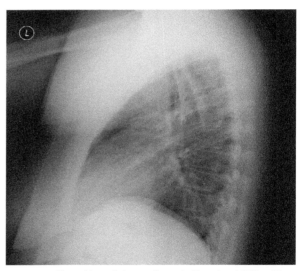

FIGURE 6-2 Normal lateral chest radiograph. Note the visibility of lung markings superimposed on the heart and spine.

natural tendency. Consider the difference between entering a room and *looking around* versus looking in that room *for* a specific item or *for* the absence of a specific item. The search pattern used to look *for* normal anatomy and *for* radiographic findings of disease is personal and variable. No set pattern is required, as long as you consistently look *for* all the fundamental features that are visible (see later section and Table 6-2) and how they normally appear so that you don't mistake them for an abnormality.

Cardiac size on chest radiography is used to help differentiate cardiac from pulmonary disease when the clinical presentation could be consistent with either. The maximum transverse diameter of the heart in a PA view should be no

TABLE 6-2 Chest Radiograph Search Pattern

What to Look AT	What to Look FOR
Heart	Is it normal in size and configuration?
Aortic arch and aorta	Present on the left, and normal in size and shape?
Mediastinum	Is it too wide?
Lung hila	Are major hilar vessels normal in size? Is there hilar enlargement or nodularity?
Peripheral pulmonary veins	Are upper lobe veins thinner than those at the lung bases?
Pulmonary nodules or masses	Can you identify any lung masses or nodules?
Pulmonary interstitial lines	Can you find any linear interstitial lines?
Ring or tram-track shadows	Do rings and parallel lines suggest thick bronchi?
Pulmonary consolidation	Is there pulmonary consolidation (e.g., silhouette sign)?
Pleural thickening	Are fissures too easy to see? Does air density touch the inner margin of the rib cage or is the pleura thick?
Costophrenic sulci	Are there sharp acute angles, or is there a pleural effusion?
Pneumothorax	Can you see a white line of visceral pleura?
Under the diaphragm	Is there free abdominal air? Is gastric air–fluid level normal? Is splenomegaly present?
Trachea	Are contours of the trachea and carina normal?
Bones	Are all visible bones normal in density and shape?
Entire region	See any foreign objects (medical devices, bullets, surgical materials)?

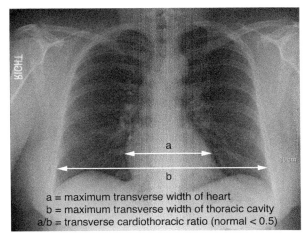

a = maximum transverse width of heart
b = maximum transverse width of thoracic cavity
a/b = transverse cardiothoracic ratio (normal < 0.5)

FIGURE 6-3 PA chest radiograph showing how the transverse cardiothoracic ratio is determined.

muffled heart sounds, may help in differentiating cardiac dilatation from pericardial effusion, and it is critical that this information is included in your radiology order. When a large pericardial effusion is suspected from clinical and radiographic findings, echocardiography is indicated, and it may be urgently needed if the patient is in distress.

In a patient without clinical or radiographic findings of pericardial effusion, an enlarged heart shadow indicates cardiac chamber dilatation. This can occur with valve disease or with heart failure. Finding cardiomegaly on chest radiography usually means referral of the patient to a cardiologist.

Important landmarks of the mediastinum are found along the left mediastinal/heart border (Fig. 6-4). Between the aortic

more than 50% of the transverse diameter of the inner margin of the rib cage at the level of the highest point of the diaphragm. This is the transverse cardiothoracic ratio. When this ratio is above 50%, there is cardiomegaly (Fig. 6-3). An enlarged or dilated heart is one that is not functioning well. By looking *for* cardiac size on the PA chest radiograph, you have investigated cardiac function. Note, however, that except with a grossly dilated heart, the cardiothoracic ratio is not reliable on an AP view, largely because of the effect of magnification in the AP projection. Also, a supine or sitting patient getting an AP chest radiograph is less able to achieve a deep inspiration than a standing patient getting a PA radiograph. Even on a standing PA chest radiograph, a limited degree of inspiration, whether because of poor patient effort or obesity, results in a high position of the diaphragm that increases the apparent transverse diameter of the heart.

A large pericardial effusion may result in an apparently "large heart" on the PA chest, but clinical findings, such as

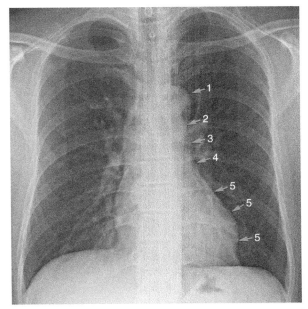

FIGURE 6-4 PA chest radiograph, with features of the left mediastinal border indicated: aortic arch (1), aortopulmonary window (2), pulmonary trunk (3), location of left atrial appendage (4), and left ventricle (5).

arch and the pulmonary artery there is a normal concavity, the aortopulmonary window, which contains one or more lymph nodes. Enlargement of these nodes may result in convexity of the mediastinal margin just below the aortic arch. Inferior to the pulmonary artery is a subtle concavity or straight segment of the mediastinal margin that is the location of the left atrial appendage (auricle). A convexity here usually indicates left atrial dilatation. The major contour of the lower left mediastinum represents the margin of the left ventricle that can become abnormally enlarged with cardiomegaly.

Mediastinal widening may occur with tumor, adenopathy, or vascular dilatation. Potential confounding issues are excessive mediastinal fat and/or a poor inspiration. Hilar enlargement may be seen with adenopathy or vascular dilatation (Fig. 6-5).

An official radiology report on chest radiography may include an appropriate recommendation for further study of non-cardiac findings of the mediastinum and hila, most commonly CT scanning. If the finding on chest radiography of vascular dilatation is specifically suspicious of aortic aneurysm, then CT arteriography is appropriate.

With mediastinal widening or hilar enlargement, your role as the clinician may be to explain the situation to your patient; to order a recommended exam, very often a contrast-enhanced chest CT; and to be sure that the patient has no contraindication to the use of intravenous contrast material. It is important, when ordering any imaging procedure that involves the use of intravenous contrast material, to be certain that your patient has no history of allergic reaction to such agents or compromised renal function, both of which generally preclude the use of these agents.

Your search pattern while inspecting chest radiographs should include the rib cage, clavicles, shoulders, thoracic spine, and upper abdomen, not just the heart and lungs. A "routine" chest radiograph may be an opportunity to diagnose unexpected disease. For example, routine PA and lateral chest radiographs (Fig. 6-6) done as part of a workup for mild dyspnea showed increased bone density in a thoracic vertebral body. The radiologist who interpreted this radiographic exam recommended a radionuclide bone scan and determination of the prostate specific antigen (PSA) level. The PSA level was very high, consistent with prostate carcinoma, and the bone

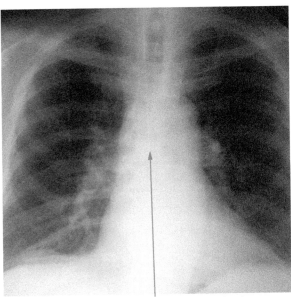

Abnormally increased vertebral bone density
(blastic bone disease)

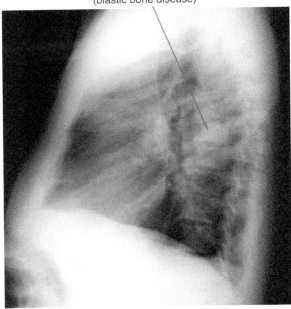

FIGURE 6-6 PA **(top)** and lateral **(bottom)** chest radiographs in which increased bone density was incidentally detected in a thoracic vertebra on a radiographic study done for dyspnea.

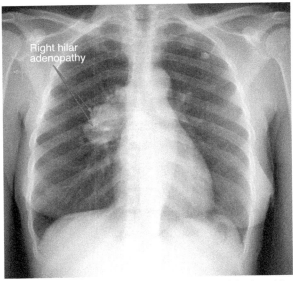

FIGURE 6-5 PA chest radiograph demonstrating right lung hilar adenopathy.

Right hilar adenopathy

scan showed widespread metastatic disease. This clinically un-suspected disease was diagnosed because the radiologist used a comprehensive search pattern while interpreting "routine" chest radiography.

The pleural spaces should be closely inspected for evidence of pleural thickening or pleural effusion. The normal costophrenic sulci are sharp, acute angles. A *blunted* costophrenic sulcus likely indicates the presence of pleural effusion (Fig. 6-7).

You must inspect the contour of the major airways. Is the trachea in the midline or is it being displaced by a mass or vascular abnormality in the superior mediastinum? Is there a deformity of the trachea or mainstem bronchus? These are findings that will rarely be obvious if you are just "looking at" a chest radiograph. You will find such abnormalities only if you look *for* them in your search pattern.

The normal lung is mostly air density. Most lung markings (soft tissue densities) represent vessels, mostly pulmonary veins, which are larger than arteries. Peripheral bronchial walls and the pulmonary interstitium contribute much less than vessels to lung density. The pulmonary hilar structures visible on radiographs include pulmonary veins, major pulmonary arteries, and often the walls of the mainstem bronchi.

The lungs must be carefully inspected for nodules or masses and abnormal lung densities. In specific geographic regions, endemic pulmonary infections (e.g., histoplasmosis in the midwestern United States) are associated with a residual spherical scar, a granuloma, which often calcifies. When calcified granulomatous disease is found on routine chest radiography, with one, several, or many calcified pulmonary nodules (often with calcified hilar and mediastinal lymph nodes), it is evidence of old disease that is not considered to be of clinical significance (Fig. 6-8).

Innumerable radiology reports over the past many decades have described abnormal pulmonary density as an **infiltrate**. You will continue to see this term used, although pulmonary radiologists have settled on the current usage of **opacity** to describe the change in radiographic density of the **pulmonary airspace**, from an air density to a water or soft-tissue density in disease. Another more current term used instead of infiltrate is **consolidation**. The traditional description for the radiographic appearance of common bacterial pneumonia, **alveolar infiltrate,** is now described as a pulmonary density or **parenchymal opacity** (Fig. 6-9). When pulmonary opacification is in the lung periphery adjacent to the diaphragm or

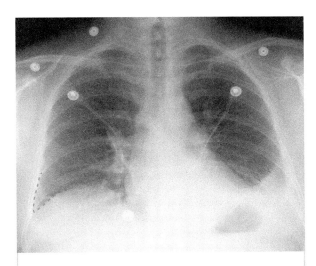

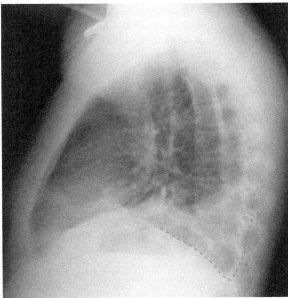

FIGURE 6-7 PA **(top)** and lateral **(bottom)** chest radiographs demonstrating the presence of a moderate left pleural effusion (short arrows) that blunts the left costophrenic sulcus; compare with normal right side outlined by blue dotted line. The round metallic densities in the PA view are gown clips and ECG electrodes.

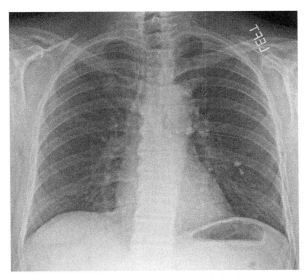

FIGURE 6-8 PA chest radiograph showing calcified pulmonary granuloma (short arrow) and calcified left hilar lymph nodes (long arrow).

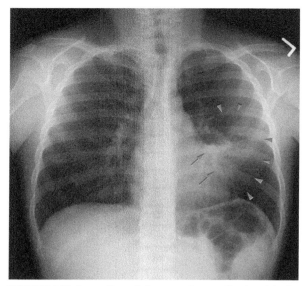

FIGURE 6-9 PA chest radiograph demonstrating opacification of the lingula of the left upper lobe secondary to bacterial pneumonia. Arrows point to segment of left cardiac border that is obscured by the pneumonia (silhouette sign); arrowheads indicate area of hazy increased pulmonary density characteristic of alveolar pneumonia. Note that the silhouette sign is the absence of an expected border or edge.

mediastinum, there is loss of the normally visible edge between soft tissue and aerated lung. This loss of a visible edge is known as the **silhouette sign.**

Pectus excavatum can cause an apparent silhouette sign of the right cardiac border on the PA view that might lead you to erroneously conclude that there is right middle lobe pneumonia. This sternal deformity (Fig. 6-10) shifts the heart toward the left, moving the right cardiac margin toward the midline. Additionally, the right infrahilar vascular structures become crowded, increasing apparent lung density (Fig. 6-11).

Collapse or partial collapse of a lung or part of a lung is called **atelectasis** and is seen as increased density with reduced volume of lung tissue (Fig. 6-12). This can occur with mechanical bronchial obstruction or a variety of pathologies that result in loss of surfactant, leading to alveolar collapse. Atelectasis can develop slowly (e.g., bronchial obstruction

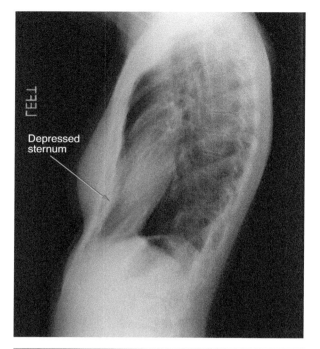

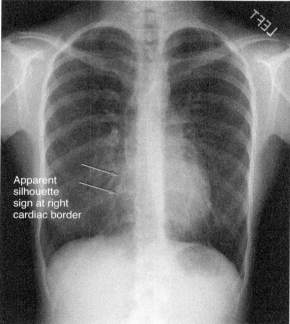

FIGURE 6-11 Lateral **(top)** and PA **(bottom)** views of a patient with pectus excavatum. There seems to be loss of the right cardiac border that suggests the silhouette sign. However, this is more apparent than real because it is caused by the geometry of the pectus deformity rather than a change in lung density. Also, there is crowding of the right infrahilar lung markings, which could erroneously be interpreted as an increase in lung density.

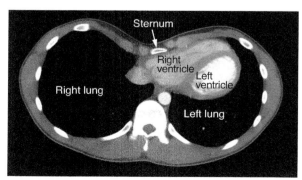

FIGURE 6-10 Axial CT showing pectus excavatum.

from a mass growing within or compressing a bronchus) or acutely (e.g., with acute pulmonary embolus).

There are many pulmonary diseases in which histologic changes are primarily found in the interlobular and intralobular septa and in the peribronchovascular interstitium. This

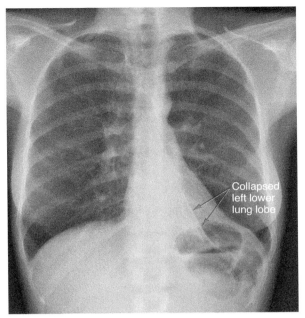

FIGURE 6-12 PA chest radiograph showing left lower lobe atelectasis (arrows).

contrasts with the filling of alveoli with inflammatory cells that characterizes pneumonia. **Interstitial lung disease** may be idiopathic, related to autoimmune disorders, or associated with specific pulmonary toxicities. With alveolar opacification, vascular lung markings are obscured, as well as adjacent mediastinal or diaphragmatic borders (silhouette sign). However, interstitial pulmonary disease is characterized by increased lung density that does not obscure pulmonary vascular markings or result in the silhouette sign. Interstitial disease may be **micronodular, reticular,** or **reticulonodular** (Fig. 6-13).

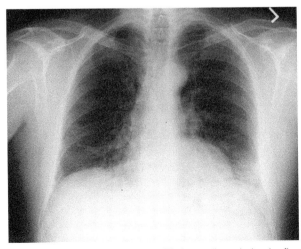

FIGURE 6-13 Interstitial lung disease. PA chest radiograph showing fine reticular increased density at the lung bases that does not obscure the margins of the diaphragm or heart border.

It may be difficult to exactly characterize an interstitial pattern, and it is not uncommon for you to receive a radiology report indicating the presence of "mild interstitial prominence."

A spherical opacity less than 3 cm in diameter is a **nodule;** when greater than 3 cm, it is properly termed a **mass.** Do not be surprised if you see in a radiology report that a 2 cm rounded opacity is considered to be a possible "mass." Strict adherence to recommended terminology is far from universal in radiology reports (Fig. 6-14).

TRAUMA

Physical examination after chest trauma should include determining any specific site(s) of point tenderness in the chest wall, which may suggest a rib fracture. Physical examination should also always include auscultation even if the patient does not have dyspnea. Post-traumatic pneumothorax or pleural effusion/hemothorax may produce distant or absent breath sounds. Pleuritic type chest pain after trauma suggests that a rib fracture has injured the pleura.

Modalities

Radiography is ideal for diagnosing rib fractures and secondary injuries that may complicate rib fractures. A **rib series** of radiographs, which uses radiographic techniques optimized for rib details, varies between institutions and practices but should always include AP (for posterior rib injuries), PA (for anterior chest wall injuries), and several oblique rib radiographs.

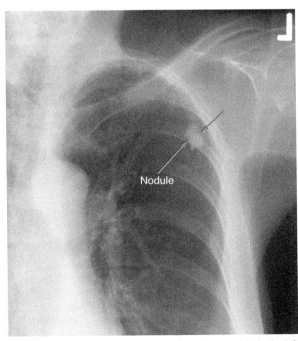

FIGURE 6-14 PA chest radiograph showing a large nodule in the left upper lobe (arrows).

When injuries to the anterior chest wall appear to involve the sternum, radiography of the sternum should specifically be requested, in addition to a routine rib series. If you suspect a sternal injury clinically and yet a fracture is not revealed on sternal radiographs, CT scanning may reveal radiographically occult fractures. However, detecting a non-displaced sternal fracture with CT may not change clinical management of the patient. Remember that no medical testing should ever be done without first deciding if the information obtained from that testing will alter clinical management of the patient.

CT is usually done in severe chest injuries. CT of the lower chest and abdomen may be appropriate in fractures of lower ribs because of the possibility of splenic or hepatic injuries, even when the patient does not seem to have suffered severe trauma. Instead of CT, an ultrasound exam can be used to rule out significant intra-abdominal injury such as splenic laceration. However, ultrasound does not have the very high sensitivity and specificity of CT scanning for organ injury.

In a patient with a subacute chest wall injury and negative radiographs, a radionuclide bone scan can provide evidence of radiographically occult bone injuries but should only be ordered if the information will change clinical management.

Interpretation

The search pattern used for evaluating chest and rib radiographs in trauma is not essentially different from that discussed earlier for routine chest radiography. However, emphasis is directed toward excluding or identifying specific findings. Ribs should be carefully inspected for any cortical discontinuities or the linear radiolucencies characteristic of any fracture. Because these findings may be subtle, the search for rib fractures is greatly aided by **skin markers** placed over locations of point tenderness. However, with multiple rib fractures, pain may be diffuse, confounding a precise alignment of skin markers with visible rib fractures; thus, markers are not always used.

A rib fracture may only be clearly visible on one of several rib series images. Sometimes rib fractures that appear non-displaced in one view appear significantly displaced in another projection. Whether or not rib fractures are displaced is the major factor determining the likelihood of complications such as pleural or pulmonary injury. In the patient case shown in Figure 6-15, the AP view shows a mildly deformed rib that could be an old or acute fracture. However, the oblique projection shows the abrupt "step-off" of rib cortex and sharp margins that indicate an acute and mildly displaced fracture. This highlights the need for multiple views.

Sometimes the only clue to a radiographically occult non-displaced rib fracture is localized thickening of the parietal

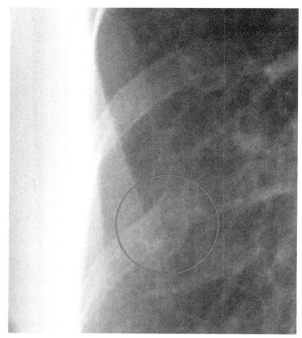

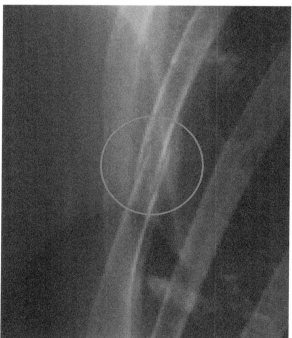

FIGURE 6-15 AP **(top)** and oblique **(bottom)** rib radiographs. It is not clear in the AP view if the rib deformity is an acute fracture; however, the oblique view clearly shows the features (e.g., sharp margins) of an acute fracture.

pleura (Fig. 6-16) that can indicate the presence of a chest wall hematoma.

Uncomplicated rib fractures are common in chest trauma and are not serious injuries. However, occasionally even minor chest wall trauma can result in complicated rib fractures with significant organ or vascular injuries. Displaced rib fractures and injuries with multiple rib fractures are frequently associated

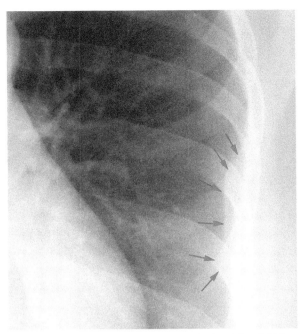

FIGURE 6-16 PA chest radiograph demonstrating focal pleural thickening (arrows), which, in a trauma case, could indicate a chest wall hematoma.

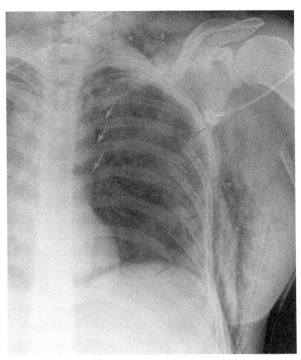

FIGURE 6-17 Multiple rib fractures (arrows) in more than a single location within each rib, resulting in an unstable segment of the thoracic wall (flail chest). Note also the presence of subcutaneous emphysema (dark streaks of air in the soft tissues) from the trauma (stars).

with respiratory compromise or pneumothorax, hemothorax, and organ injury. Therefore, imaging is done not only to establish a diagnosis of rib fracture but also to differentiate between complicated and uncomplicated rib fractures.

Fractures of the first ribs are associated with a high incidence of major vascular injuries. Hemorrhage from such injuries often widens the superior mediastinum and causes extrapleural thickening over a pulmonary apex, called an **apical cap.** These are usually found in severely injured patients who are most likely being cared for in an ED.

As mentioned earlier, common complications of rib fracture are pulmonary contusion, pneumothorax, and hemothorax. For these reasons, a radiographic rib series always includes at least a PA chest radiograph if the patient can stand, or an AP chest if a standing PA chest cannot be done. A lateral chest radiographic view is not always done for rib injuries and not usually necessary for clinical management, but may reveal a small pleural effusion that may not be evident on other views.

A clinically important common finding is the presence of multiple fractures within each of three or more adjacent ribs, or three anterior ribs and sternum or costal cartilages. This may result in a segment of the chest wall that paradoxically moves inward with inspiration, called **flail chest** (Fig. 6-17). This will compromise respiration and is associated with atelectasis and pneumonia.

Immediately after blunt trauma to the chest that results in rib fracture, a pulmonary contusion may be evident on radiographs as a hazy pulmonary opacity. This usually resolves

quickly, often within days. Note, however, that in a patient who initially showed no abnormal pulmonary density after injury, a developing pulmonary opacity suggests pneumonia.

A displaced rib fracture may lacerate an intercostal artery, leading to hemorrhage into the pleural space—a hemothorax. The amount of blood in the pleural space can be much greater than is often appreciated on routine rib and chest radiographs. If such a pleural effusion/hemothorax is shown on available radiographs, a lateral view (if not yet done) of the chest may provide better indication of the size of a hemothorax. A **decubitus** chest radiograph, done with a horizontal x-ray beam and a patient lying on his side, may be even more revealing but is often painful with rib injuries. CT scanning is more easily tolerated than decubitus radiographs and is often appropriate in the severely injured patient (Fig. 6-18).

The incidence of pneumothorax as a complication of rib fractures increases with the number of ribs that are fractured and with the presence of displaced rib fractures. Pneumothorax is identified as an air density between the pleural surface of the lung and the chest wall. Look carefully for the very thin white line representing the visceral pleura that separates the air within the lung from the pneumothorax. It is very important to identify the visceral pleural white line to differentiate a pneumothorax from a large paraseptal (subpleural) **bulla** (Fig. 6-19).

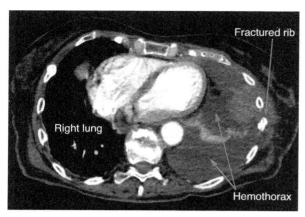

FIGURE 6-18 Axial CT demonstrating left hemothorax.

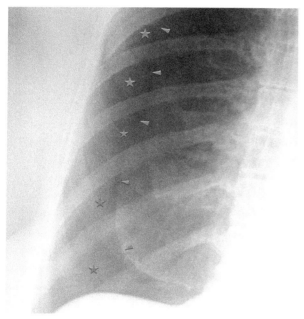

FIGURE 6-19 Pneumothorax. The arrowheads indicate the visceral pleural line, which is not normally visible; the red stars indicate the pneumothorax, air in the pleural space. Diagnosis of pneumothorax requires both identification of the white line that represents the visceral pleura and the absence of lung markings between that white line and the chest wall.

DYSPNEA

You will see patients whose chief complaint of dyspnea covers a range of discomforts, from the overweight and sedentary patient who is disturbed by being "short of breath" when climbing stairs, to the patient who is severely dyspneic and hypoxemic at rest. The characteristics and history of this common symptom, along with findings on physical exam, often lead to a clinical impression of cardiac or pulmonary disease as the underlying cause.

Modalities

Chest radiography is almost universally the appropriate initial diagnostic imaging procedure in dyspnea, not only to

help in providing support for the preliminary clinical diagnosis but also to aid in judging severity of disease.

Standing PA and lateral radiographic views of the chest should be obtained in patients with dyspnea whenever possible. If a patient is wheelchair-bound and unable to stand, then a sitting AP radiograph may be all that is attainable. For the severely ill and bedridden patient, a portable or "bedside" AP radiograph is done.

 In children presenting with dyspnea and clinical signs that the dyspnea may be from disease of the upper airway, "soft tissue neck" radiographs are needed and may be far more appropriate than chest radiography.

When clinical and radiographic evidence indicates cardiac disease as the underlying cause of dyspnea, as discussed later in this chapter, an array of imaging studies may be used during a cardiac "workup. For patients whose initial clinical evaluation and radiographic studies indicate pulmonary disease, further imaging is almost always done with CT. For example, suspected tumor is usually evaluated with contrast-enhanced chest CT. For suspected interstitial pulmonary disease, the indicated protocol is a non-contrast high resolution CT scan (**HRCT**) in which very thin slices are acquired, often in full inspiration and in full expiration. In patients with unexplained chronic cough and/or wheezing, dynamic expiratory CT (scanning during exhalation) is done to look for collapse of the airway (tracheobronchomalacia). For acute dyspnea that presents with clinical features suspicious for pulmonary embolism, the procedure of choice is a CT pulmonary arteriogram (**CTPA**). This differs from a routine contrast-enhanced chest CT in the rate of injection of intravenous contrast material and in the timing of the CT scan after the injection is started. The specific CT protocol may depend on the clinical information that you provide on the radiology order. In some institutions, a ventilation/perfusion radionuclide study (**V/Q scan**) is used for diagnosis of pulmonary embolism. This study is less often used than CT because of the higher sensitivity and specificity of CT. However, the V/Q scan is useful in patients who have renal compromise or history of major reaction to intravenous contrast material.

CASE UPDATE

The 52-year-old nicotine user complaining of breathlessness shows findings of "mild diffuse interstitial prominence" on chest radiography. You correctly interpret this to suggest the presence of interstitial lung disease, consistent with the history of gradual and progressive onset of symptoms. On your order for this patient to have pulmonary HRCT, you state, "No meds known to cause interstitial disease, no occupational exposures or autoimmune diseases, normal labs."

When dyspnea is from chronic or frequently recurrent asthma, the imaging workup may include non-pulmonary studies. A significant number of patients with asthma may be found to have gastroesophageal reflux disease (GERD; see Non-Traumatic Chest Wall and Pleuritic Pain later in this chapter). Another common disease in patients with asthma is otherwise clinically silent sinusitis; CT scanning of the paranasal sinuses is then often done (see Chapter 5).

Interpretation

When a patient presents with relatively acute onset of dyspnea with cough and fever, the chief clinical concern is to rule out bacterial pneumonia, which is apparent on radiographs as a hazy pulmonary opacity or consolidation. Such increased pulmonary density may result in the previously discussed silhouette sign in which an expected border, such as the edge of the heart, cannot be seen because of the adjacent lung disease (see Fig. 6-9). In some cases, a segmental pulmonary consolidation may outline a fissure, as in this case (Fig. 6-20) in which bacterial pneumonia in the right upper lobe clearly outlines the lateral aspect of the minor fissure.

Another visual feature of alveolar pulmonary consolidation is the **air bronchogram sign,** in which the opacified lung outlines distal bronchi that would not normally be seen (Fig. 6-21).

Viral bronchitis may cause some subtle prominence of central bronchial markings but does not result in the increased

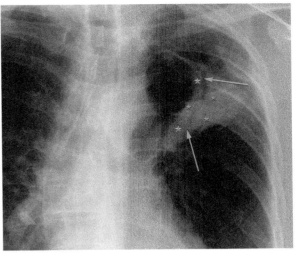

FIGURE 6-21 Air bronchogram sign. Bronchus (arrow) outlined by opacified lung (stars).

pulmonary density found in bacterial pneumonia, except for some limited pulmonary density surrounding bronchi that is often referred to as **peribronchial cuffing.** With infectious bronchitis, thickening of bronchial walls and peribronchial cuffing may result in visible ring shadows and parallel lines called **tram tracks** (Fig. 6-22).

There is concern about overuse of antibiotics in cases of respiratory infection, and this may result from over-interpretation of chest radiographs. Objective radiographic signs should be identified to make a radiologic diagnosis of bacterial pneumonia.

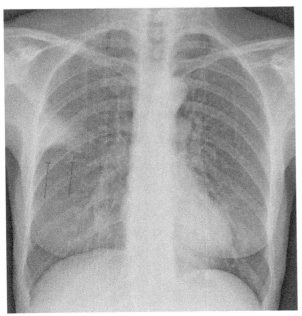

FIGURE 6-20 PA chest radiograph in which the position of the minor fissure (arrows) is clearly outlined by an alveolar consolidation in the right upper lobe.

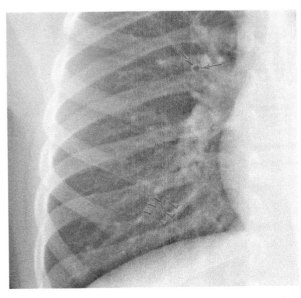

FIGURE 6-22 PA and lateral chest radiographs showing a ring shadow (arrows) and parallel lines ("tram tracks") that suggest thickened bronchi (arrowheads). The bronchi become visible when inflamed because of thickened walls and surrounding thin zone of increased pulmonary parenchymal density, which is called "peribronchial cuffing."

As a generalization that is especially true for children, infectious bronchitis is almost always viral, while pulmonary parenchymal infection is bacterial. Therefore, the presence or absence of alveolar pulmonary opacity on chest radiographs may determine whether or not a patient with cough and fever is given antibiotics.

However, radiography is not 100% sensitive for detection of bacterial pneumonia, especially if radiographs are not ideal because of patient factors, such as poor inspiratory effort and/or obesity. In a patient with dyspnea, high fever, and leukocytosis, treatment for bacterial pneumonia may be appropriate even if no pneumonia is clearly shown radiographically.

 In children from 6 months to 6 years of age, croup, an acute viral infection of the upper airway, causes narrowing of the subglottic trachea and dyspnea; it has a characteristic "steeple sign" on neck radiographs (Fig. 6 23).

A more serious pediatric bacterial disease resulting in dyspnea is epiglottitis, which is most often seen in children ages 2 to 7 years (but may also be seen in adolescents and sometimes even in adults). Acute epiglottitis can be rapidly life threatening. A main role for radiography in these cases is to differentiate croup from acute epiglottitis. The classic appearance of a swollen epiglottis on a lateral soft tissue neck radiograph (Fig. 6-24) should result in prompt efforts to provide urgent care of the patient by personnel qualified to secure the airway, if deemed necessary.

Occasionally, patients who present with acute dyspnea will have suffered a spontaneous pneumothorax. The radiographic finding of such a pneumothorax (see Fig. 6-19) is no different than when pneumothorax is secondary to trauma.

Although chest radiography is often normal in asthma, it is commonly obtained to exclude an underlying process, such as pneumonia. In acute asthma, radiographs may show bronchial thickening, pulmonary hyperinflation, and focal areas of atelectasis. An old aphorism that "all that wheezes is not asthma" applies to this use of chest radiography. Wheezing may be a symptom of major airway compromise, such as tracheal tumor, and these can be detected by careful inspection of "plain" chest radiography.

High resolution computed tomography is fundamental in evaluating and diagnosing interstitial lung disease. The imaging findings in interstitial lung disease are numerous and complex. The appearance of interstitial lung disease on radiography or CT is generally described as **reticular** if the visual pattern is that of fine lines, **micronodular** if the pattern consists of many small nodules (often too small to perceive radiographically), or the combined pattern of **reticulonodular** interstitial lung disease. Nodules may be clustered around bronchovascular bundles; for example, the peribronchovascular disease

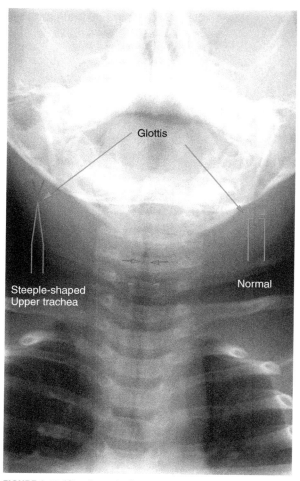

FIGURE 6-23 AP radiograph of the soft tissues of the neck of a child with croup. Note the steeple-shaped upper airway (arrows), which is caused by subglottic edema. A drawing shows the outline of the more squared-off shape of the upper airway in a normal child.

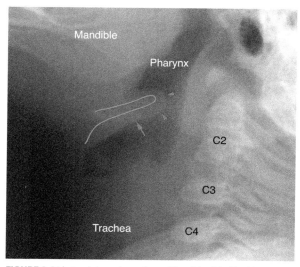

FIGURE 6-24 Lateral view of a patient with epiglottitis. The blue outline shows the appearance of the normal epiglottis (resembles a slender finger) superimposed upon the swollen epiglottis (arrows), which looks like a fat thumb.

commonly seen in pulmonary sarcoidosis. Nodules may be centrilobular, such as in hypersensitivity pneumonitis and smoking-related bronchiolitis/interstitial lung disease. **Ground glass opacity,** a hazy increase in lung density, may cause indistinctness of vessel margins but is not as dense as pulmonary consolidation.

Definitive diagnosis of interstitial lung disease may be made on imaging but often requires close clinical, laboratory, and radiologic correlation, and may require lung biopsy. Clinical history is important; interstitial lung disease may be idiopathic but is often associated with environmental exposures, medications, and autoimmune disorders, such as scleroderma. A major value of HRCT for clinical triage is the differentiation between lung fibrosis such as seen with **honeycombing** (Fig. 6-25), which does not respond readily to medical treatment, from the finding of ground glass opacity (Fig. 6-26), which often indicates pathology that will respond to treatment with steroids.

CASE UPDATE

The 52-year-old nicotine user complaining of breathlessness had the HRCT that you ordered. With the aid of the clinical data that you provided on the order, a radiologic diagnosis of respiratory bronchiolitis–interstitial lung disease (RB-ILD) was made. The radiology report, sent to you and the pulmonologist to whom you referred the patient, indicated the presence of significant ground glass opacity on the HRCT.

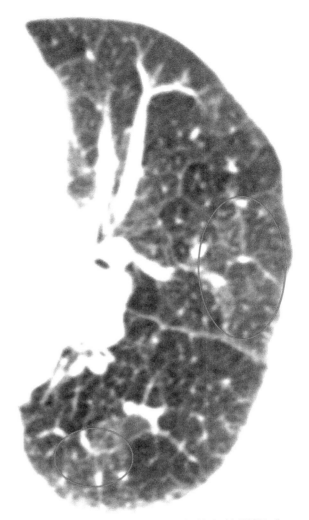

FIGURE 6-26 Areas of ground glass opacity (circles) in HRCT indicating active interstitial pulmonary disease.

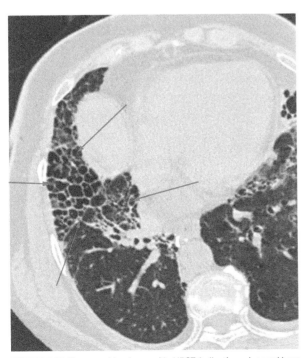

FIGURE 6-25 Honeycombing (arrows) in HRCT, indicating advanced lung fibrosis.

HRCT may demonstrate significant bronchial abnormalities. Thickened bronchi suggest chronic bronchitis. **Bronchiectasis,** dilatation of bronchi, may be the result of chronic infection or may be secondary to traction bronchial walls by adjacent lung fibrosis (Fig. 6-27).

Emphysema is visible on HRCT as the absence—destruction—of lung parenchyma caused by chronic airway disease. In smokers, this destruction of lung tissue is often centrally placed within the structural unit called the secondary pulmonary lobule and is called **centrilobular emphysema** (Fig. 6-28, top). When this process is more advanced, whole secondary pulmonary lobules may become a single air sac, **panlobular emphysema** (Fig. 6-28, bottom). Centrilobular and panlobular emphysema often coexist.

Another form of emphysema shown on CT is **paraseptal emphysema** (Fig. 6-29), which is usually subpleural. The presence of these **bullae** may predispose a patient to suffering a spontaneous pneumothorax.

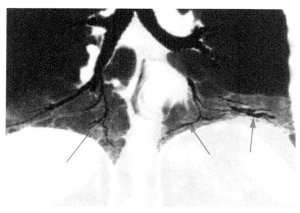

FIGURE 6-27 Bronchiectasis (arrows) secondary to retraction of surrounding lung fibrosis, shown in special CT reconstruction focused on this portion of the bronchial tree. These bronchi are dilated by retraction of surrounding pulmonary fibrosis.

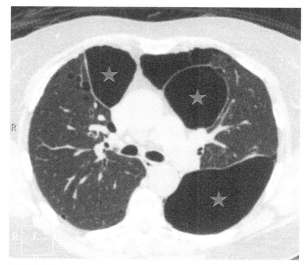

FIGURE 6-29 Paraseptal emphysema (stars within the large subpleural bullae) in an axial CT.

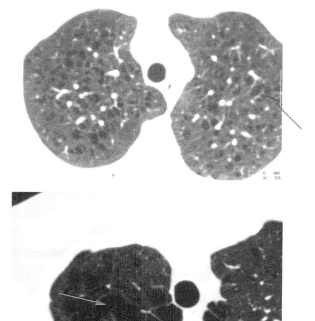

FIGURE 6-28 **Top:** Arrow points to one of many foci of missing tissue in the center of lobules that is characteristic of centrilobular emphysema. **Bottom:** Arrow indicates the more extensive destruction of lung tissue characteristic of panlobular emphysema.

In severe bullous emphysema, large pulmonary bullae may overexpand, compressing adjacent relatively normal lung parenchyma and producing progressively severe dyspnea. These patients may benefit from surgical bullectomy.

Chronic obstructive pulmonary disease (COPD) is the widespread chronic disease of the airways that is usually caused by smoking. COPD consists of reduced air flow through the airways and the destruction of alveolar walls (emphysema), which can be shown with HRCT. The functional limitation of the airways in COPD is not generally evaluated with radiologic imaging; **pulmonary function testing** is the primary method of evaluating COPD patients.

Acute dyspnea, especially with tachypnea, pleuritic chest pain, decreased arterial oxygen saturation, and tachycardia, raises clinical suspicion of pulmonary embolism. Pulmonary emboli most commonly originate from deep leg veins, so signs of lower extremity deep venous thrombosis in a patient with these chest symptoms and signs raise the likelihood of pulmonary emboli. Such patients often undergo lower extremity venous sonography to search for thrombi (see Chapter 2). Laboratory testing for D-dimer levels is also often done, elevated levels correlating with the presence of thrombi. The characteristic imaging finding is the direct visualization of emboli within pulmonary arteries on CTPA (Fig. 6-30).

HEMOPTYSIS

Hemoptysis may result from infectious and malignant disease; can occur with bronchiectasis and in chronic bronchitis; and rarely can occur from vascular abnormalities, such as a pulmonary arteriovenous malformation (AVM). In the acute setting of severe infectious bronchitis, with or without pneumonia, and with severe coughing from acute respiratory illness, hemoptysis may be benign and self-limited. However, the presence of hemoptysis is usually considered a worrisome sign of a malignancy involving the tracheobronchial system, especially when the patient is a cigarette smoker. Although many patients with persistent hemoptysis will need definitive diagnosis by bronchoscopy, imaging is still fundamental in patient evaluation.

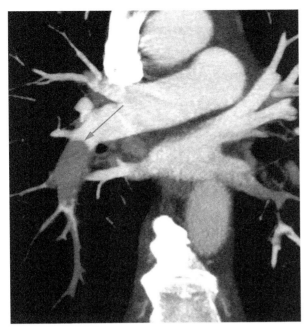

FIGURE 6-30 Pulmonary embolism (arrow) in the right pulmonary artery in CTPA.

Modalities

Chest radiography should be done for the initial radiologic evaluation of hemoptysis. If chest radiography is normal or shows evidence of infectious bronchitis (see Interpretation) in a non-smoker, no further imaging may be needed. However, hemoptysis usually requires further evaluation of the chest with contrast-enhanced CT. When hemoptysis is explained by an imaging finding of pulmonary malignancy or proven by biopsy, staging is often done with PET scanning.

Interpretation

With acute infectious bronchitis, chest radiographs may be normal. Sometimes, however, thickened bronchi are visible as parallel lines or as ring shadows when seen en face ("looking down the barrel"). Patients who present with dyspnea, fever, and cough often show this finding (see Fig. 6-22) in chest radiography done for possible pneumonia. In a patient with chronic airway disease due to cigarette smoking or asthma, these features may appear chronically. It is very common to find a variety of slightly prominent lung markings on chest radiography that could be either chronic or indicate acute disease. As mentioned frequently in this book, comparison with any available prior imaging studies may be crucial. An important part of gathering patient history is determining if there are any prior imaging studies that should be obtained for comparison with a current exam. Patients do not always accurately recall what diagnostic procedures they have had, and sometimes "history taking" requires that you contact your patient's prior health care

providers. Attributing hemoptysis to acute infectious bronchitis would not be appropriate if all of the radiographic findings are chronic and stable. There may be a cause for hemoptysis not visible on chest radiography.

Small endobronchial tumors may result in no radiographic findings. Although these tumors may be seen on CT, bronchoscopy is almost always needed for diagnosis. Endobronchial tumors causing hemoptysis may obstruct a bronchus, leading to atelectasis that is evident on radiography. For example, the left lower lobe atelectasis shown in Figure 6-12 could be the result of a tumor in the left lower lobe bronchus, and if that patient presented with hemoptysis, there would be very high suspicion for the presence of endobronchial tumor. Larger bronchogenic tumors may be visible as masses, or large nodules, and may be associated with hilar and/or mediastinal adenopathy and with a malignant pleural effusion.

Occasionally, a patient with severe bacterial pneumonia may present with hemoptysis, and the radiographic findings may just be a typical appearance of a fluffy alveolar opacity or consolidation, perhaps with a silhouette sign (Fig. 6-31) or air bronchograms.

CT scanning for hemoptysis may reveal a pulmonary mass (or masses), pleural effusion, and hilar and/or mediastinal adenopathy (Fig. 6-32).

In addition, because a substantial portion of the liver is visible on a chest CT scan, hepatic metastases from lung cancer may be detected. A common location of metastatic disease from lung cancer is the adrenal gland, and the adrenals are usually also in the scanning range of chest CT. Finally, in addition to viewing chest CT with lung and soft tissue window settings, bone window images should be viewed to search for skeletal metastatic disease.

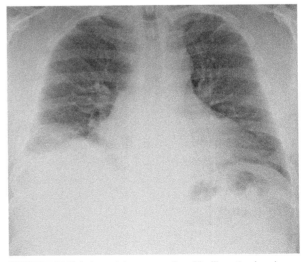

FIGURE 6-31 Right lower lobe pneumonia, with silhouette sign obscuring the right hemidiaphragm on a PA chest radiograph.

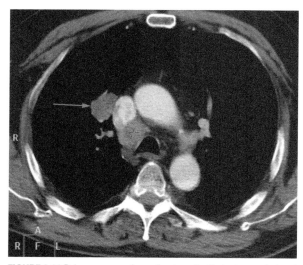

FIGURE 6-32 Pulmonary mass (arrow) and mediastinal adenopathy (star) in axial CT.

NON-TRAUMATIC CHEST WALL AND PLEURITIC PAIN

Non-traumatic chest wall pain may arise from the musculoskeletal components of the chest, pleural disease, a thoracic radiculitis, or shingles. Usually, a careful history and physical exam provide relatively clear evidence for a particular cause. When a patient presents with characteristic pleuritic pain, chest radiography is usually done to search for pleural effusion or lung disease that involves the pleura.

Modalities

Anterior chest wall pain, especially when it is symmetric and associated with tenderness of the anterior rib cage, may indicate the presence of costochondritis. Usually, the diagnosis can be made clinically and no imaging is needed. Radionuclide bone scans are sometimes done on patients with suspected costochondritis. However, if clinical management depends on documentation of the presence or absence of costochondritis, then CT has been shown to be a better exam.

Chest wall masses, with or without pain, are usually best evaluated with CT. However, a clinically suspected subcutaneous lipoma may be satisfactorily diagnosed with ultrasonography. Masses that are less mobile and firmer than a lipoma on physical exam are usually examined with CT. As with many clinical situations that are somewhat unusual, discussion of the particulars of a case with a radiologist may be very appropriate for guidance to the most ideal imaging exam.

When a patient with an oncologic history presents with chest wall pain, rib radiographs, in addition to chest radiography, are indicated. High clinical suspicion of skeletal metastatic disease or positive findings on radiography

usually results in the patient getting a radionuclide bone scan. Oncologists are increasingly requesting PET scanning for evaluation of suspected metastatic disease and staging of malignancy.

When the clinical presentation suggests a thoracic radiculitis, thoracic spine radiography should be considered, and MRI may be indicated if the patient does not respond to conservative management.

Interpretation

When pleuritic chest wall pain is caused by infectious pleural disease, an effusion may be rather small in relation to the sometimes severe pleuritic pain. When there is a free-flowing pleural effusion, the superior margin of the fluid has a characteristic curved "meniscus" shape (see Fig. 6-7) on standing chest radiography. However, when fluid in the pleural space is loculated, it may produce a water or soft-tissue density that has its base along the chest wall and a convex inner margin. This raises concern of possible empyema. Loculated pleural effusions may be more difficult to aspirate and/or drain without image guidance, and CT may be appropriate for further study (Fig. 6-33).

The most common finding on a radionuclide bone scan for costochondritis is increased activity at the costochondral junctions, often symmetric. However, such increased activity may also be seen in normal individuals and is therefore not specific. CT may reveal swollen, abnormally low density, or eroded costal cartilages.

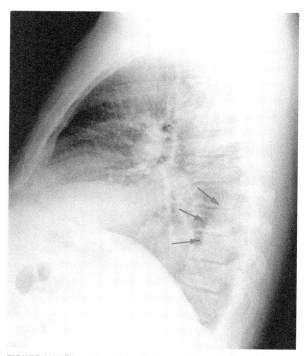

FIGURE 6-33 Pleural-based density (arrows) shown in lateral chest radiograph with a configuration suspicious for loculated pleural effusion.

CT done for evaluation of a chest wall mass will demonstrate abnormal soft tissue, often with involvement of an adjacent rib or of the sternum (Fig. 6-34).

The radiographic findings of rib metastases may be very subtle. Radiographs may show lytic (destructive) or blastic (abnormally increased bone density) lesions, but radiography is far from 100% sensitive in detecting active skeletal disease, and many lesions may be radiographically occult. For most malignancies, a radionuclide bone scan will show foci of markedly increased activity at the sites of rib metastases (Fig. 6-35).

CARDIAC DISEASE: GENERAL CONSIDERATIONS

Patients presenting with chest pain and congestive heart failure are discussed in detail later in this chapter. In the following section we address general issues of cardiac imaging.

Modalities

Most cardiac imaging is done within an evaluation of a patient by a cardiologist. Procedures such as echocardiography, **cardiac catheterization and angiography, radionuclide myocardial perfusion** studies (i.e., stress SPECT sestamibi scans), cardiac MRI, and cardiac CT are frequently performed, supervised, interpreted, or ordered by cardiologists.

Although referral to a cardiologist is standard when a primary care provider suspects cardiac disease, primary care providers can work with a radiologist in the initial imaging of patients with, and screening for, cardiac disease.

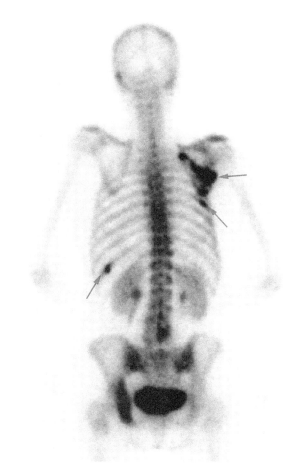

FIGURE 6-35 Radionuclide bone scan, revealing foci of rib and scapular metastases (arrows).

Risk factors for coronary disease, such as hypertension, family history of coronary disease, cholesterol levels, and use of tobacco, are used among other factors to measure coronary risk, based upon data from the Framingham Heart Study. A newer tool for coronary risk assessment is the **coronary calcium score** ("screening heart scan"). This non-invasive, widely available, and inexpensive test, done in either an electron beam CT scanner or the more common multi-detector CT scanner, provides an assessment for the risk of coronary disease that stands independently from the Framingham risk assessment indicators. A very low dose CT scan is done that is optimized to measure calcified coronary artery plaque (Patient Communication Box 6-1).

Another procedure for evaluating a patient for coronary artery disease that is often requested by primary care providers is the cardiac or coronary CT arteriogram (**CCTA**). This is a much more elaborate exam than the calcium score. Multidetector CT (MDCT) scanners that acquire up to 320 slices in a single rotation of the x-ray tube and detector array are used for the CCTA exam. This study provides a non-invasive visualization of the coronary arteries using an intravenous injection of iodinated contrast material and advanced image

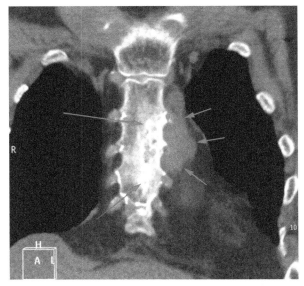

FIGURE 6-34 Coronal CT image revealing a soft tissue mass (short arrows) in the anterior chest wall that was proven by biopsy to represent local recurrence of breast cancer several years after mastectomy. Increased bone density in the sternum (long arrows) secondary to tumor infiltration of bone with blastic response.

You should discuss with your patients the difference between a risk assessment tool such as the coronary calcium score and a definitive diagnostic examination. They should understand the value of risk assessment in guiding their medical care. A high-risk calcium score, for example, may affect a decision to place a patient on statins but may also require more elaborate and definitive coronary testing.

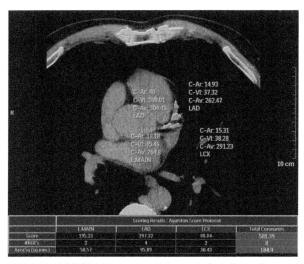

FIGURE 6-36 MDCT calcium score study report of a patient with a total score of 581.39 (moderate disease). This report not only gives the total score but also separate scores for some of the coronary arteries: Left main (195.23); left anterior descending (297.32), and left circumflex (88.84). (*C-ar, C-vl,* and *C-av* on the image refer to the scoring algorithm and are not critical for understanding the report.)

processing. The radiation dose to which patients are exposed during CCTA has been drastically reduced and now may be lower than the traditional workup, which often includes both a radionuclide myocardial perfusion study and cardiac catheterization. Because up to one third of patients who undergo cardiac catheterization are found to have no significant coronary stenosis, and because CCTA has a high sensitivity for coronary disease, many patients could avoid myocardial perfusion studies and coronary catheterization if CCTA was done first.

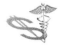

COST-EFFECTIVE MEDICINE
CCTA is far less expensive than cardiac catheterization.

Optimum patient selection for this exam is being actively studied, and is an evolving process.

Interpretation

A low or zero calcium score is associated with a very low (but not zero) risk for the presence of occlusive or stenotic coronary artery disease and low incidence rates of sudden cardiac events. There are several scoring systems that vary somewhat in absolute numbers given. Numerical calcium "scores" are meaningful only in broad ranges. Moderate levels of calcified plaque (approximately 80–400) may indicate increased risk for the presence of significant coronary disease. A high score (sometimes well over 1,000) predicts a high probability that there is coronary artery stenosis or occlusion and strong incidence rates for acute myocardial infarction (Fig. 6-36). In patients with relatively modest risk for coronary disease, the calcium score can be used to guide risk factor modification, such as exercise programs, smoking cessation, and use of statins. Calcium scores may also influence clinical decisions about further diagnostic procedures, such as treadmill testing, myocardial perfusion scanning, CCTA, or coronary catheterization.

CCTA is an excellent screening test because of its very low false-negative rate. When CCTA displays the absence of significant coronary artery disease (Fig. 6-37), stenotic coronary artery disease is essentially ruled out.

When CCTA shows severe left main or triple vessel coronary artery disease, the patient is not usually a candidate for coronary stenting but might be considered for coronary artery bypass surgery. However, many patients with potentially flow-limiting coronary stenosis are candidates for stenting. For example, a 55-year-old general surgeon had postprandial angina. CCTA demonstrated a severe stenosis

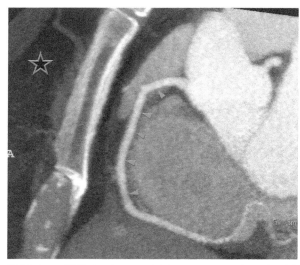

FIGURE 6-37 CCTA showing normal right coronary artery (arrowheads). Image appears "grainy" because this was done on an obese patient; note the thick layer of presternal fat (star).

in a large marginal branch of the left circumflex coronary artery (Fig. 6-38). Cardiac catheterization was done, during which initial angiography confirmed the CCTA finding (Fig. 6-39); the stenosis was dilated (Fig. 6-40), and the vessel was stented. The patient had immediate relief of symptoms. He went home the afternoon after the procedure, had a large dinner, and for the first time in months had no postprandial chest pain (which he had attributed to GERD).

ACUTE CHEST PAIN

Acute chest pain is a medical emergency that requires prompt and coordinated medical attention for rapid patient assessment and triage. Imaging is often part of this process.

Modalities

When a patient presents with acute chest pain but the clinical suspicion is low for an acute coronary event, standing chest

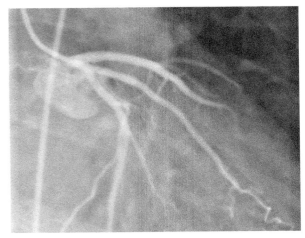

FIGURE 6-40 Repeat arteriogram of the same artery as shown in Figure 6-37 after balloon dilatation.

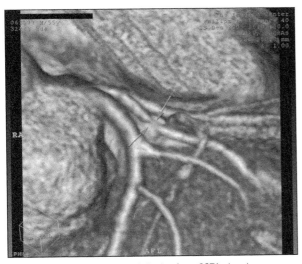

FIGURE 6-38 Volume rendered display from CCTA showing a severe stenosis (arrows) of a large marginal branch of the left circumflex coronary artery.

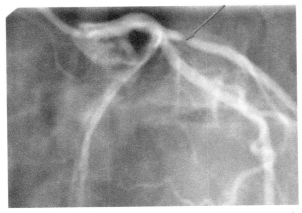

FIGURE 6-39 Coronary arteriogram confirming the severe stenosis (arrow) shown on the CCTA in Figure 6-38.

radiography is appropriate. However, when clinical history, ECG, and other indicators are suggestive of either an aortic dissection or acute coronary occlusion, an immediately available bedside portable chest radiograph should be done, but only if it does not delay a more definitive radiologic examination.

In cases of suspected aortic dissection, the procedure of choice is usually CT angiography (**CTA**) of the chest and abdomen. As an alternative to CTA—for example, in patients who are allergic to iodinated contrast material—MRI/MRA may be considered. However, MR scanning should never be given preference if it would delay diagnosis and should not be used in patients who are hemodynamically unstable. Except in rare clinical environments, MRI is too time consuming for evaluation of a clinical situation that could become catastrophic very quickly. Furthermore, monitoring unstable patients is very difficult in most MR scanners.

Transesophageal echocardiography can be used for a rapid diagnosis of aortic dissection, but, again, only in rare clinical environments is it possible to get such an examination as rapidly as CTA. The use of immediate invasive, intra-arterial catheter angiography is now much less common because of the widespread availability of fast multi-detector CT scanners.

When there is intermediate to high probability for coronary occlusion or acute high-grade stenosis, immediate SPECT myocardial perfusion imaging is often the most appropriate test.

When a patient presents with clear signs of an acute coronary event, such as ST segment elevation on electrocardiography (ECG), elevated troponin levels, or elevated creatine kinase–MB levels, the standard of care is immediate coronary catheterization. Not all patients with acute coronary symptoms present with significantly elevated enzymes or ST segment elevation. In these patients who are considered at low to intermediate risk, CCTA is becoming more widely used.

There is growing interest in using a slightly modified injection and scanning timing protocol for chest/coronary CTA as a "triple rule out" in patients who present with a confusing clinical picture that could represent either a pulmonary embolism, aortic dissection, or acute coronary occlusion.

Interpretation

Chest radiography in the setting of acute chest pain is used to seek an alternative diagnosis to cardiac causes for chest pain. Other sections in this chapter discuss such alternative causes for chest pain: An acute pleural inflammatory process may cause a pleural effusion (see Fig. 6-7). Pneumonia may irritate a pleural surface enough to cause significant chest pain. In some cases of pulmonary embolism (Fig. 6-41), peripheral segmental or subsegmental pulmonary infarction may cause severe pleuritic chest pain that may be a more dominating symptom than dyspnea. In such patients, a peripheral wedge-shaped pulmonary opacity would suggest a pulmonary infarction.

Acute aortic syndromes causing chest pain, such as aortic dissection and penetrating atherosclerotic ulcer, are readily shown on CTA. Aortic dissections are characterized by their location and extent, involvement of major aortic branches, presence of thrombus, and any associated aortic leak or rupture. Evaluation often requires study of numerous post-processed multiplanar images of large image data sets. Figure 6-42 is an example of a segment of the aorta with a dissection in which the true lumen is separated from the false lumen by the elevated intima.

The obvious advantage of direct catheter coronary angiography for acute coronary occlusion is the opportunity for immediate transcatheter revascularization. Patients with ST

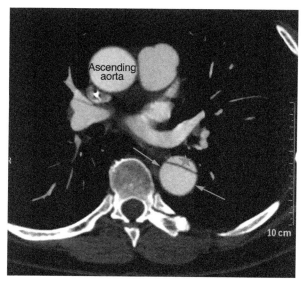

FIGURE 6-42 Aortic dissection shown in a CTA; true (arrows) and false (red star) channels of descending aorta separated by the elevated intima (dark line).

segment elevation myocardial infarction (STEMI) are usually taken directly to coronary catheterization whenever possible.

When the major vascular causes for acute chest pain have been ruled out and there is no evident acute pulmonary or pleural process, GERD is usually considered as a possible cause. GERD usually has a classic chronic history but sometimes can present with an acute onset and clinical history that is not clear on initial patient evaluation. The imaging of GERD is discussed in Chapter 8.

CHRONIC CHEST PAIN

Many patients who have chronic chest pain of cardiac origin are under the care of a cardiologist or are under the care of a primary caregiver after consultation with a cardiologist. A patient with chronic stable angina who is well managed medically would not normally need special diagnostic imaging unless there is a change in clinical status.

Modalities

Patients without documented cardiac disease may present to you with a complaint of chronic chest pain. Chest radiography in this situation, as in the acute situation, is appropriate for initial examination. Ischemic cardiac disease is usually the main clinical concern to rule out as a cause of chronic chest pain. Referral to cardiology may result in stress echocardiography or radionuclide stress myocardial perfusion imaging. Alternatively, as described earlier, cardiac or coronary CTA (CCTA) that is conducted in a radiology facility or department may be ordered by a primary care provider to rule out coronary disease. Increasingly, CCTA is also now being done

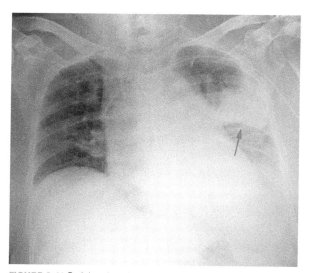

FIGURE 6-41 Peripheral wedge-shaped opacity (arrows) in a portable AP radiograph that may represent a pulmonary infarction. Patient has a central venous line (curved white line over upper left chest).

within cardiology practices. Non-coronary chest CTA or CT pulmonary angiogram (CTPA) is considered an appropriate exam if the clinical history or chest radiography findings suggest the possibility of chronic, recurrent pulmonary embolism or thoracic aortic aneurysm or dissection. Cardiac MRI is an appropriate exam but is not widely available and is a longer examination that may be more difficult for a patient than CT.

If coronary disease has been ruled out or is very unlikely from the clinical history, GERD is usually considered in the differential diagnosis for chronic chest pain and occasionally for acute chest pain. Also, biliary disease may cause referral of pain to the chest. Appropriate studies for these disorders are discussed in Chapter 8.

Interpretation

Chest radiography in the setting of chronic chest pain is used as a survey for possible cardiac, lung, or pleural disease. All the points related to interpreting routine chest radiography, discussed earlier in this chapter, apply to chronic chest pain.

Stress echocardiography and radionuclide myocardial perfusion imaging cannot image the coronary arteries directly. These are functional examinations of the epicardial coronary artery system that may display evidence of insufficient blood flow to regions of the myocardium either at rest or with stress. The limitations of these studies with respect to sensitivity and specificity are very well known. Even at the highest level of quality in the performance of these studies, and with the most informed and conscientious cardiology practice, it has been difficult to decide, from these non-invasive studies, which patients should undergo coronary catheterization. Nearly one third of patients undergoing invasive coronary angiography are found to have no significant coronary stenosis.

Chest CTA is very reliable for diagnosis or exclusion of thoracic aortic disease such as aortic dissection, whether in the chronic or acute situations, with close to 100% sensitivity and specificity. CTPA is not quite as accurate for detection of pulmonary emboli as CTA is for aortic disease. However, although small subsegmental pulmonary emboli may escape detection with CTPA, such small emboli may not have any clinical significance. In fact, normal individuals may from time to time have tiny pulmonary emboli that have no consequences. Therefore, a negative CTPA essentially removes pulmonary embolism from your differential diagnosis for a patient with chronic chest pain.

CONGESTIVE HEART FAILURE

Although the symptomatology and radiologic findings in congestive heart failure (CHF) overlap some of the information presented earlier, we provide here a separate section on it because of its frequent occurrence and high morbidity and mortality in our society. CHF is the consequence of any cardiac abnormality that results in the inadequate pumping function of the heart. However, it is not primarily the amount of blood being pumped out through the aorta that results in radiographic findings. It is the failure of the heart to pump all the blood returned to it from the pulmonary and systemic circulation that results in elevated pulmonary venous and systemic venous pressure. These elevated pressures cause the clinical and radiologic findings of CHF.

It will certainly happen in the outpatient setting that you will see a patient complaining of dyspnea and your initial clinical evaluation will reveal evidence of chronic or even acute congestive heart failure. The classic clinical findings are tachypnea; a history of orthopnea (dyspnea worse when the patient is recumbent); elevated venous pressure resulting in ankle edema (especially pitting edema) and even visible distention of jugular veins; cough; and rales found on pulmonary auscultation. In severe cases with pulmonary edema, the patient may be cyanotic.

Modalities

Chest radiography is the indicated imaging procedure, either standing PA and lateral views done on an ambulatory patient who may be in mild CHF, or a portable AP exam in a severely distressed patient.

Interpretation

The first finding usually evident on chest radiography is cardiomegaly, usually from dilatation of the left ventricle secondary to cardiomyopathy, ischemia, or any other cause. Dilatation of the left atrium is often found in CHF. Differentiation of specific chamber dilatation is not needed in the initial evaluation of a patient in active CHF.

With elevated left atrial pressure, the pulmonary venous pressure is elevated. In chest radiography of a healthy standing patient, or one sitting upright, the pulmonary veins at the lung bases are more distended than the upper lobe veins, simply because the hydrostatic pressure gradient caused by gravity. In active CHF, the upper lobe vessels are conspicuously distended. This reversal of the pulmonary venous pattern is called **cephalization** of the pulmonary venous pattern, or simply pulmonary venous congestion.

With elevated pulmonary venous pressure, fluid accumulates in pulmonary interstitial spaces, first evident in the immediate subpleural space as thickening of the fissures, and in the interlobular septa at the lung bases. These are seen as **Kerley-B lines,** short white lines at the lung bases that are perpendicular to, and meet, the pleural surface at the lateral aspect of the lung in the costophrenic sulcus on

---

frontal radiographs (AP or PA). (**Kerley-A** and **C lines** may also be reported in CHF but are less common, and not critical to look for or to understand the condition). Small pleural effusions may be present (Fig. 6-43).

In severe CHF, fluid leaks into the alveoli, and arterial oxygenation falls because of the pulmonary edema. The characteristic appearance of pulmonary edema is a **batwing**-shaped distribution of pulmonary opacity (Fig. 6-44).

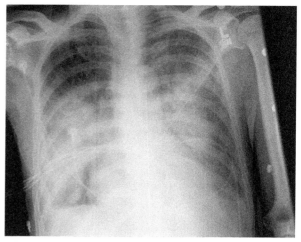

FIGURE 6-44 Severe CHF shown in a portable chest radiograph; note pulmonary edema (hazy central pulmonary opacities) and ECG leads in this patient in extreme distress.

CASE UPDATE

Your patient, a 52-year-old nicotine user, has now seen the pulmonologist. Additional examination included pulmonary function tests. The pulmonary specialist agrees with the radiologic diagnosis of smoking-related respiratory bronchiolitis-interstitial lung disease, and, because of the substantial amount of ground glass opacity shown on HRCT, has placed the patient on corticosteroids. You are now following the patient as the steroids are being tapered off, and managing the patient's efforts to stop smoking.

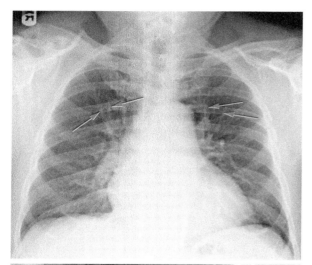
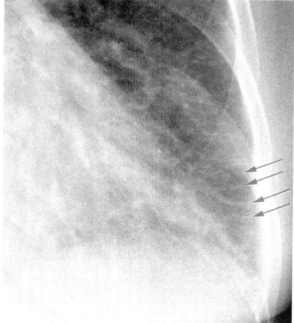

FIGURE 6-43 Features of CHF shown in PA chest radiographs. **Top:** Mild cardiomegaly and distended upper lobe pulmonary veins (arrows). **Bottom:** Magnified view showing Kerley-B lines in lower left lobe (arrows).

Chapter Review

Chapter Review Questions

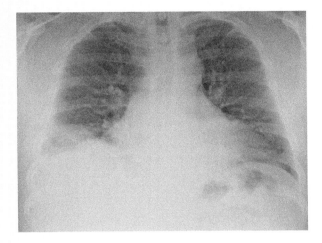

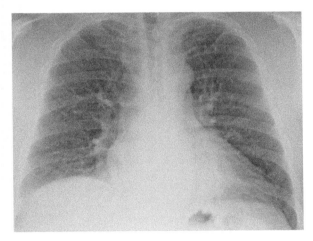

1. Answer the following question based on the images above.

   In examining this PA chest radiograph of a patient whom you suspect has pneumonia, you notice that the patient has not taken in a deep breath, and this is not an ideal radiograph.

   You compare it with the prior PA chest radiograph on this patient, looking for a finding that represents an objective change.

   You see that both hemidiaphragms on the prior chest x-ray (bottom) and the left hemidiaphragm on the current x-ray (top) are sharply seen, but the right hemidiaphragm is not well seen on today's PA chest radiograph. Which of the following is this an example of?

   A. Pneumonia sign

   B. Silhouette sign

   C. Middle lobe sign

   D. Pleural effusion sign

   E. Positive bacteria sign

2. Which of the following is not correct pertaining to CT of the chest?

   A. It should be done in a patient who smokes heavily and has hemoptysis

   B. It may reveal hepatic or splenic injuries in a patient with lower rib fractures

   C. It is always done when there are rib fractures

   D. It may reveal radiographically occult sternal fractures

   E. It may explain apparent cardiomegaly that is caused by a chest wall deformity

3. Which of the following is correct about rib fractures?

   A. They always involve fractures in at least two parts of a rib

   B. They always involve injury to deeper structures such as pleura and lung

   C. They are more likely to be associated with vascular injuries if in the lower ribs than in upper ribs and require a vascular imaging study

   D. They typically require radionuclide bone scan for firm diagnosis

   E. If they fracture in more than one location in individual ribs, paradoxical respiratory movements of the chest wall accompanied by respiratory distress may result

4. Your patient with scleroderma has progressive dyspnea. You order chest radiography. The report is non-specific, indicating only some possible "interstitial prominence." What do you order next?

   A. Routine contrast-enhanced chest CT

   B. Chest MRI

   C. HRCT of the chest

   D. Follow-up radiography in 3 months

   E. V/Q radionuclide study

5. Which of the following is the least likely condition to be revealed by radiography?

   A. Pleural effusion

   B. Pneumothorax

   C. Costochondritis

   D. Atelectasis

   E. Pneumonia

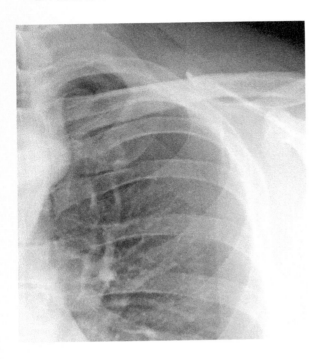

6. A patient comes into your clinic with complaint of sudden, atraumatic onset of dyspnea. You obtain chest radiography in your office, and you see the very important finding shown above:

   A. Pleural effusion that is probably viral

   B. Spontaneous pneumothorax

   C. Evidence of a poor inspiration

   D. Pneumonia

   E. Pulmonary edema

7. *Coronary calcium scoring* refers to:

   A. The metabolic test done after radiography shows calcified plaque in the thoracic aorta

   B. An estimate of coronary calcium deposits based upon a serum lipid profile

   C. A statistical term in population studies that cannot help you with an individual patient

   D. The discovery of calcium deposits in the coronary arteries using PET scanning

   E. A measurement of calcified atherosclerotic plaque in the coronary arteries using CT

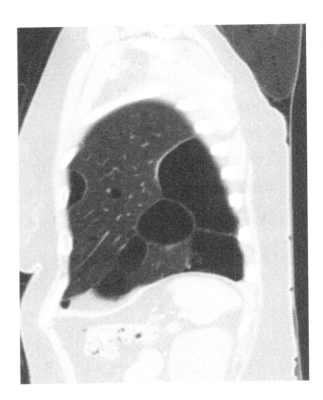

8. Based on the image above, the patient has:

   A. paraseptal emphysema.

   B. pulmonary fibrosis.

   C. little chance of ever needing any surgical treatment.

   D. ground glass opacity that indicates possible clinical improvement with steroids.

   E. an excellent demonstration of a pneumothorax.

9. CCTA reveals some fatty atherosclerotic plaque in coronary arteries, but there is no coronary artery stenosis. The patient is now likely to need:

A. ECG, cardiology consultation, and treadmill testing with myocardial rest and stress perfusion imaging.

B. coronary catheterization to confirm the absence of coronary stenosis.

C. echocardiography.

D. cardiac MRI.

E. counseling about cardiac risk factor modification, such as smoking cessation, and possible medical treatment if lipid levels are elevated.

10. Which of the following is the least likely to be ordered for a patient who has an acute aortic dissection and who is hemodynamically unstable?

A. Aortic CTA

B. Transesophageal ultrasound

C. Immediate aortic angiography

D. Portable chest radiography

E. Magnetic resonance angiography (MRA)

7 BREAST

FUNDAMENTALS OF BREAST IMAGING

Prior to the advent of mammography (radiography optimized for the breast), a diagnosis of breast disease was made by physical examination. This resulted in both over-diagnosis (low specificity of testing) and under-diagnosis (low sensitivity of testing) for breast cancer. The low sensitivity was reflected in the large percentage of cases in which women were diagnosed with breast cancer in advanced stages, and the uncommon diagnosis of early breast cancer. The low specificity of the physical exam resulted in as many as 85% of surgical biopsies of the breast finding only benign tissue.

Medical imaging of the breast is still not perfect, and there are rare occasions when a patient's physical exam is accurately suspicious for cancer, while imaging does not reveal the presence of cancer. However, usually the diagnosis of breast cancer, or the confident diagnosis that a palpable lump is benign, is an imaging diagnosis.

The risk from the radiation used in mammography is remarkably low. One recent study estimated that a woman undergoing yearly screening mammography beginning at the age of 40 might suffer a fatal radiation-induced cancer once every 76,000 to 97,000 years! This low risk does not prevent the promotion of unscientifically exaggerated fear of this medical radiation exposure. (See Patient Communication Box 7-1.)

BREAST CANCER SCREENING

Screening mammography is done on women who do not have a palpable breast mass. Women with signs and/or symptoms of breast cancer are referred for diagnostic mammography.

The potential primary downside of any kind of screening mammography is that it may result in a "false positive." With breast cancer screening that may mean additional studies and perhaps a biopsy that does not reveal cancer.

Three points are critical for you to understand and to explain to your patients about the issue of false positive results from screening:

1. Radiologists in the clinical practice of breast diagnosis find that the overwhelming number of patients are not significantly upset about the occasional special mammography views or ultrasound study needed to clarify a potential concern seen on screening mammography. The usual response from those patients is appreciation of the conscientious effort to find early breast cancer.

2. The vast majority of breast biopsies done in modern medical practice are minimally invasive, image-guided core needle biopsies, usually done with stereotactic mammographic, ultrasound, or MRI guidance. The morbidity of these needle biopsies is minimal. The phrases *negative biopsy* and *false positive* may exaggerate the impression of risk because the word *biopsy* is often taken to mean surgery. A reasonable percentage of needle biopsies that are negative for cancer seems to be a small price to pay for finding many very early cancers.

3. Screening mammogram programs consistently monitor their "call back" rates as well as their true positive and false positive rates. Thus, imaging facilities are continually trying to modify their procedures and interpretations to maximize the value of screening for their patients based on currently available technologies.

Patient Communication Box 7-1

One of your clinical responsibilities, one that you may face regularly, is to have a good response when one of your patients expresses exaggerated fear of radiation exposure during mammography based on something she saw on TV or read on the Internet.

Women at average risk for breast cancer should begin screening mammography at the age of 40, and should then have a screening mammogram yearly. These guidelines for breast cancer screening in women who are at average risk for breast cancer are those of the American Cancer Society, the American College of Radiology, and the Society of Breast Imaging.

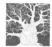 You may be faced with a difficult question: At what age should a woman *stop* getting her yearly mammogram? This is actually a complex question to answer, because it varies so much with the individual characteristics of each patient. An elderly woman in good health who might easily live well for another 10 years may benefit from the early detection of breast cancer. However, a frail 88-year-old woman with severe cardiovascular disease and emphysema is not likely to have either the quality of her life improved or the length of her life extended through screening mammography.

Some patients may ask you about the role of ultrasound in breast cancer screening. Although each mammogram image shows essentially the whole breast, each breast ultrasound image is a cross-section, only showing a thin "slice" of the breast. Surveying the entire breast by ultrasound can be done, but reliability and reproducibility of results for screening is difficult with ultrasonography because the transducers are handheld. Ultrasonography is best used to investigate a potential problem in a specific location of the breast rather than as a screening tool. Automated whole breast ultrasound scanners have been developed but have not been widely adopted for a variety of practical reasons.

Another issue that your patients may raise is the role of screening MRI. For women at increased risk of developing breast cancer, as discussed later in this chapter, screening breast MRI is assuming a rapidly growing role. You may also be asked about the role of a variety of alternative technologies other than mammography, ultrasound, and MRI. For some of these other technologies, such as breast-specific gamma imaging (BSGI), studies to determine efficacy are being conducted and they may become accepted by the medical community for more widespread use in the future.

Other alternative techniques for examining the breast, such as thermography, have failed to show efficacy but are still being promoted by those who profit from their use.

The Screening Mammogram Modalities

The basic radiographic views obtained during screening mammography consist of craniocaudal (CC; Fig. 7-1, A and B) and mediolateral oblique (MLO; Fig. 7-1, C and D) views of each breast.

In the CC view, the x-ray beam traverses the breast from superior to inferior, with a detector at the inferior aspect of the breast. The standard image presentation is that the lateral portion of the breast is "up," so that in the CC views in Figure 7-1, the lateral aspect of each breast is toward the top of the page. In the MLO view, the x-ray beam traverses the breast from the superomedial to inferolateral aspects of the breast and includes as much of the pectoralis muscle and axilla as possible. By convention, the MLO views are presented with the axillary region "up," as shown in Figure 7-1.

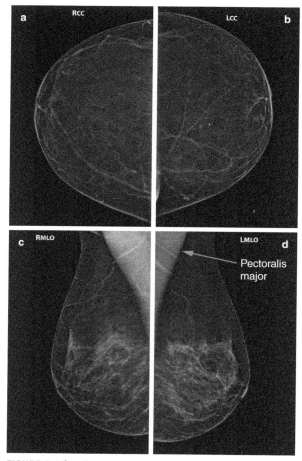

FIGURE 7-1 Standard screening mammography views showing fatty breast parenchyma of one patient in CC views (**A** and **B**) and scattered fibroglandular densities in the MLO views of a different patient (**C** and **D**).

Most imaging facilities display the right-left orientation of breast images as shown in Figure 7-1 (same as a chest radiograph or an axial CT or MR image, with the patient's right to the viewer's left).

Interpretation

Findings on mammography are standardized by a lexicon published by the American College of Radiology, although not all official mammography reports use language that strictly adheres to those guidelines.

The radiographic density of the breasts should be described as mostly fatty (see Fig. 7-1), scattered fibroglandular densities (see Fig. 7-1), heterogeneously dense (Fig. 7-2), or extremely dense (Fig. 7-3); and the symmetry or asymmetry of breast tissue density may be reported. The ideal is for this description to be based on a quasi-quantitative analysis; fatty breasts contain less than 25% non-fatty tissue; breasts with scattered fibroglandular

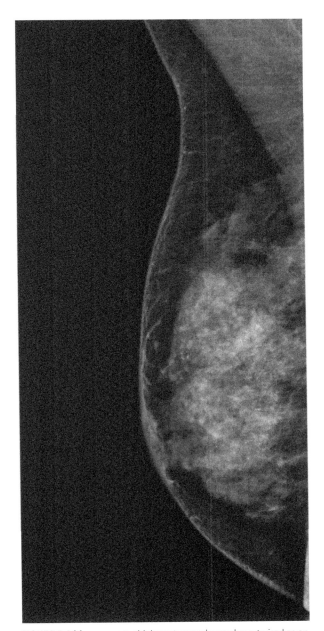

FIGURE 7-3 Mammogram with breast parenchyma characterized as extremely dense.

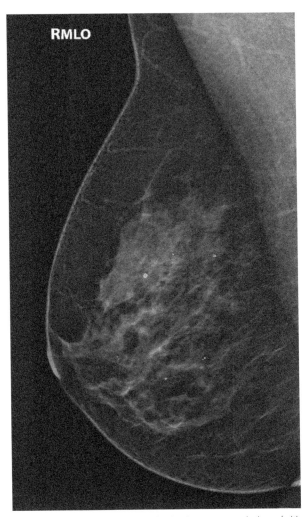

FIGURE 7-2 Mammogram characterized as heterogeneously dense (with incidental benign calcifications; see Fig. 7-5).

density contain 25% to 50% non-fatty tissue, and so on. However, because this estimation is a subjective one by the radiologist, you may not always obtain the identical description of breast density from different radiologists reporting on the same patient.

The mammographic density of the breast has implications for a patient's risk of breast cancer and for your clinical management. Breast cancer risk may increase with increasing density just because a woman has more fibroglandular tissue in her breast than fatty tissue. False negative mammography (cancer not visible on a mammogram) is less likely with fatty breast density simply because a soft tissue mass has a higher radiographic density than fat and is thus more conspicuous in a fatty breast compared to a breast characterized primarily by fibroglandular tissue.

A basic potentially significant finding on a mammogram is a visible change from a prior examination. Therefore, if your patient has relocated or otherwise is getting screening mammography at a different facility than she did previously, you can avoid potential delays in diagnosis by making arrangements for prior mammograms to be available for comparison. If a mammogram shows a new mass or developing density (especially if it has a spiculated margin), as in Figure 7-4, it is suspicious for cancer. The small developing density (later proven to be an invasive cancer, Fig. 7-4) is obviously very subtle and may not have been detected if prior mammography was not available for comparison.

To the contrary, a new water or soft tissue density mass that is perfectly round and has circumferentially sharp margins, especially in a woman with known fibrocystic changes, is more likely to be a new cyst than a cancer. Sometimes a distinct mass may not be apparent, but a progressive "developing density" or "developing asymmetry" may indicate the presence of a mass that is difficult to see as a discreet structure because its margins are obscured by adjacent or overlying fibroglandular tissue density.

Some breast cancer may be detected by a distortion of the breast architecture. This may be seen as a stellate arrangement of fine linear markings that radiate from a locus, without a distinct mass as in Figure 7-5.

A wide variety of commonly found breast calcifications have an appearance that allows the radiologist to be confidant that they are benign, such as those with radiolucent centers. Characteristically benign breast calcifications can be dismissed as incidental findings (Fig. 7-6). Breast calcifications that are not clearly benign require additional study (Fig. 7-7).

At the conclusion of all official breast imaging reports, the interpreting physician must assign a numerical assessment, a Breast Imaging—Reporting and Data System (BI-RADS) category (Table 7-1), which provides a framework for assessing the accuracy and appropriateness of breast imaging interpretation.

It is not uncommon for a mammogram to be coded as BI-RADS 0 (see Table 7-1), indicating that additional imaging is appropriate; upon further study, the potential finding would then receive a final BI-RADS assessment.

THE PALPABLE BREAST MASS OR POSITIVE FINDINGS ON SCREENING MAMMOGRAPHY

Any possible breast lump raises concern. Your role is to guide the patient to appropriate procedures that will establish if a mass is really present or whether it is a benign lump that can be ignored or a suspicious lesion that may require biopsy.

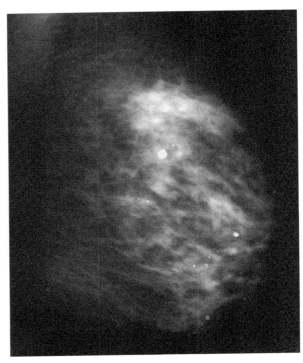

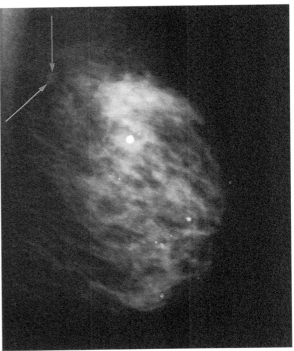

FIGURE 7-4 Left MLO views from prior **(top)** and most recent **(bottom)** yearly screening mammography on the same patient. Arrows point to a developing asymmetric density.

This discussion specifically addresses palpable masses, not breast pain, because generalized breast pain, and even relatively localized pain and tenderness, is rarely a symptom of breast cancer, especially when there is no palpable mass. Normal breast tissue is commonly tender. Benign fibrocystic changes may increase breast tenderness; breast cysts may occasionally become inflamed and very painful. When breast

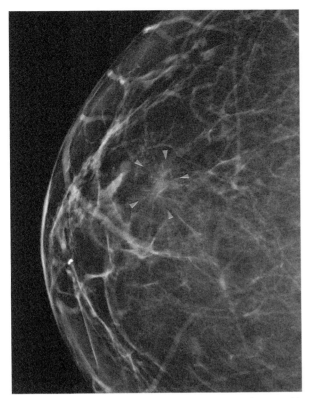

FIGURE 7-5 Mammogram with area of architectural distortion (arrowheads).

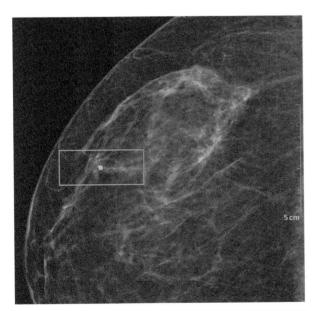

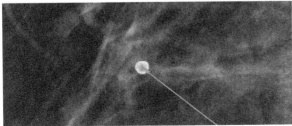

FIGURE 7-6 Screening mammogram showing a benign breast calcification; lower image is a magnified view of the outlined region in the top image containing the calcification. Note the radiolucent center that is one of the characteristics of benign breast calcification (arrow).

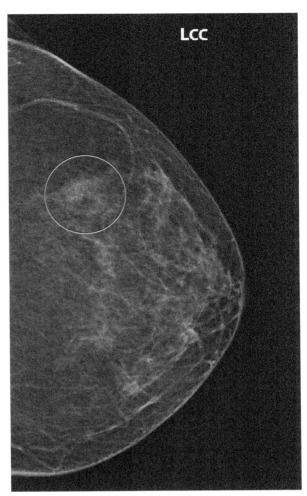

FIGURE 7-7 On this routine screening view, there were some punctate calcifications (within the circle) that were barely visible even on the high resolution monitors used for mammography interpretation. (These may not be visible in this printed format.) Coded as BI-RADS 0. Patient was notified and was scheduled for diagnostic mammography to evaluate the potential finding of the screening exam (see Fig. 7-14).

cancer is palpable, it is usually a painless mass. Often, it is characterized on physical examination as a lump or localized tissue firmness that is much less mobile than lumpy (but normal) breast tissue.

One of the surprising lessons from many years of clinical experience with breast diagnosis is how lumpy even normal breast tissue can be, typically because of the uneven distribution of (usually softer) adipose tissue and (usually firmer) fibroglandular tissue. An important point related to the section earlier on Screening Mammography is that most breast cancer diagnosed today is not palpable or symptomatic in any way (hence the need for screening). Your counseling of a patient on these matters may be as important as your requisition for imaging.

One of the greatest values of imaging can be to demonstrate, definitively, that some lumpy breast tissue is normal, avoiding unnecessary procedures that puncture the skin such as a "blind" attempted aspiration of a non-existent cyst. In addition to patient discomfort, attempted aspiration without

TABLE 7-1 BI-RADS Classification

BI-RADS Category	Definition	Follow-Up Recommendation
0	Findings that are uncertain or not clearly benign in appearance	Immediate or scheduled additional studies that are specified in radiology report: special mammographic views, ultrasonography, or MRI
1	Negative (normal) study	Routine yearly screening mammography
2	Findings that are characteristically benign on imaging or have been proven to be benign by biopsy or aspiration	Routine yearly screening mammography
3	Findings that are very likely benign; low risk of significant change before follow-up exam	Repeat exam (ultrasound, mammogram) typically in 6 months (patients may need assurance that biopsy not needed at this time)
4	Findings that are suspicious for cancer	Image-guided core needle biopsy
5	Findings that are highly suspicious for cancer	Image-guided core needle biopsy
6	Findings of a known malignancy	Imaging done with a known malignancy that has not been excised (e.g., MRI to assess response to neoadjuvant chemotherapy)

imaging may create tissue changes that would then complicate or confuse findings on subsequent imaging. Also, it is a common experience that a patient presents with a palpable abnormality that is shown on imaging to be normal tissue or a benign finding such as a simple cyst, but some other potentially more significant pathology is found. Except for the uncommon case of a clinically obvious large cancer, patients benefit from imaging as the initial procedure when the clinical presentation is that of a potentially significant breast lump.

Modalities

Diagnostic mammography is done for palpable masses and when screening mammography shows a suspicious mass (Fig. 7-8). The additional views and modalities used to evaluate palpable masses may reveal that an apparent finding is not significant (Fig. 7-9).

Not only does diagnostic mammography often require special and additional views beyond those used in routine screening, it also requires the direct supervision of a radiologist. When done for a palpable suspected mass, a radiopaque marker is placed on the skin overlying the mass.

The quality of the diagnostic process for palpable masses begins with your physical examination and continues with a properly written order for diagnostic mammography. This must include a (brief) description of the nature of the mass on physical examination (e.g., mobile vs. immobile, tenderness, and an estimate of size) and location within the breast as shown in Table 7-2.

This minimal effort in communication ensures that diagnostic imaging is focused upon the specific clinical concern. Women older than approximately 30 years of age who have a suspicious mass should be evaluated first by diagnostic mammography, followed by ultrasonography if necessary. Younger women should be first evaluated with ultrasonography, supplemented with mammography when needed.

Interpretation

When benign palpable lumps, such as cysts or fibroadenomas, are visible on mammography, they often have well defined (sharp) margins. Another common description is that they are well circumscribed. Such features suggest benign histology. Often, definitive diagnosis is then established with ultrasonography as shown in Figure 7-10.

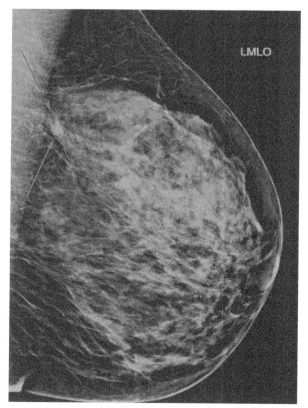

FIGURE 7-8 Screening mammogram showing a possible developing density (arrows). Coded as BI-RADS 0. The patient was notified and was scheduled for diagnostic mammography to evaluate the potential finding of the screening exam (see Fig. 7-9).

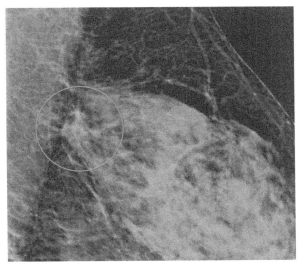

FIGURE 7-9 Spot compression mammogram showing that the apparent new density or mass (blue circle) suggested on the screening mammogram was not a persistent imaging finding; additional views also showed no mass. The apparent finding on screening was caused by overlapping densities. Coded as BI-RADS 1.

TABLE 7-2 **Sample Diagnostic Mammography Requisition Information**

Modality	Body Region	Clinical Data/History
Diagnostic mammography	Right breast	Non-tender 2–3 cm mass in upper outer right breast, not freely mobile. No prior screening.

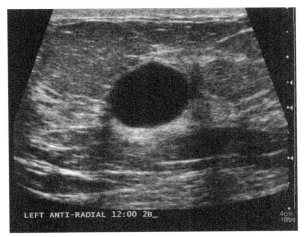

FIGURE 7-10 Ultrasound of a palpable mass that has characteristic features of a simple breast cyst; it is anechoic, with acoustic enhancement deep to the cyst. Coded as BI-RADS 2.

CASE UPDATE

The 39-year-old patient with the breast mass was referred for diagnostic mammography and breast ultrasound. The imaging order indicated that physical examination revealed a freely mobile, slightly tender mass in the far lateral left

breast in the 3:00 position. The patient had very nodular breast parenchyma on her diagnostic mammogram. At the location of the finding on physical exam, there was a water density or soft tissue density mass that had some sharp margins, but this lesion was not completely sharply marginated. Furthermore, some of the margins of the lesion were obscured by adjacent dense breast tissue. Because the mass did not meet mammographic criteria for a definitely benign lesion, ultrasonography was done, which revealed numerous simple benign breast cysts, the largest of which was the palpable mass. It was explained to the patient that cysts are not precancerous, may often decrease in size on their own, and do not require any intervention.

Solid masses that meet ultrasound criteria for benign fibroadenoma (see later section) do not have to be biopsied. Fibroadenomas are common solid breast tumors that have no malignant potential. They may be assigned BI-RADS 3, typically followed by repeat ultrasound in 6 months (Fig. 7-11). The patient shown in Figure 7-11 returned for follow-up sonography, at which time the lesion was found to be perfectly stable, and the imaging finding was reassigned to BI-RADS 2.

Adipose tissue can be locally quite firm and can give the impression of a mass or lump. When mammography shows entirely fatty tissue in the region of the breast where there is a possible mass, the presence of non-adipose structures (cysts or tumors) is very unlikely. Simultaneous palpation and sonography can show that a palpable lump is nothing more than a discreet adipose lobule (Fig. 7-12).

As noted earlier, the uneven distribution of different kinds of tissue can contribute to the impression of a breast lump. It is quite common that an apparent lump can be shown on ultrasound (Fig. 7-13) to be caused by locally thick fibroglandular tissue, sometimes referred to as a "fibrous ridge."

Breast cysts are very common, usually need no intervention, and are not premalignant. They often decrease in size on their own. When ultrasound reveals that a palpable lump is a cyst (see Fig. 7-10), there is no need for aspiration if the cyst is not painful; all that is needed is patient education.

If there is concern about a possible breast mass, you and your patient should get an answer that goes beyond "No cancer is seen" on the radiology reports. Ideally, a satisfactory explanation for a possible lump will be provided, such as a firm adipose lobule or focal collection of fibroglandular tissue, even when there is no specific benign pathologic structure, such as fibroadenoma or cyst.

Diagnostic mammography may reveal calcifications that are suspicious for breast cancer (Fig. 7-14) and in these cases, stereotactic biopsy is planned (Fig. 7-15).

Usually, the mammographic finding of a mass or architectural distortion is followed by ultrasonography for confirmation and to determine if an ultrasound-guided needle biopsy can be performed. When mammographic and sonographic findings are almost certain to represent a cancer, then a BI-RADS 5 may be assigned.

In some cases with uncertain findings on "conventional imaging" (mammography and ultrasound), or with unexplained discrepancy between imaging and physical examination, MRI can be used for further evaluation of a clinical concern. In MRI, breast cancers usually show significant enhancement with gadolinium-based contrast agents (Fig. 7-16).

Solid masses in the breast may be cancers or may be benign fibroadenomas. When a possible fibroadenoma has atypical features on sonography (and are assigned BI-RADS 4, rather than BI-RADS 3 with recommendation for follow-up), an ultrasound-guided needle biopsy is a minimally invasive way to establish the diagnosis (Fig. 7-17). Fibroadenomas do not become malignant and usually can then be ignored after tissue diagnosis.

Occasionally, lesions suspicious for cancer may only be visible on MRI. Many imaging departments and facilities now offer MRI-guided needle biopsies for those lesions.

When solid masses or calcifications are found in the breast that are mildly to highly suspicious for cancer, image-guided large core needle biopsy provides more than just a diagnosis of malignancy. A sufficient amount of tissue is provided to the pathologist for grading of the cancer and for testing of hormonal receptor status that provides a great deal of prognostic information and aids in surgical planning.

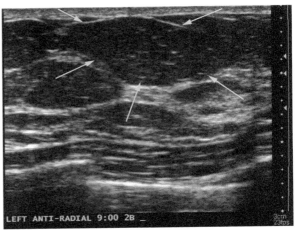

FIGURE 7-12 Ultrasound showing adipose lobule (arrows) at the location of a palpable mass.

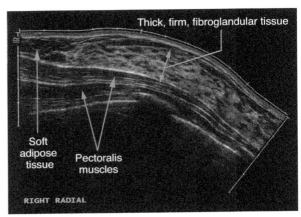

FIGURE 7-13 Ultrasound showing thick collection of normal brightly echogenic fibroglandular tissue where physical examination found locally firm tissue believed to be suspicious for a mass.

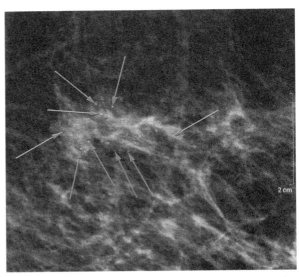

FIGURE 7-14 Image from diagnostic mammogram that was done after indeterminate calcifications were seen on screening study (see Fig. 7-7). The magnification view shown here displays calcifications (arrows) that are suspicious for malignancy far more clearly than on the routine screening views. This study was coded as BI-RADS 4.

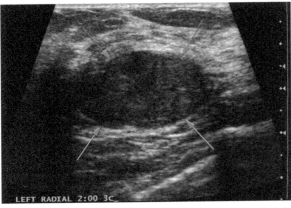

FIGURE 7-11 Ultrasound showing a solid mass (arrows) characteristic of fibroadenoma. Coded as BI-RADS 3.

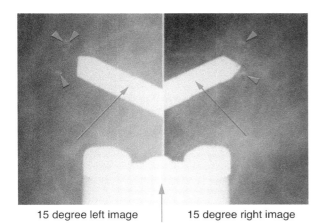

15 degree left image | 15 degree right image
Needle holder

FIGURE 7-15 Digital radiographic images obtained during stereotactic breast biopsy show the biopsy needle (arrow) in proper position within a suspicious cluster of microcalcifications (arrowheads).

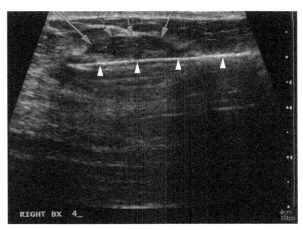

FIGURE 7-17 Ultrasound image showing biopsy needle (arrowheads) within a solid breast mass (arrows) during ultrasound-guided needle biopsy that established the benign diagnosis of fibroadenoma.

CASE CONCLUSION

It was explained to your patient that if the cyst should ever become painful, ultrasound-guided cyst aspiration would be recommended.

For symptomatic breast cysts, ultrasound-guided aspiration ensures complete cyst aspiration and allows for aspiration (Fig. 7-18) of adjacent cysts with a single skin puncture.

BREAST CANCER SCREENING IN THE HIGH-RISK PATIENT

There is widespread misunderstanding about what constitutes a high-risk personal and family history for breast cancer, as well as the importance of risk assessment in recommending breast cancer screening. In some cases, women may feel no need to undergo recommended screening because they have no family history of breast cancer. You must explain to patients that the majority of breast cancer is diagnosed in women with no family history or other high risk factors. In other situations, a woman may seek screening mammography at an inappropriately young age because she believes she has a "family history of breast cancer" based on breast cancer in her mother's third cousin, who was diagnosed at the age of 80.

Modalities

If one of your patients has a family history that includes a first degree relative who was diagnosed with premenopausal breast cancer, then she should begin yearly screening

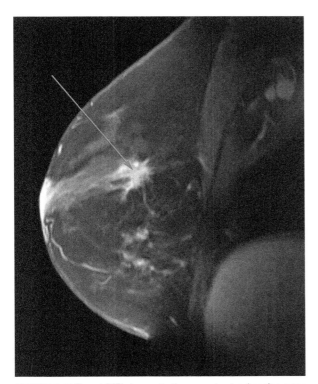

FIGURE 7-16 Breast MRI demonstrating a contrast-enhancing mass (arrow) suspicious for cancer.

COST EFFECTIVE MEDICINE

Image-guided needle biopsies are not only very well tolerated by patients and usually have minimal morbidity, but they are far less expensive than surgical biopsies.

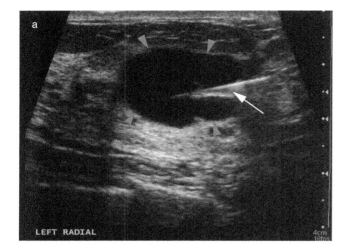
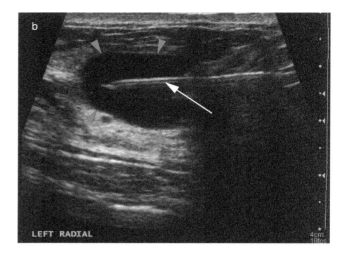
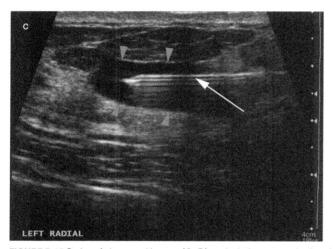
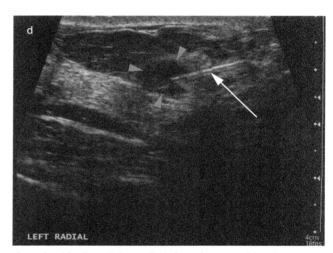

FIGURE 7-18 Series of ultrasound images **(A–D)** made during cyst aspiration. As the cyst (arrowheads) collapsed, the needle tip (arrow) was repositioned to assure that it stayed within the progressively decreasing fluid space.

mammography at an age 10 years younger than the age at which her relative was diagnosed. For patients with genetic risk for breast cancer, such as those with BRCA-1 and BRCA-2 mutations, referral to genetic counseling and/or to a comprehensive breast cancer program may be indicated. At the very least, discussion of your patient's situation with a radiologist is recommended if there is any question about when to start screening. In general, for women with a lifetime risk for breast cancer above a threshold value (typically 20%), an ideal screening program would be yearly breast MRI in addition to yearly screening mammography. A common recommendation is to stagger these studies at 6-month intervals.

One tool that can be used to determine an individual woman's risk for breast cancer is the Breast Cancer Risk Assessment Tool provided on the website of the National Cancer Institute (http://www.cancer.gov/bcrisktool/)

Interpretation

The objective interpretation of breast imaging in the high-risk patient is identical to those used in screening mammography (see earlier section). However, the "index of suspicion" for borderline or questionable imaging findings is elevated in the high-risk patient, and it may be appropriate to pursue borderline or questionable imaging findings more aggressively in these patients.

Chapter Review

Chapter Review Questions

1. A 50-year-old patient felt a lump in her breast during her shower yesterday morning. You order:
   A. screening mammogram.
   B. diagnostic mammogram (with ultrasound to follow, if indicated).
   C. breast ultrasound.
   D. breast MRI.
   E. breast-specific gamma imaging.

2. False negative mammography:
   A. is more likely in a fatty breast.
   B. refers to when two radiologists disagree on a diagnosis of breast cancer.
   C. refers to cancer not diagnosed on mammography when a cancer is present.
   D. is a good reason for not doing screening mammography.
   E. refers to identifying a mass as cancer when it is not.

3. Which of the following is true about the BI-RADS classification system?
   A. There are 10 categories ranging from 0 to 10 with 0 indicating a normal breast and 10 indicating metastatic disease
   B. Assignment of a BI-RADS category is recommended by the American Cancer Society but not mandatory for all breast radiology reports
   C. The BI-RADS assignment always results from mammography and not ultrasound exams
   D. BI-RADS 4 or 5 indicates the need for image-guided core needle biopsy
   E. BI-RADS categories 0 and 1 are for women at low risk for breast cancer

4. You have a patient with a BRCA-1 mutation, indicating a very high risk of breast cancer. It is likely that this patient would be advised to:
   A. have monthly screening mammograms.
   B. alternate screening mammograms and breast MRI at 6- month intervals.
   C. be examined monthly for palpable lumps with annual screening mammograms.
   D. have exploratory surgery of her breasts to look for and remove any cancer.
   E. have all her axillary lymph nodes removed to prevent any spread of cancer via the lymph system.

5. Which of the following is not true about breast lumps?
   A. They may be composed of only adipose tissue or a collection of normal fibroglandular tissue
   B. They may be cystic
   C. They may be benign fibroadenomas that never become malignant
   D. They are typically painful if they are cancer
   E. They are typically less mobile than normal breast tissue if they are malignant

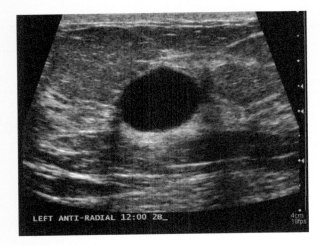

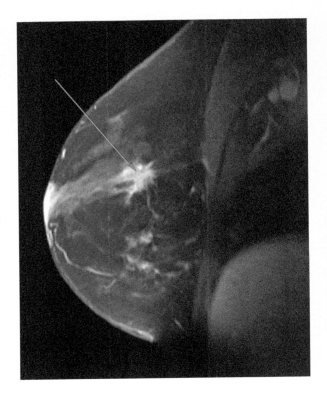

6. This ultrasound shows a palpable breast mass. What is it based on the image above?

   A. Solid mass

   B. Simple cyst

   C. Shadowing lesion suspicious for cancer

   D. Indeterminate lesion that determines MRI for further evaluation

   E. Adipose lobule

7. The arrows on the image above indicate:

   A. Benign calcifications

   B. Normal adipose tissue

   C. Enhancing mass in breast MRI

   D. Fibrous ridge

   E. Breast cyst

8 ABDOMEN

CASE STUDY

A 40-year-old-male comes into your clinic reporting increasing abdominal pain over the last 24 hours. You learn that the pain is mainly anterior in the midline, but that the patient also has some back pain. He reports no fever or respiratory symptoms. He has some nausea, but there has been no diarrhea. He does not seem to ascribe the onset of these symptoms to anything that he ate or drank. The medical history prior to this episode that is obtained may have gaps because the patient is new to your practice and is "not a good historian." You remember that the patient is not the "historian," you are. You realize that "taking" a good history sometimes means using email, telephone, and fax machines to get credible information. You remember that a solid history is fundamental to diagnosis prior to ordering an abdominal CT scan.

FUNDAMENTALS OF ABDOMINAL IMAGING

The large number of internal structures in the abdomen that can contribute to symptoms requires that a careful history, thorough physical examination, and laboratory findings guide the use of medical imaging. Pain is often "referred" to a location distant from a diseased organ, and understanding the varied patterns of clinical presentation must always inform your clinical impression.

Radiography is often an initial procedure for acute abdominal pain and for suspected bowel obstruction. CT scanning has become a fundamental initial diagnostic imaging tool when

significant abdominal disease is suspected and diagnosis is not established by other means, such as endoscopy. Abdominal ultrasound is widely available, commonly used, and the procedure of choice for certain abdominal conditions and trauma. MRI is assuming an important role in definitive characterization of specific abdominal conditions, but usually not in the acute setting. In oncologic imaging, PET scanning has become integral in the staging of patients who may have abdominal malignancies or cancers that have metastasized to the abdomen and/or retroperitoneum (Table 8-1).

TRAUMA

Acute penetrating or blunt abdominal trauma is almost always seen in the ED, so unless you are practicing in that environment, your involvement with such cases may be very limited, perhaps to providing follow-up care after such an episode. Nevertheless, we are providing detailed information on the imaging modalities and interpretations used in abdominal trauma here because you should be aware of these procedures when you are providing such follow-up care.

Modalities

For severe abdominal trauma seen in a hospital ED, ultrasound and contrast-enhanced CT have become more important than radiography. In the unstable patient who should not be transported to CT from the ED, portable radiographs are often obtained of the chest and abdomen. Ultrasonography can be performed simultaneously with resuscitation and stabilization of the patient. The Focused Assessment with Sonography in Trauma (FAST examination) is part of the standard

TABLE 8-1 **Sample Abdomen Radiology Requisition Information**

Modality	Body Region	Clinical Data/History
Radiography	Abdomen	Abdominal pain and distention, active bowel sounds; R/O obstruction
CT without and with contrast	Abdomen—pancreas protocol	Weight loss, vague abd pain, jaundice, dilated CBD on US; R/O pancreatic mass
CT without and with contrast	Abdomen and pelvis	Elevated liver enzymes, hx of stage IIIB lung ca; R/O mets
Ultrasound	Limited abdomen—right upper quadant	Acute right upper quadrant pain; R/O gallstones, cholecystitis
MRI with contrast	Abdomen	Uncertain nature of hepatic mass seen on ultrasound

Advanced Trauma Life Support (ATLS) protocol. Ultrasound is very specific: free fluid in the traumatized abdomen is almost certainly hemorrhage, and the patient can be triaged for immediate surgery. However, ultrasound does not have the extremely high sensitivity or specificity of contrast-enhanced (this phrase always refers to IV contrast material injection) CT and cannot completely replace the need for abdominal CT in the injured abdomen. The CT protocol used in blunt abdominal trauma typically includes an early arterial phase scan for CT angiography, and then a delayed scan, typically 60 to 70 seconds, to best reveal parenchymal injuries.

 Children, similar to adults, suffer hepatic, pancreatic, and splenic injuries with blunt abdominal trauma, but are more likely than adults to develop a duodenal hematoma. Blunt trauma to the anterior abdominal wall in a child may compress the duodenum between the anterior abdominal wall and the vertebral column, resulting in a duodenal wall hematoma. Symptoms may develop or progress during the subacute period after trauma. These may be evaluated by sonography and, if that is inconclusive, by CT scanning with oral contrast administration. This is often a dilute barium suspension but may be a "negative contrast agent," such as whole milk, that is seen as hypodense in the gastrointestinal lumen.

Severe abdominal trauma that results in abdominal bleeding occasionally requires arteriography with possible therapeutic embolization of the bleeding vessel, obviously an in-hospital procedure.

Renal injury is discussed in the genitourinary chapter of this book (see Chapter 9), although this separation is arbitrary; trauma patients may have any combination of abdominal and retroperitoneal injuries.

Interpretation

For both penetrating and blunt injuries to the abdomen, clinical stability of the patient and CT findings of relatively minor internal injuries may result in conservative management. However, when the FAST exam shows free abdominal fluid (Fig. 8-1) and the clinical picture is one of ongoing hemorrhage, the patient is most likely to need immediate surgery.

When the FAST exam is equivocal or negative and the clinical evaluation strongly suggests significant internal injury, contrast-enhanced CT scanning may reveal internal organ injuries not visible on a FAST exam, such as the hepatic laceration shown in Figure 8-2.

ABDOMINAL PAIN

Abdominal pain is common, often self-limiting, unrelated to serious illness, and certainly does not always require imaging. In this section, we discuss more serious abdominal

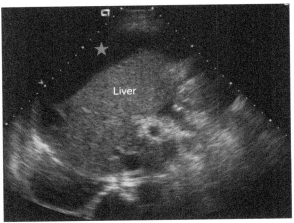
FIGURE 8-1 FAST exam showing intraperitoneal fluid (star). In the trauma setting, this is presumed to be blood.

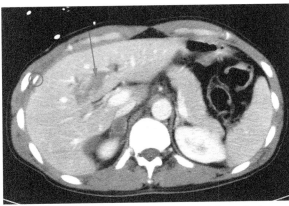
FIGURE 8-2 Contrast-enhanced CT showing hepatic laceration (arrow), the irregular hypointensity within the contrast-enhanced liver. Note the small displaced fragment of a fractured rib (circled).

pain that may require medical imaging for definitive diagnosis.

Modalities

The history and character of serious abdominal pain often provides clues to organ of origin. However, overlap of symptoms can be quite broad, hence the need for laboratory findings, imaging studies, and endoscopy. Laboratory findings such as presence or absence of leukocytosis, elevated bilirubin, anemia, or elevated hepatic or pancreatic enzymes must be correlated with radiographic findings. Radiography may be the initial imaging procedure done in the evaluation of some acute abdominal pain, especially when the clinical presentation suggests an acute small bowel obstruction.

 COST-EFFECTIVE MEDICINE
Radiography is a far more cost-effective means to rule out bowel obstruction than CT and, in the appropriate clinical setting, may be all the imaging that is needed.

An "acute abdominal series" includes a PA chest radiograph and supine and upright abdominal radiographs. However, a chronic presentation that suggests intermittent or partial small bowel obstruction is best examined with CT or MRI.

A standing PA chest radiograph is part of an acute abdominal series for three reasons: (1) Because basilar lung diseases such as pneumonia can cause referred pain to the upper abdomen; (2) to search for free abdominal air inferior to the diaphragm (well seen on the standard upright PA radiograph); and (3) a patient with severe abdominal pain may have a surgical emergency, and chest radiography is typically requested prior to general anesthesia.

Supine abdominal radiography is obtained to identify soft tissue masses, the intestinal gas pattern, calcifications, and abnormal gas collections.

When the clinical presentation suggests gastric/duodenal inflammatory mucosal disease or GERD, radiographic upper GI examination or endoscopy may be appropriate when the patient does not respond quickly to the usual medical treatment. The standard radiographic upper GI exam (including the esophagus, stomach, and duodenum) consists of radiographs obtained during a fluoroscopic examination. The patient typically swallows effervescent crystals to distend the upper GI tract with CO_2, and also a dense barium suspension that coats the GI mucosa. It is best to not order this as a "barium swallow," which could be misinterpreted as a dynamic swallowing study done for pharyngeal dysfunction.

As noted in Chapter 6, GERD often presents with chest pain, but symptoms may be centered at the epigastric region of the abdomen. A radiographic upper GI exam, or just an esophogram, may be an appropriate part of the workup for GERD.

When the clinical presentation of right upper quadrant abdominal pain suggests hepatobiliary disease, right upper quadrant abdominal sonography is the initial imaging procedure of choice. Patients with chronic unexplained right upper quadrant pain may have a functional biliary issue that can be evaluated with cholescintigraphy (also known as a HIDA scan), which measures gallbladder ejection fraction. Patients who are found to have a poorly contracting gallbladder may have relief of their symptoms by cholecystectomy.

When a patient presents with right lower quadrant abdominal pain, especially with fever and leukocystosis, and there is significant clinical concern for acute appendicitis, CT or ultrasonography is appropriate. Individual patient factors are often the most important aspects to consider when selecting between these two diagnostic procedures, as described below. If you remain uncertain about which procedure to choose for an individual patient, consultation with a radiologist is worthwhile.

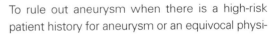

COST-EFFECTIVE MEDICINE
Ultrasonography (with graded compression over the right lower quadrant) can be highly effective in establishing a diagnosis of acute appendicitis and is preferred in pregnant and in pediatric patients. In addition to avoiding ionizing radiation, ultrasound is much less expensive than CT.

However, ultrasonography is less effective in adults and much less effective in the obese. Therefore, CT scanning is more widely used than ultrasonography for the adult (nonpregnant) patient who may have acute appendicitis. There is some variation in radiologic practice with respect to administration of oral and intravenous contrast enhancement when performing CT in this clinical situation. You should consult with a radiologist if you are uncertain about this issue when ordering an exam.

A pulsatile abdominal mass is suspicious for abdominal aortic aneurysm and can be diagnosed readily with ultrasonography, except in the very obese patient. Rapid ultrasound diagnosis of an abdominal aneurysm in the ED in a hemodynamically unstable patient whose aneurysm may have ruptured is obviously preferable to transporting such a patient for CT. For the stable patient, contrast-enhanced CT provides more information for preoperative planning than ultrasonography. Catheter angiography with stenting may be used for non-surgical treatment of an aneurysm.

COST-EFFECTIVE MEDICINE
To rule out aneurysm when there is a high-risk patient history for aneurysm or an equivocal physical exam, or to follow up on a small aneurysm, ultrasonography is far less expensive than CT. A one-time screening exam is recommended for all male smokers age 65 to 75. As part of the Welcome to Medicare physical exam, men in this category and all men and women with a family history of abdominal aortic aneurysm qualify for a one-time no–co-pay ultrasound screening exam.

Criteria for surgery may vary slightly between surgical practices and for individual patients, but generally an abdominal aortic aneurysm is not considered for repair until it has reached 5.0 to 5.5 cm in diameter or shows enlargement greater than 1 cm in a year. Until that point, ultrasound is sufficient, but then CT arteriography should be done for planning of stenting or surgical grafting.

If the physical examination suggests that a palpable abdominal "mass" in a patient with a distended or uncomfortable abdomen might be a dilated loop of bowel with a GI obstruction, then abdominal x-ray can be a fast and simple approach to a diagnosis.

Routine abdominal CT scans for suspected abdominal masses usually involve a single scan done with oral and IV contrast enhancement (resulting in lower patient radiation exposure than scanning "without and with" IV contrast). Acquisition of unenhanced CT in addition to IV-enhanced CT is best done only for very specific clinical conditions, such as when renal or pancreatic disease or possible hepatic steatosis is suggested by clinical history. For pancreatic disease, a common pancreatic protocol would include late arterial phase (30–35 seconds after starting the IV injection) and portal venous phase (approximately 65 second delay) scans.

Occasionally, studies such as CT, MRI, or cholescintigraphy, are indicated in patients with right upper quadrant abdominal pain—usually only when ultrasound reveals a very complicated case or an unexpected finding, such as possible tumor, or when ultrasound fails to provide an explanation for the right upper quadrant pain. CT is readily available and easy for the patient to tolerate. MRI has the advantage of improved visualization of the biliary and pancreatic ductal systems, an issue that will be discussed in more detail in the section on Jaundice later in this chapter.

Interpretation

Figure 8-3 shows free abdominal air inferior to the diaphragm on a standing PA radiograph, indicating the presence of a

perforated viscus. In a decubitus abdominal radiograph, the air would appear in the patient's flank.

In examining abdominal radiographs for bowel abnormalities, the mucosal folds provide an important clue as to the location of the abnormality. When mucosal folds traverse the entire width of an air-filled loop of bowel, as in Figure 8-4, that segment of the GI tract is identified as small bowel. These folds are more conspicuous in the jejunum than in the ileum. Air-filled loops of large bowel have characteristic partial-width folds (haustrations) as shown in Figure 8-5.

Upright abdominal radiography demonstrates gastrointestinal air–fluid levels. The appearance of "stepladder" air–fluid levels in small bowel loops, with an airless (or almost airless) colon, suggests the presence of an acute small bowel obstruction (Fig. 8-6). Air–fluid levels without this pattern may indicate a

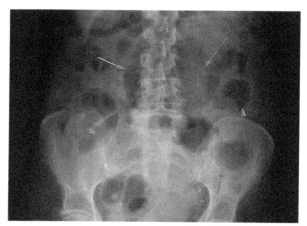

FIGURE 8-4 Supine abdominal radiograph showing dilated small bowel loops (arrows).

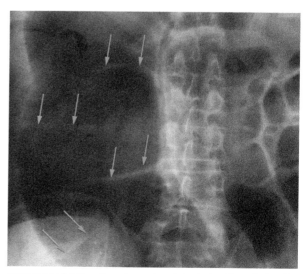

FIGURE 8-5 Small portion of a supine abdominal radiograph showing dilated ascending colon secondary to a distal large bowel obstruction. Note the haustral folds (arrows), which, unlike mucosal folds in the ileum, do not extend across the entire lumen.

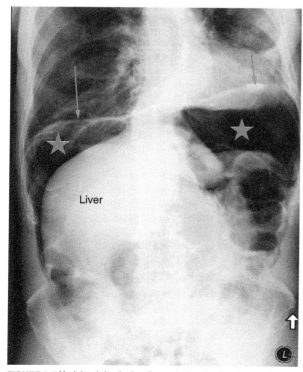

FIGURE 8-3 Upright abdominal radiograph showing free intraperitoneal air (stars) beneath diaphragm (arrows) from perforated viscus.

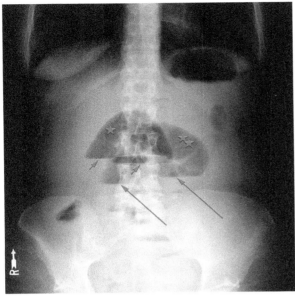

FIGURE 8-6 Small bowel obstruction showing stepladder configuration of two distended small bowel loops that are superimposed in the AP projection. Within each loop (one indicated with one star, the other with two stars) there are air–fluid levels at different heights (arrows).

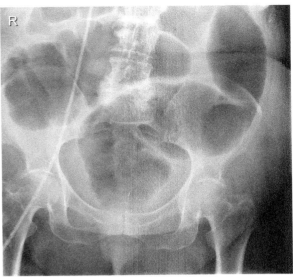

FIGURE 8-8 Supine abdominal radiograph showing a dilated large bowel that extends to the rectosigmoid colon, secondary to an obstructing rectal carcinoma.

"paralytic ileus" (Fig. 8-7), meaning the loss of normal peristalsis secondary to an inflammatory or ischemic process.

When you see any part of the large bowel to be greatly dilated, as is the rectosigmoid colon in Figure 8-8, you should suspect a large bowel obstruction; in this case, the patient had an obstructing rectal cancer.

A special case of distal large bowel obstruction is the sigmoid volvulus, a twisting of the sigmoid colon that can occur with a redundant sigmoid mesocolon (Fig. 8-9). Although unusual, cecal volvulus can also occur.

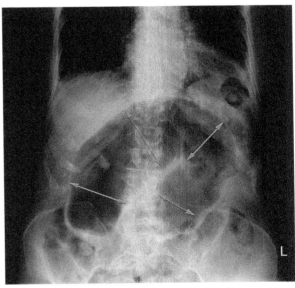

FIGURE 8-9 Abdominal radiographs showing a dilated loop of sigmoid colon (double-headed arrows) caused by sigmoid volvulus.

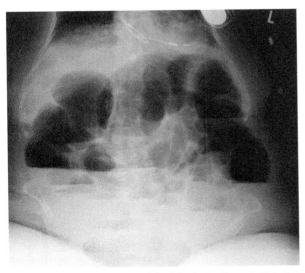

FIGURE 8-7 Paralytic ileus on upright abdominal radiograph. Note that air–fluid levels are at the same height within each dilated loop of bowel (no stepladding).

There are a variety of extraluminal gas collections that do not result in free intra-peritoneal air, such as in an abscess or pneumatosis coli (air or gas in the bowel wall; Fig. 8-10). A finding of pneumatosis coli suggests mesenteric vascular occlusion with ischemia or infarction of the bowel.

Characteristic calcifications may refine radiographic diagnosis in the patient with an acute abdominal condition. Most gallstones are not calcified (low sensitivity of radiography), but the presence of faceted calcifications in the right upper quadrant of the abdominal radiograph shown in Figure 8-11 is definitive for cholelithiasis. A calcification

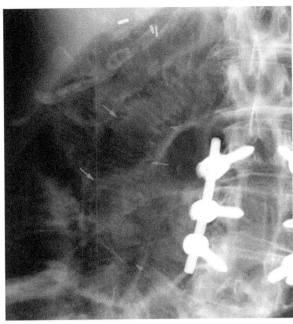

FIGURE 8-10 Magnified section of AP abdominal radiograph showing pneumatosis of a small bowel loop (arrows). Note internal fixation hardware in the lumbar spine and surgical clips in the right upper quadrant (probably prior cholecystectomy).

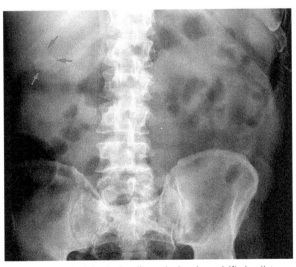

FIGURE 8-11 AP abdominal radiograph showing calcified gallstones (arrows).

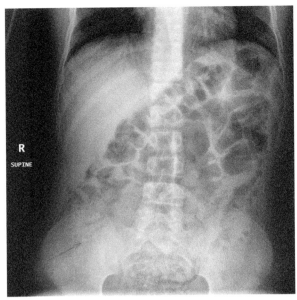

FIGURE 8-12 Appendicolith (arrow) visible on abdominal radiograph.

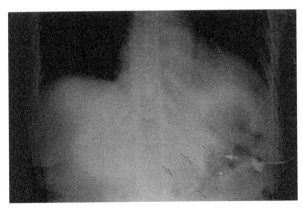

FIGURE 8-13 Radiograph showing calcifications in pancreas (chronic pancreatitis).

in the right lower quadrant of the abdomen in a patient with acute right lower quadrant pain may represent an appendicolith supporting a diagnosis of appendicitis. These are more commonly visible on CT scanning for acute appendicitis than on radiographs (Fig. 8-12). In the patient shown in Figure 8-13, calcifications in his pancreas are evidence of chronic pancreatitis, which, if associated with acute abdominal pain, would increase your diagnostic suspicion of recurrent pancreatitis.

CASE UPDATE

Your patient with abdominal pain is not severely ill. Laboratory results show mildly elevated amylase and lipase but are otherwise not remarkable. The "poor historian" patient did relate that he has had his gallbladder removed, but you wanted details rarely available from a patient and you get a faxed surgical report, as well as available clinical notes from a facility where the patient had been seen previously. You also get a faxed report from abdominal x-rays the patient had elsewhere, which revealed pancreatic calcifications.

Esophagitis can be diagnosed on an upper GI study by the presence of mucosal edema, a nodular mucosal pattern, or visible erosions or ulcertations. As is common, the patient shown in Figure 8-14 had GERD and a sliding hiatus hernia, which is easily demonstrated on a radiographic upper GI exam (Fig. 8-14).

Hypertrophic gastric mucosal folds and mucosal erosions found in gastritis/ulcer disease of the stomach can be demonstrated with the upper GI exam, and these findings often correlate with a positive test for *Helicobacter pylori*.

As evident in Figure 8-15, mucosal ulcerations in the gastic and duodenal mucosa are visible as collections of barium that "puddle" within such lesions.

Gallstones are clearly shown as brightly echogenic structures within the gallbladder lumen that cause acoustic

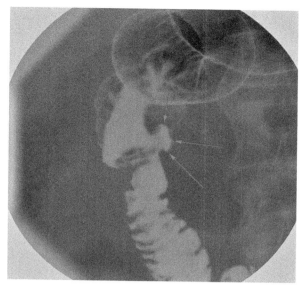

FIGURE 8-15 Duodenal ulcer (postbulbar ulcer just beyond the duodenal bulb) shown on radiographic upper GI exam (arrows).

shadowing on right upper quadrant ultrasound exam (Fig. 8-16). In the patient with acute cholecystitis shown in Figure 8-16, the gallbladder wall is edematous on ultrasound; in severe cases, there may be fluid around the gallbladder.

A finding that strongly suggests acute cholecystitis on cholescintigraphy is the failure to see activity in the gallbladder, indicating mechanical or functional obstruction of the cystic duct. Ultrasound finding of dilatation of the biliary system indicates the presence of an obstruction. In a patient with biliary colic, a small impacted calculus in the distal common bile duct (choledocholithiasis) may explain the presence of a dilated common bile duct. However, this may be very difficult

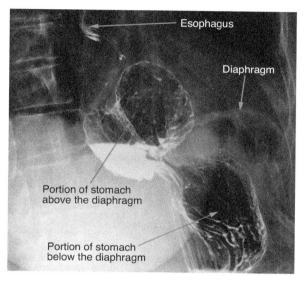

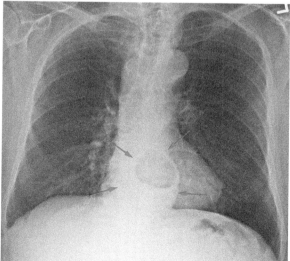

FIGURE 8-14 Top: Hiatus hernia shown on upper GI exam; radiograph done while the patient was standing. Note pool of barium collecting in the dependent aspect of the part of the stomach herniated above the diaphragm. **Bottom:** A large hiatus hernia (arrows) is occasionally obvious on a routine chest radiograph. Note the normal gastric air–fluid level above the diaphragm in this case.

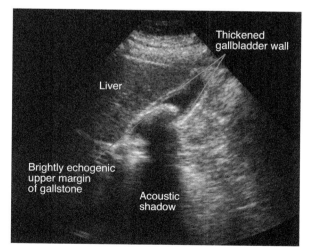

FIGURE 8-16 Right upper quadrant abdominal ultrasound demonstrating the presence of cholelithiasis and a thickened gallbladder wall that suggests acute cholecystitis.

to visualize on ultrasound, and other modalities such as CT or MRI with MR cholangiopancreatography (MRCP), may be necessary.

An ultrasound image of a liver, such as in Figure 8-17, that shows bright echogenicity of the liver in the near field and poor transmission of the ultrasound beam suggests hepatic steatosis. This diagnosis may be supported by elevated liver enzymes and upper quadrant discomfort (Fig. 8-17).

Incidental simple benign liver cysts may be found on right upper quadrant sonography. The brightly echogenic hepatic mass shown for the patient depicted in Figure 8-18, who does not have an oncologic history, is most likely a benign cavernous hemangioma.

Pancreatitis can be caused by a small biliary calculus impacted at the ampulla of Vater (hepatopancreatic ampulla). Even if the choledocholithiasis itself is difficult to see, an ultrasound exam on a patient such as the one shown in Figure 8-19, who has acute pancreatitis and the presence of many small gallbladder calculi or "biliary gravel" (indicated by arrows in the figure), strongly suggests this etiology.

In severe cases of acute pancreatitis, CT scanning is used to evaluate potential surgical complications, such as pancreatic necrosis and the development of pancreatic pseudocysts.

CASE UPDATE

Your patient with the abdominal pain and the history of pancreatic calcifications did not return for follow-up and you haven't seen the patient for 6 months. He comes in again with a complaint of abdominal pain. You learn that he was admitted to the hospital 2 months ago after being seen in the ED for abdominal pain, and was discharged after 1 week. You get records from the hospitalization, including the radiology report, which indicated an edematous pancreatic body and tail but no pancreatic necrosis or discrete fluid collection. You order laboratory studies, including amylase and lipase levels.

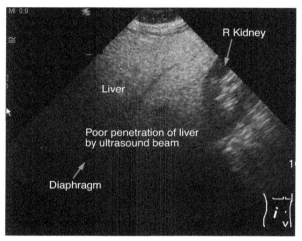

FIGURE 8-17 Ultrasound image of a liver with steatosis that results in bright echogenicity of the liver in the near field and such poor transmission of the ultrasound beam through the steatotic liver that it is often extremely difficult to see the diaphragm.

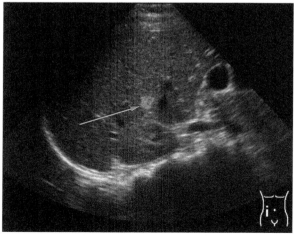

FIGURE 8-18 Hepatic ultrasound image showing a hyperechoic mass (arrow). Most lesions with this sonographic appearance are proven, by CT or MRI, to be benign cavernous hemangiomas.

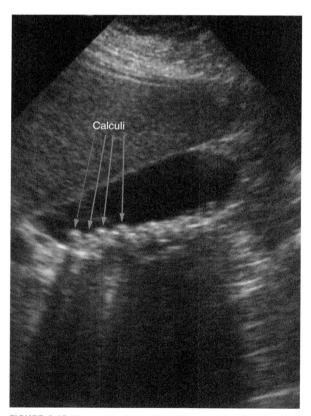

FIGURE 8-19 Ultrasound of a gallbladder containing "small stone" cholelithiasis or "biliary gravel."

Ultrasonography cannot always exclude a diagnosis of acute appendicitis but may help establish that diagnosis when it reveals a distended and non-compressible appendix with a diameter greater than 6 to 7 mm (Fig. 8-20). A conspicuously thickened appendiceal wall and fluid surrounding the appendix support that diagnosis.

CT reveals similar findings for a diagnosis of acute appendicitis often, as is the case in Figure 8-21, with the additional imaging finding of increased density of fat in the region of the appendix. This represents evidence of inflammatory change. In addition, calcified concretions of fecal material may form fecoliths, which may be called appendicoliths if in the appendix. A normal appendix and normal periappendiceal fat on CT excludes the presence of appendicitis. In advanced, subacute cases of perforated appendix, an abscess may develop as shown by the long arrows in Figure 8-22.

When a patient presents with left lower quadrant abdominal pain, fever, and leukocytosis and the clinical concern is for diverticulitis, the CT demonstration of diverticulosis with associated colonic mural thickening and pericolonic inflammatory changes supports a diagnosis of diverticulitis, which can often be treated medically. In more severe cases, peridiverticular abscesses are clearly demonstrated. In that case, CT findings may lead to percutaneous drainage or surgery. Figure 8-23 shows divericulitis in its most common location, the sigmoid colon. Note the inflammatory changes (increased density) in the sigmoid mesocolon (arrowhead).

Mesenteric ischemia may present with subacute symptoms in a stable patient. The bowel wall thickening associated with GI mural ischemia is sometimes nodular, resulting in an appearance that you may see described in a radiology

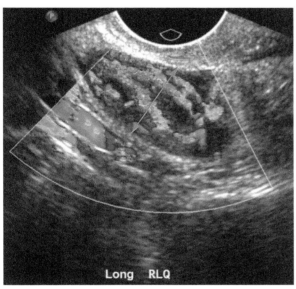

FIGURE 8-20 Ultrasound image in the right lower quadrant of the abdomen, long axis view, of a thickened and distended appendix (double-headed arrow) well above the maximum normal diameter of 7 mm. Color flow Doppler signal shows hyperemia. This ultrasound finding was at the location of point tenderness in the RLQ.

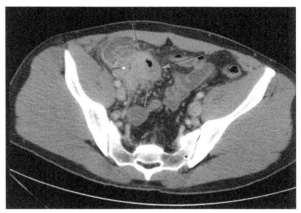

FIGURE 8-22 Axial CT showing peri-appendiceal abscess (arrows) and appendicolith (arrowhead).

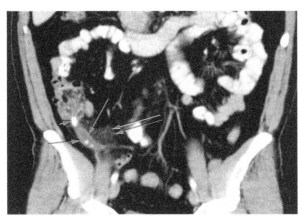

FIGURE 8-21 Coronal CT with fluid-distended appendix (long arrows), appendicolith (short arrow) and peri-appendiceal mesenteric edema (double arrow), indicating acute appendicitis.

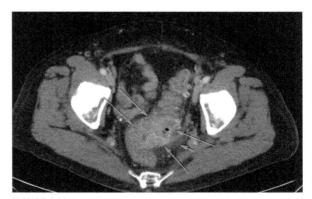

FIGURE 8-23 Axial CT that shows a thickened segment of the sigmoid colon (long arrows) and increased density in the sigmoid mesocolon (short arrow). Normally, fat adjacent to the colon is very dark. Inflammatory disease in the bowel results in tissue edema, and lymphatic and vascular engorgement in adjacent mesenteric or retroperitoneal fat, increasing its density and resulting in the appearance of "streaky" linear densities in pericolonic fat.

172

Chapter 8

report as thumbprinting. This nodular appearance of GI mural thickening can be also be seen with intramural hemorrhage. Elderly patients may present with an abdominal catastrophe of acute mesenteric vascular occlusion and intestinal infarction. A radiographic sign worrisome for such bowel infarction is intramural pneumatosis. In advanced cases of bowel infarction, gas may be seen in mesenteric and portal veins. The most specific finding for mesenteric vascular insufficiency is the presence of arterial stenosis (Fig. 8-24) or intraluminal arterial clot. Mesenteric venous thrombosis causing intestinal ischemia is rare.

JAUNDICE

Severe liver failure may cause jaundice. It is often clear from laboratory studies that this is the case, rather than obstruction of the biliary tract. However, when patients present with jaundice and the liver function studies do not suggest severe diffuse liver disease, the differential diagnosis must include obstruction of the biliary system. Causes of obstructive jaundice include choledocholithiasis and malignant obstructions of the biliary tract, either maligancies of the biliary tract itself, ampullary tumors, or pancreatic tumors.

Modalities

For clinically suspected obstructive jaundice, the initial imaging procedure is usually ultrasonography, both to confirm the pathophysiology by demonstrating obstructive dilatation of the biliary tract and often to demonstrate what is causing the obstruction. Commonly, definitive diagnosis of the specific cause for biliary obstruction is established with

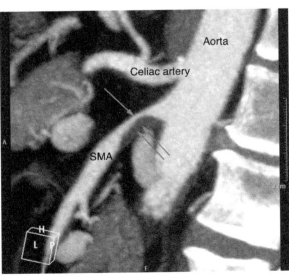

FIGURE 8-24 Sagittal CT that shows a stenosis (arrow) of the superior mesenteric artery (SMA) cause by mural thrombus/fatty atherosclerotic plaque (double arrow).

contrast-enhanced CT or MRI after ultrasound diagnosis of an obstructed biliary system.

COST-EFFECTIVE MEDICINE
When a patient more than 50 years of age presents with painless obstructive jaundice, especially if there is a history of weight loss and vague back pain, the clinical differential diagnosis should have pancreatic tumor at the top of the list and it is appropriate to proceed directly to CT, bypassing ultrasonography. Although ultrasound is less expensive than CT, one imaging examination is always less expensive than two procedures done when the first procedure is unable to provide a definitive diagnosis and comprehensive evaluation.

When laboratory studies indicate non-obstructive jaundice, ultrasonography may be appropriate to search for evidence of liver disease, such as tumor or steatosis. When diagnosis of hepatic parenchymal disease is not established by laboratory data and ultrasonography, more definitive imaging of hepatic parenchyma is obtained with CT or MRI.

It is important to consider the variety of abdominal CT scanning protocols and provide appropriate clinical history on orders for CT scans associated with jaundice. For obstructive jaundice, a "pancreas protocol" contrast-enhanced abdominal CT scan is ideal. This usually includes initial unenhanced CT scanning to identify calcifications, scanning during the optimal phase of pancreatic parenchymal enhancement, and scanning with the optimal timing for hepatic opacification. This scanning protocol is not only ideal for identifying the most common pancreatic neoplasms, but also provides a moderately good visualization of the common bile duct.

Abdominal contrast-enhanced MRI with MRCP may be needed for ideal depiction of the biliary and pancreatic tracts and is an excellent alternative to endoscopic cholangiopancreatography.

Interpretation

Dilatation of the intrahepatic biliary system on ultrasonography (Fig. 8-25) confirms a clinical and laboratory diagnosis of obstructive jaundice.

The finding of intrahepatic biliary dilatation without dilatation of the common bile duct raises the suspicion of intrahepatic tumor, such as cholangiocarcinoma. The finding of dilated intrahepatic ducts in both the left and right hepatic lobes and the absence of a dilated common bile duct may indicate the presense of malignancy at the confluence of the right and left major hepatic ducts, known as a Klatskin tumor.

More commonly, a patient with obstructive jaundice will be found to have dilated intrahepatic and extrahepatic ducts.

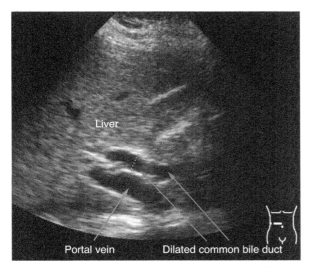

FIGURE 8-25 Ultrasound image showing a dilated common bile duct. Note the short dashed line in the duct that is the electronic caliper measurement of the duct.

The finding of cholelithiasis in the gallbladder may increase the likelihood that a benign process, choledocholithiasis, is causing the obstruction. The suspicion that obstruction of the CBD is caused by a calculus is increased if the patient has many tiny calculi ("biliary gravel") in the gallbladder that are more likely pass through the cystic duct into the common bile duct (see Fig. 8-19).

When there is a dilated common bile duct and no cholelithiasis is visible, the differential diagnosis becomes one of pancreatic or ampullary tumor. These tumors can often be seen on ultrasound, but usually contrast-enhanced CT is done, as shown in Figure 8-26, either for tumor detection or preoperative planning. MRI is also excellent for demonstration of pancreatic cancer.

Contrast-enhanced MRI is excellent for demonstrating biliary and pancreatic tumors. MRCP (a fluid-sensitive MR sequence that does not require any contrast material) demonstrates bililary strictures, malignant obstructions, and the intraluminal filling defects of common bile duct calculi (Fig. 8-27).

GI BLEEDING

When a patient has hematemesis, the presumption is made of an upper GI source of bleeding. When there is no hematemesis, the presence of black stool, age greater than 50 years, and elevated blood-urea-nitrogen (BUN) levels suggest upper GI bleeding. Common causes include esophageal varices and gastric and duodenal ulcers. Up to 25% of occult GI blood loss may be from the small bowel. The most common cause of lower GI bleeding is diverticulosis, followed by angiodysplasia. The number of pathologic

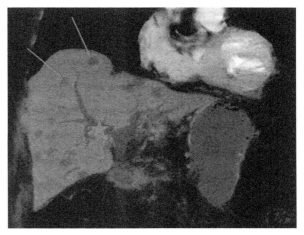

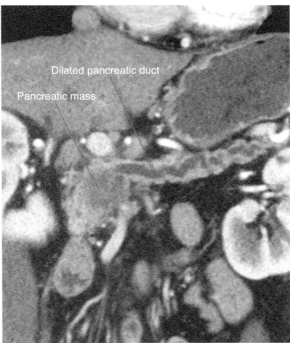

FIGURE 8-26 Contrast-enhanced CT abdomen, coronal minimum intensity projection display **(top)** showing dilated biliary system (star) and metastatic tumors in the liver (arrows). Oblique coronal reconstruction **(bottom)** from the same CT scan showing a pancreatic mass and a dilated pancreatic duct. This CT study was done shortly after ultrasonography showed a dilated biliary system.

conditions that can cause GI bleeding is quite large, and the mainstay of initial diagnosis is either fiberoptic or capsule endoscopy. However, imaging is often needed if endoscopy is not diagnostically or therapeutically difinitive.

Modalities

If endoscopy is negative in a patient with active upper GI bleeding, IV contrast-enhanced abdominal CT scanning and "negative oral contrast" (dark intraluminal contrast such as whole milk rather than bright barium or iodine) or no oral contrast material is recommended. In stable patients with

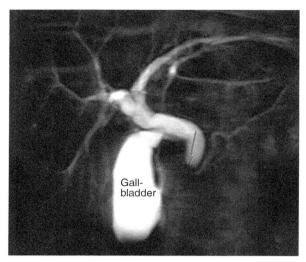

FIGURE 8-27 MRCP demonstrates a dilated biliary system (bright branching tubular structures) secondary to a calculus inpacted at the distal end of the common bile duct. The arrow points to the upper margin of the impacted calculus.

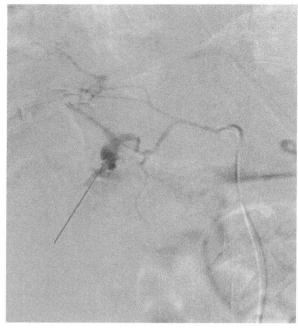

FIGURE 8-28 Abdominal angiogram. Selective catheterization of a branch of the SMA shows extravasation (arrow), locating the source of bleeding. Embolotherapy can then be done through the same catheter.

slow bleeding, a Tc-99m–labeled red blood cell radionuclide bleeding study or angiography is appropriate. This radionuclide bleeding study is sometimes useful in the diagnosis of intermittent lower GI bleeding if endoscopic diagnosis is elusive.

When endoscopy reveals a source of bleeding that does not respond to endoscopic treatment, catheter angiography is indicated. If the source of bleeding is found to be esophageal varices, the patient is usually referred to interventional radiology for a possible transjugular intrahepatic portosystemic shunt (TIPS) procedure.

CT is sometimes useful as a secondary procedure in patients with GI bleeding from varices—for example, in treatment planning. If the source of GI bleeding is a malignancy, CT or MRI may be used for staging.

Interpretation

Both catheter angiography and CT angiography may directly show extravasation into the lumen of a part of the GI tract if the study is done during active bleeding (Fig. 8-28). Catheter embolotherapy may provide definitive treatment.

If GI bleeding is at least 0.5 to 1 mL per minute, it may be detected by a radionuclide bleeding study, in which the radioactively tagged RBCs will accumulate in the segment of the GI tract where bleeding is occurring, localizing the source, which is the case shown in Figure 8-29.

Esophageal, abdominal, retroperitoneal, and abdominal wall varices are easily demonstrated on contrast-enhanced CT, especially with special image reconstruction techniques that highlight vascular structures, as demonstrated in Figure 8-30.

NON-SPECIFIC ISSUES, SUCH AS WEIGHT LOSS, VOMITING, AND ABNORMAL LABORATORY STUDIES

Besides the specific conditions discussed earlier in this chapter, there are many other indications for abdominal imaging. Routine laboratory study may suggest liver disease in an asymptomatic patient. Unexplained weight loss and other non-specific symptoms may prompt the search for an otherwise asymptomatic malignancy. In patients with a known malignancy, imaging is done for staging, follow-up to gauge treatment effectiveness, and to evaluate new clinical problems suspected of being caused by metastatic disease. In one special case, colorectal cancer screening, an abdominal imaging procedure is appropriately used for screening the asymptomatic patient.

Abdominal imaging is sometimes done as follow-up for small lesions found on prior imaging, such as small (<1 cm), solitary liver lesions and incidentally found adrenal masses.

Modalities

Virtual colonoscopy (CT colonography) is a low-dose CT scan performed while the colon is distended with air or CO_2, and the lumen of the colon is examined by a radiologist at a graphics workstation using advanced processing of the CT data. At the time of writing this chapter, conflicting opinions exist on the relative roles to be played by colonoscopy and virtual colonoscopy for colorectal cancer screening. Certainly,

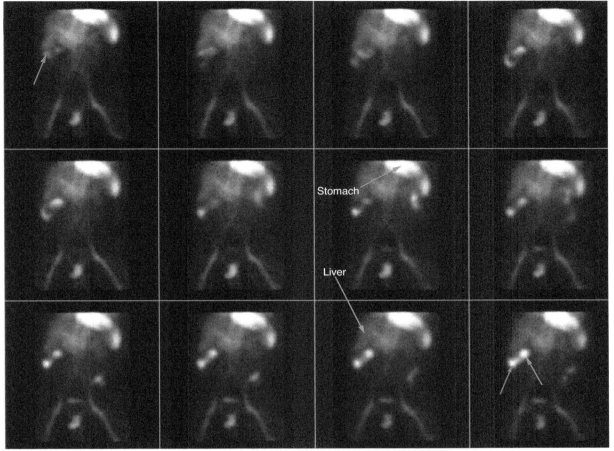

FIGURE 8-29 Radionuclide GI bleeding study that localizes GI bleeding to the ascending colon as an abnormal collection of activity (red arrows) in the right side of the abdomen on these sequential images recorded every five minutes after injection of radioisotope labeled RBCs.

colonoscopy has the advantage of allowing biopsy of any suspicious lesion that is found. However, a very large number of very small mucosal polyps (which are often biopsied) are benign hyperplastic lesions that are the mucosal equivalent of "skin tags."

COST-EFFECTIVE MEDICINE

Virtual colonoscopy is less expensive and has a lower complication rate than colonoscopy. Neither examination is perfect. The two studies are very comparable in sensitivity and specificity in the detection of clinically significant colon polyps.

During a radiographic barium enema exam, radiographs are obtained while the colon is either filled with barium (single contrast exam) or distended with air while barium coats the mucosa (an air-contrast or double contrast exam). This exam is now only used when a patient has an unsuccessful endoscopic exam or virtual colonoscopy.

When laboratory data suggest liver disease, right upper quadrant abdominal ultrasound, abdominal MRI, or abdominal CT is often appropriate, depending upon clinical history and severity of abnormal serum chemistry data. If CT is done, unenhanced scanning would be needed to properly assess the presence of hepatic steatosis. Abdominal MRI should be done with special imaging sequences optimized for detection of steatosis. Clinical data given on the order may be critical to the patient being scanned with the ideal protocol in either CT or MRI. Right upper quadrant abdominal ultrasound can identify hepatic steatosis and hepatic masses, although with somewhat lower sensitivity and specificity than CT or MRI.

If a mass is found on CT that has reliable characteristics of a benign lesion, such as a cavernous hemangioma, no further procedure is needed. However, if more definitive lesion characterization is needed after detection of a mass on abdominal CT or ultrasound, then contrast-enhanced MRI is the procedure of choice.

Patients at high risk for hepatocellular carcinoma (such as those with cirrhosis, chronic hepatitis, and hemochromatosis) are often followed with screening ultrasonography. When a mass is detected on initial imaging, contrast-enhanced CT or

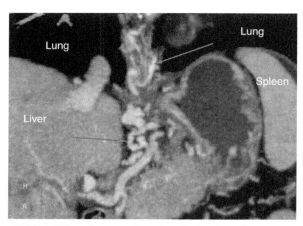

FIGURE 8-30 Coronal maximum intensity projection display from contrast-enhanced abdominal CT showing retroperitoneal and esophageal varices (arrows).

MRI is needed for further lesion characterization, and testing for serum alpha-fetoprotein (AFP) should be done.

When a patient with a known malignancy is suspected of having hepatic metastases, or is being staged, contrast-enhanced CT or MRI is appropriate. If the known malignancy may be a hypervascular hepatic metastatic tumor, such as pancreatic islet cell, renal cell, or thyroid cancer, the radiologist should be alerted so that an arterial phase scan is done, in addition to the routine portal venous phase scan.

For a growing number of malignancies, FDG PET-CT scanning is indicated for staging and evaluating response to cancer treatment.

Countless abdominal CT scans done each year result in the incidental finding of a small adrenal mass.

COST-EFFECTIVE MEDICINE
In patients with no known malignancy that might metastasize to an adrenal gland, the chance of malignancy in a smoothly marginated, small (>3–5 cm), incidentally found adrenal mass is extremely remote, and primary adrenal maligancies are rare. More important than any additional imaging would be appropriate laboratory tests to be sure that an adrenal mass is not a functioning adenoma causing hormonal issues, such as Cushing syndrome, or that the mass is not a pheochromocytoma.

Large bowel inflammatory disease is usually examined endoscopically, although occasionally CT may have an important role in complicated cases. Patients with suspected or known Crohn's disease are appropriately studied by contrast-enhanced CT or MRI (routine abdominal protocols, or CT or MR enteroclysis). The radiographic small bowel follow-through (a series of radiographs done after oral adminstration of barium suspension) is still widely used for small bowel disease, although capsule endoscopy may rapidly diminish the role of radiography.

In pediatric patients with Crohn's disease, abdominal ultrasonography may be useful but is highly dependant on the skill of the examining sonographer and/or radiologist.

Interpretation

After one of your patients undergoes virtual colonoscopy (CT colonography), you may have one of those professional pleasures of informing your patient that no worrisome findings were detected and that another similar screening exam for colorectal cancer should be done in 5 years.

When a polyp is detected, the radiologist not only reports its size, but may characterize the finding as pedunculated and smooth (likely benign histology) or sessile (flat), and describe whether or not it has an irregular shape or appears to be ulcerated (likely a malignant or premalignant lesion). However, morphology alone cannot accurately predict histology, and therefore the size as well as the shape of polyps found is generally used to decide if further study with endoscopy and biopsy is indicated. There is no universal agreement on such criteria. However, polyps under 5 mm pose such low risk that follow-up virtual colonoscopy in 5 years is considered appropriate. Above this size threshold, endoscopy and biopsy are typically recommended.

CT scanning done for non-specific issues such as weight loss or unexplained anemia or as a search for a primary tumor in a patient who presented with metastases from an unknown primary malignancy may reveal an otherwise clinically silent mass, such as the pancreatic islet cell tumor shown in Figure 8-31.

Abdominal imaging done for elevated liver enzymes in a patient with early or mild liver disease may reveal evidence

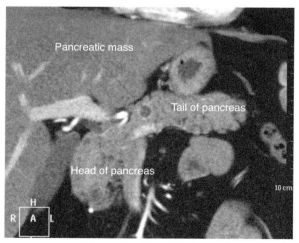

FIGURE 8-31 Coronal contrast-enhanced CT showing the presence of a small low-density pancreatic mass with rim enhancement in a patient who had metastatic disease from an unknown primary malignancy. Biopsy revealed an islet cell tumor.

Abdomen

of diffuse hepatic steatosis. With ultrasonography, the characteristic finding is that of hyperechoic parenchyma with very poor transmission of the ultrasound beam through the liver (see Fig. 8-17). In unenhanced CT, the "fatty liver" has reduced attenuation—that is, it is visually less dense than the spleen (Fig. 8-32). If the hepatic attenuation of liver parenchyma is so low that intrahepatic blood vessels are easily seen on unenhanced CT, then there is severe steatosis. Special MRI sequences are very sensitive to detecting steatosis. The presence or absence of steatosis should be explicitly stated on the radiology reports that you receive.

With chronic and advanced liver disease, as in the patient shown in Figure 8-33, the liver becomes fibrotic and has increased CT density. A cirrhotic liver has not only increased density but a nodular margin. With severe cirrhosis, ascites may be present (Fig. 8-33).

Patients with inherited forms of severe cystic kidney disease may also have a large number of large hepatic cysts that are evident on CT. However, most incidental benign hepatic cysts reported on CT can generally be ignored, as can the characteristically benign hepatic cavernous hemangioma, unless they are very large such as the one shown in Figure 8-34.

The characterization of liver masses is complex, but when the imaging workup (including contrast-enhanced MRI) leads to the conclusion that a mass is likely to be malignant, then image-guided core needle biopsy or surgical referral is needed.

Benign adrenal adenomas, such as the one shown in Figure 8-35, are typically small, smoothly marginated, and have low CT density on unenhanced CT.

Abdominal imaging evaluation for suspected metastatic disease may reveal multiple liver lesions, abdominal or retroperitoneal adenopathy, and adrenal or other organ metastases. Oncologic imaging is very demanding because there is no limit to the wide variety of disease that may be

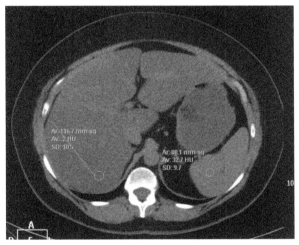

FIGURE 8-32 Axial unenhanced CT of the abdomen. The liver is visually less dense than the spleen, indicating hepatic steatosis. Density measurements in HU, shown on the image in green, were obtained to quantify the disorder.

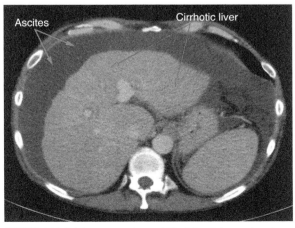

FIGURE 8-33 Axial contrast-enhanced CT of the abdomen that shows ascites and a cirrhotic liver with a nodular margin.

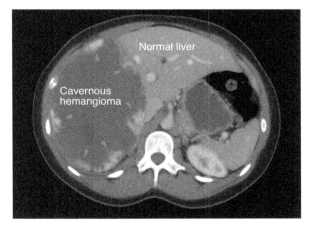

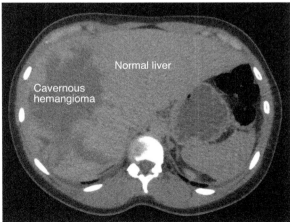

FIGURE 8-34 Axial multiphase contrast-enhanced CT. Portal venous phase scan (top) showing beaded peripheral enhancement of the large mass occupying virtually the entire right hepatic lobe. Ten-minute delay scan (bottom) showing the progressive centripetal (from periphery inward) enhancement that is characteristic of benign cavernous hemangioma.

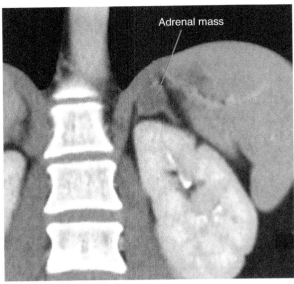

FIGURE 8-35 Coronal contrast-enhanced CT showing a small, smoothly marginated, low-density adrenal mass, most likely to be a benign adenoma.

encountered. An abdominal/pelvic CT scan, for example, may detect suspicious nodules at a lung base, abdominal or retroperitoneal neoplasm, and lytic or blastic bone disease in the portion of the visible skeleton.

The impression of gastrointestinal mural thickening is not reliable for a segment of gut that is contracted. However, the perception of mural thickening in a segment of gut that is at least moderately distended is a reliable sign of disease. In addition to mural thickening, visualization of tissue layers within the wall because of edema and hyperenhancement of the wall of a viscus are signs of inflammation (Fig. 8-36).

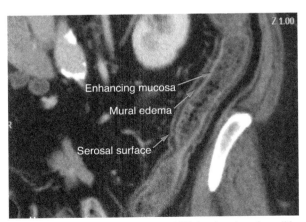

FIGURE 8-36 Coronal contrast-enhanced CT showing ulcerative colitis. Note the thickened colon wall, with mural edema and hyperenhancement of the mucosa.

CASE CONCLUSION

Your patient with the recurrent, chronic abdominal pain clearly has had chronic pancreatitis for a long time, evident to you from the moment you saw the old radiology report indicating the presence of pancreatic calcifications. Conservative medical treatment was essentially successful in treating your patient through an episode of acute pancreatitis during his most recent hospitalization. However, the persistent pain and anorexia prompted you to do appropriate serum blood chemistry studies; results showed mildly elevated or borderline serum lipase and amylase levels. You ordered a CT scan because of your clinical suspicion of a complication of pancreatitis. A pseudocyst (Fig. 8-37) of the body of the pancreas was found. You referred the patient to a surgeon.

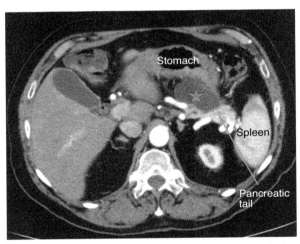

FIGURE 8-37 CT pancreatic pseudocyst (star) that developed after episode of acute pancreatitis.

Chapter Review

Chapter Review Questions

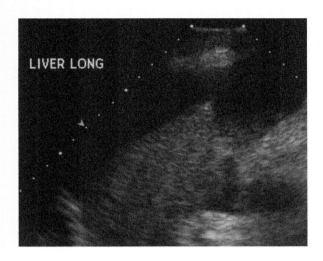

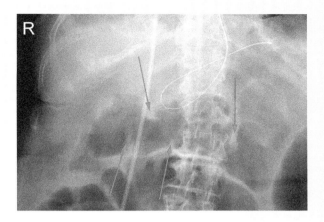

1. The image above was taken in an ED after an MVA. Which of the following is correct based on the anechoic areas shown in the image?

   A. The patient should be discharged

   B. The patient is likely to proceed immediately to surgery

   C. The patient should have a CTA

   D. The patient should have catheter angiography

   E. The patient should have a radionuclide study

2. In a pediatric patient with right lower quadrant abdominal pain, fever, and leukocytosis, the imaging "procedure of choice" is:

   A. abdominal MRI.

   B. abdominal CT.

   C. RLQ ultrasound.

   D. abdominal radiographic series.

   E. cholescintigraphy.

3. In the abdominal radiograph shown above of a patient complaining of abdominal distention and constipation, the loop of bowel with the prominent folds (arrows) is:

   A. characteristic of a dilated segment of jejunum.

   B. a sign of a small bowel obstruction.

   C. a distended segment of large bowel.

   D. an indication of the presence of a paralytic ileus and probable peritonitis.

   E. showing a good region of the abdomen to examine with ultrasound.

4. A radiology report on your patient mentions "thumbprinting" of bowel loops. Your patient may have:

   A. mesenteric ischemia.

   B. appendicitis.

   C. a duodenal ulcer.

   D. diverticulitis.

   E. polyps.

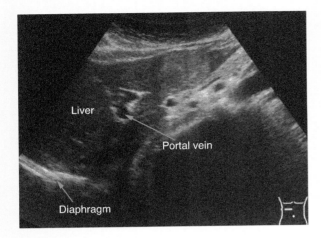

Liver

Portal vein

Diaphragm

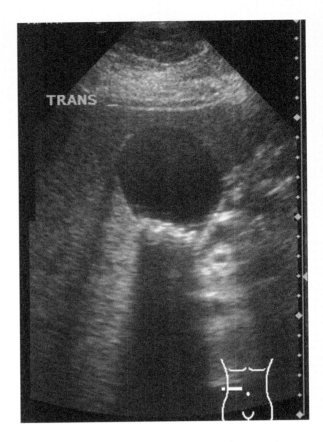

TRANS

5. During abdominal sonography (transverse image shown above), a mass is seen in the left lobe of the liver.

  A. It is hypoechoic to the rest of the liver and is likely to be malignant

  B. It is a normal variant

  C. The finding is what is causing the patient's pain. Surgical referral is indicated

  D. It is most likely a benign cavernous hemangioma

  E. A dilated biliary system

6. Pertaining to virtual and endoscopic colonoscopy:

  A. they are similar in cost.

  B. virtual colonoscopy has significantly less sensitivity than endoscopic colonoscopy.

  C. virtual colonoscopy has a lower complication rate than endoscopic colonoscopy.

  D. during endoscopic colonoscopy, only malignant polyps are biopsied.

  E. virtual colonoscopy cannot be done in patients with a pacemaker.

7. Which of the following imaging modalities cannot be used to identify hepatic steatosis?

  A. Radiography

  B. Ultrasound

  C. MRI

  D. CT

8. For a patient with pancreatitis, the image above would suggest:

  A. associated hepatic cancer.

  B. associated liver steatosis.

  C. associated choledocholithiasis.

  D. portal hypertension.

9. Your 60-year-old patient has left lower quadrant pain, tenderness to palpation, and leukocytosis. You order abdominal CT and it shows mural thickening of the sigmoid colon, with an edematous sigmoid mesocolon "consistent with acute diverticulitis." What do you do?

  A. You discuss the findings with the interpreting radiologist in order to get a recommendation for a good surgeon for your patient

  B. You discuss the findings with the interpreting radiologist in order to clarify whether or not there is any sign of abscess that may not respond to medical treatment (antibiotics)

  C. You refer the patient to interventional radiology for percutaneous drainage

  D. You order ultrasound to confirm the diagnosis

  E. You explain to the patient why immediate colonoscopy must be done to confirm the diagnosis

9 MALE AND FEMALE URINARY TRACT AND MALE GENITAL TRACT

CASE STUDY

A 49-year-old male presents with the acute onset of colicky left flank pain that started suddenly and is quite severe when it crescendos, which is characteristic of renal colic. Your suspicion of an acute obstructive uropathy caused by a ureteral calculus is supported by the finding of microscopic hematuria. You order an unenhanced helical CT of the urinary tract, renal stone protocol.

FUNDAMENTALS OF IMAGING THE MALE AND FEMALE URINARY TRACT AND MALE GENITAL TRACT

The imaging needed for the clinical management of urologic disorders ranges from very simple procedures for determining if there is a urinary tract obstruction to advanced imaging to evaluate urologic trauma and cancer (Table 9-1).

Imaging of the kidneys, ureters, and bladder follows a common clinical approach in both the male and the female. Ultrasonography can be used in specific clinical situations, as discussed later, as a relatively inexpensive procedure for basic visualization of the renal cortex, collecting systems, and bladder that avoids the use of contrast agents and does not expose a patient to ionizing radiation. However, more definitive examination of the renal cortex is achieved with CT and MRI, and ideal visualization of the renal collecting systems, ureter, and bladder depend upon filling those structures with contrast material that can be seen on radiographs or CT.

Anatomic differences result in specific issues for the male and female genital tracts. The imaging issues related to the female genital tract are discussed in Chapter 10. Imaging of the male urethra requires opacification with contrast material that can be seen on radiographs or CT. The prostate gland, testes, and related structures are visualized very well with ultrasonography, which is often a final, definitive imaging procedure.

TRAUMA

When there has been blunt trauma to the torso and the only finding during patient evaluation is microscopic hematuria, the indication for imaging is limited, often dependent upon patient factors, such as the presence or absence of other injuries, as well as individual practitioner practices and institutional policies.

With more severe blunt trauma to the torso and/or pelvis, there is often multisystem injury including to the urinary tract. The appropriate imaging in these circumstances is discussed in the abdominal trauma section of Chapter 8.

Modalities

When a patient has no signs of abdominal injury but has hematuria after blunt trauma, radiographs, contrast-enhanced CT of the abdomen and pelvis, and/or FAST exam (see Chapter 8) may be appropriate. However, with relatively minor trauma, the diagnostic yield from imaging is low.

When severe blunt trauma or penetrating injury to the torso raises clinical concern for major injury to the urinary tract, the procedure of choice is contrast-enhanced abdominal and pelvic CT. Institutional policies with respect to scanning protocols vary, but CT scanning in the trauma evaluation can be done with a multi-scan acquisition that includes an early arterial phase scan to detect vascular injury, as well as appropriately timed scanning for the best depiction of parenchymal injury. Portable abdominal radiographs are sometimes used in evaluating a trauma patient but should not delay a more definitive CT scan.

TABLE 9-1 Sample Uroradiology Requisition Information

Modality	Clinical Data/History
CT urinary tract, no contrast (renal stone exam)	Left flank pain, hematuria; R/O calculus
Renal and bladder ultrasonography	87-year-old male with progressive rise in BUN & creatinine; R/O obstructive uropathy
Renal ultrasound with Doppler	25-year-old male with hypertension
CT abdomen and pelvis without and with contrast (CT urography)	Family history medullary sponge kidney; may have passed several calculi (by history) but no prior workup
VCUG	8-year-old female; hx of numerous UTIs
Scrotal sonography	Painless mass (L); testicular?

In many EDs, it is routine to perform a FAST exam on all patients with trauma to the torso (see Chapter 8). This is most useful when there is severe blunt trauma to the torso accompanied by clinical signs of intra-abdominal injury, and is done rapidly "at the bedside." However, the FAST exam may not be needed when the mechanism of injury and clinical evaluation indicates only retroperitoneal injury, with no abdominal (intra-peritoneal) injury.

In the evaluation of bladder and/or urethral injuries, cystography or urethrography may be needed if CT scanning is not definitive for these injuries.

Interpretation

Severe trauma may result in a shear injury to the renal vascular pedicle. More commonly, renal injury involves parenchymal laceration, as shown by the red arrows in Figure 9-1, without or with disruption of the urinary collecting system. There has been an increasing trend to manage renal trauma patients non-operatively when they are hemodynamically stable. For the hemodynamically unstable patient with active bleeding, an alternative to surgery for renal injury is immediate catheter angiography with embolotherapy, as shown in Figure 9-2.

Pelvic injuries may cause disruption of the urinary bladder, especially if trauma occurred when the bladder was full. This can be seen on cystography or CT, as shown in the top and bottom images in Figure 9-3. When CT of the pelvis shows pubic fracture or wide diastasis of the pubic symphysis, there is high risk of associated urethral injury. In these cases, in order to avoid complications from transurethral catheterization, **urethrography** is performed before attempting insertion of a catheter into the bladder. If urethrography shows disruption of the urethra, as in Figure 9-4, suprapubic catheterization is usually done for urinary drainage, with delayed surgical repair of the urethra.

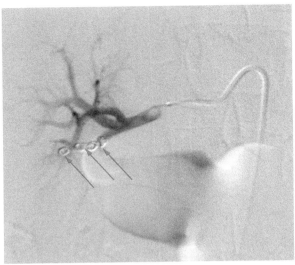

FIGURE 9-2 Angiogram after placement of coils (arrows) into a lower pole branch renal artery, successfully occluding the artery, which was bleeding. The patient injured the kidney in an MVA.

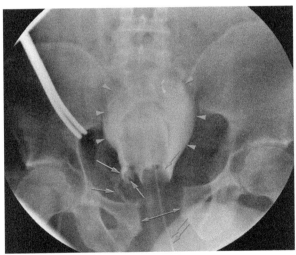

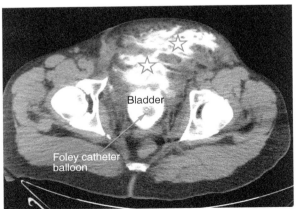

FIGURE 9-3 **Top:** Extravasated urine (red arrows) from a bladder rupture shown on a retrograde cystogram that was done on a patient who had been in an MVA. Note the diastasis of the pubic symphysis (double-headed red arrow). Contrast material was injected through a Foley catheter (double blue arrow), distending the bladder with opacified urine (arrowheads). The catheter is kept in place by inflation of a balloon near the tip of the catheter (blue arrow). **Bottom:** Axial CT showing extravasated urine (stars) from bladder rupture after trauma.

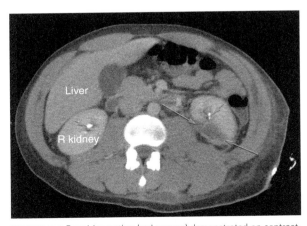

FIGURE 9-1 Renal laceration (red arrows) demonstrated on contrast-enhanced CT. Note the intense contrast enhancement of urine within intrarenal collecting structures (blue arrows) but no extravasation was shown. Therefore, the injury was limited to the renal parenchyma, without disruption of the collecting system.

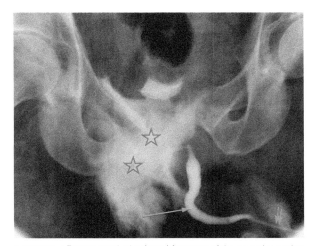

FIGURE 9-4 Extravasated urine (stars) from tear of the posterior urethra shown on retrograde urethrogram after pelvic trauma. Contrast material was injected through a catheter (double arrow) inserted a short distance into the anterior urethra (arrow).

SUSPECTED RENOVASCULAR HYPERTENSION

Unlike essential hypertension, in which medical imaging is not appropriate, when there is clinical suspicion of renovascular hypertension (hypertension caused by unilateral or bilateral renal artery stenosis), imaging is needed for diagnosis and for treatment planning.

Modalities

Renal ultrasonography with Doppler imaging of renal arterial flow for suspected renovascular disease is sometimes diagnostic, but the sensitivity and specificity of this exam is variable because it is highly dependent on operator skill and patient factors such as obesity. Instead of revealing a vascular cause of renovascular hypertension, renal sonography may find a renal or adrenal mass that could be the cause of hypertension.

Both CTA and MRA are effective in visualizing the renal arteries. Choosing between them depends on locally available equipment, expertise, and patient factors. For patients with mildly to moderately compromised renal function, the use of gadolinium-based contrast media in MRI has less renal risk than the use of iodine-based contrast agents (variably nephrotoxic) for CT. Therefore, CTA is avoided in these patients.

In patients with advanced renal failure, the use of gadolinium risks the complication of nephrogenic systemic fibrosis. This systemic complication has been mainly limited to acutely and severely ill patients in advanced renal failure who have had multiple exposures to gadolinium-based contrast agents in a short period of time (multiple contrast-enhanced MR scans within a few days). For a patient in advanced renal failure who is already on dialysis, the risk of renal toxicity from iodine-based contrast material is not an

issue. Therefore, CTA can be safely chosen over MRA in this situation. Patients with advanced renal failure who are not yet on dialysis may be examined with Doppler sonography (discussed earlier), or with angiotensin-converting enzyme **(ACE) inhibitor renal scintigraphy**. In some cases in which renal failure is a relative or absolute contraindication to using either iodine-based or gadolinium-based contrast agents, a successful angiogram may be possible with unenhanced flow-sensitive MRI techniques. Another highly specialized procedure that can be considered in these difficult cases is angiography done by injecting CO_2 through an intra-arterial catheter, visualizing the renal artery lumen with "negative contrast" during radiographic angiography.

Interpretation

During renal sonography, a search is first made for renal (and adrenal) masses and the presence or absence of obstructive dilatation of the urinary collecting system. Renal size is recorded, because chronic renal arterial insufficiency may result in renal atrophy.

Doppler measurement of peak systolic renal artery velocity above 180 cm/sec and renal artery/aorta velocity ratio above 3.5 have been considered diagnostic of hemodynamically significant renal artery stenosis. However, there is disagreement relative to the sensitivity and specificity of these measurements. Doppler waveforms and the calculated resistive index are also used for the diagnosis of renal artery stenosis, but patient factors and the operator dependence of this exam results in variable reliability. An example of a renal Doppler study that is diagnostic of renal artery stenosis, because of an abnormally high peak renal systolic velocity, is shown in Figure 9-5.

Both MRA and CTA can directly demonstrate potentially hemodynamically significant stenoses, greater than 50% of main and segmental renal arteries. It is not always clear if a stenosis in the range of 50% to 70% is flow limiting to the

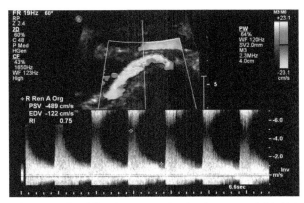

FIGURE 9-5 Renal Doppler sonography showing a remarkably high renal artery peak systolic velocity (indicated as PSV on the image) of 489 cm/sec. This patient's hypertension may be cured or vastly improved after renal artery balloon dilatation and stenting.

extent that it results in hypertension. There is little doubt that stenoses above 70% are an indication for intervention, either surgery or angioplasty and stenting. Figure 9-6 consists of three images showing a CTA of a patient with renal artery stenosis (top), the subsequent catheter angiogram that confirmed this finding (middle), and the post-stenting angiogram that documents successful dilatation of the stenosis (bottom). This patient's hypertension resolved.

ACUTE ONSET FLANK PAIN

The presence of a ureteral calculus usually causes a characteristic spasmodic or colicky acute flank pain and microhematuria. Imaging is directed toward documenting the presence or absence of a ureteral calculus and in determining the size of a ureteral calculus with respect to the need for intervention. During this evaluation the presence of intrarenal calculi that could result in future episodes of ureterolithiasis is also noted.

Modalities

In most cases, the appropriate procedure is an unenhanced CT of the abdomen and pelvis. Many facilities offer a limited x-ray dose, renal stone protocol CT procedure.

For the pregnant patient and the rare pediatric cases with suspected ureterolithiasis, ultrasonography can be used to search for urinary tract dilatation that is evidence for a distal obstruction caused by a calculus (ultrasound cannot usually show the stone itself). However, when a calculus becomes impacted in a ureter, the proximal ureter and renal collecting system may not immediately result in perceptible dilatation in some patients, limiting the sensitivity of ultrasonography for this diagnosis. Furthermore, hormonal changes in pregnancy that relax ureteral mural muscle tone and extrinsic pressure on the ureter from the gravid uterus almost always cause some ureteral dilatation, which is typically not clinically significant.

When there is compelling reason to avoid x-ray exposure and ultrasonography is not definitive, MR urography can be done in which a dilated (fluid-filled) ureter proximal to the level of an obstructing calculus can be shown on a T2 weighted image sequence. Although the calculus itself is not visible, the shape of an abrupt contour change of the ureter at the level of a calculus can be characteristic.

When a patient has a history of urinary tract calculi or a known acute ureteral calculus (diagnosed on CT), a supine abdominal radiograph (kidneys, ureter, and bladder [**KUB**]) can be useful. The radiographic visibility of a calculus depends upon the size and calcium content, body mass, position (a calculus overlying the sacrum is more difficult to see), and presence of stool in the large bowel, which can obscure a small calculus.

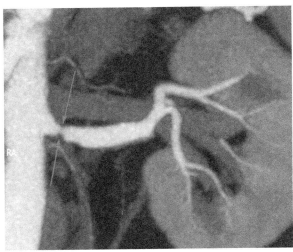

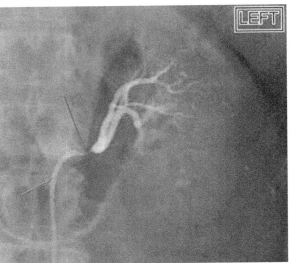

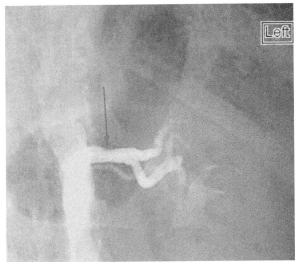

FIGURE 9-6 Top: Renal artery stenosis (arrows) shown on a coronal MIP image from CTA done on a hypertensive patient. **Middle:** Transfemoral catheter angiogram; contrast material injected through a catheter (blue arrow), the tip of which has been placed at the origin of the left renal artery, confirming the finding of a stenosis (red arrow) on the CTA shown above. **Bottom:** Angiographic image after balloon dilatation and stenting of the left renal artery stenosis (arrow).

Interpretation

Urinary tract calculi are visible in CT as focal high-density objects, as shown in Figure 9-7. In the pelvis, it can be difficult to differentiate a ureteral calculus from a phlebolith (spherical calcifications in veins) in a pelvic vein close to the expected course of the distal ureter, especially if there is no gross dilatation of the ureter. A useful clue is that when a calculus is impacted in a ureter, the ureteral wall is edematous and you can usually see a thin rim of soft tissue surrounding the calculus, as shown in Figure 9-7, bottom. Generally, phleboliths do not show a surrounding perceptible soft tissue density, as illustrated in Figure 9-8.

The CT density of urinary tract calculi is variable. If only a contrast-enhanced abdominal CT scan is done, the density of a calculus could be identical to the density of opacified excreted urine in the renal collecting systems and ureters and therefore might not be visible.

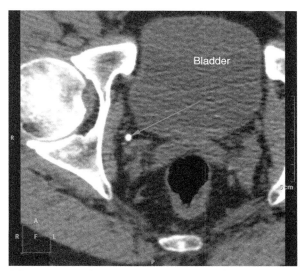

FIGURE 9-8 Axial CT showing a phlebolith (arrow) near the urinary bladder.

Small calculi (up to several millimeters in diameter) may pass with the conservative treatment of increasing fluid intake. Follow-up imaging for the acute episode is not needed if the calculus is recovered in a strainer. However, if symptoms persist and a calculus is not recovered, a radiograph may show that it has moved distally in the time period since the original CT, and continued conservative management may be indicated. Large calculi (and even small calculi that are very irregular in shape) often need intervention. Figure 9-9

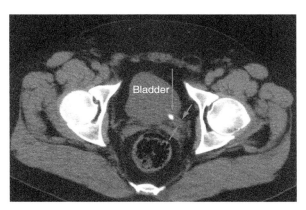

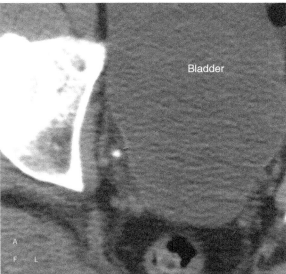

FIGURE 9-7 **Top:** Axial CT showing a calculus at the ureterovesical junction (long arrow). Note the distended distal ureter (short arrows). **Bottom:** Axial CT showing a small calculus in the distal ureter very close to the urinary bladder (arrow). Note the hazy soft tissue density surrounding the calculus. Differentiate this appearance from that shown of the phlebolith in Figure 9-8.

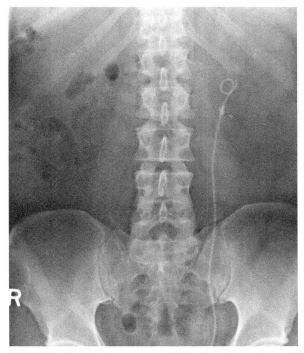

FIGURE 9-9 AP abdominal radiograph (KUB) after placement of a left ureteral catheter. The coiled proximal end of the catheter has been placed above the left UPJ to keep it in place. Urine flows through the catheter to the bladder, bypassing an obstructing calculus in the ureter (arrow).

is a radiograph of a patient whose left ureteral obstruction was relieved by placement of a ureteral catheter until lithotripsy could fragment the calculus.

ACUTE SCROTAL PAIN AND SCROTAL MASSES

Clinical scrotal issues usually involve trauma, pain due to inflammatory disease, vascular compromise of the testicle, and palpable masses. Severe infectious processes are rare, usually only seen in the immunocompromised patient.

Modalities

Ultrasonography is used to identify hydroceles, characterize testicular injury, evaluate testicular blood flow, characterize intrascrotal masses, and identify epididymitis, which is the most common inflammatory process in the scrotum. **Transillumination** is widely used for the diagnosis of hydrocele, but false positive results may occur and this modality is not as comprehensive as ultrasonography.

Interpretation

Hydrocele is obvious as free intrascrotal fluid, as shown in Figure 9-10. Ultrasound done for trauma to the scrotum can reveal testicular injury ranging from a small hematoma to frank rupture of the testicle, as shown in Figure 9-11, which may be considered a surgical emergency if the tunica albuginea is disrupted.

The differential diagnosis for hemiscrotal pain of acute epididymitis versus acute testicular torsion is easily clarified with Doppler sonography. In acute epididymitis (treated medically), there is conspicuously increased flow in the affected epididymis, as shown in Figure 9-12. In acute testicular torsion (treated surgically), there is decreased or absent testicular Doppler signal. In both these conditions, the contralateral asymptomatic side is used for comparison (Fig. 9-13).

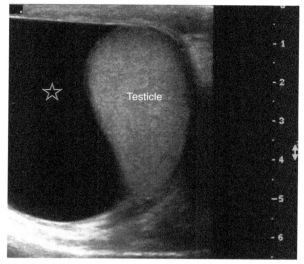

FIGURE 9-10 Scrotal sonography showing a large hydrocele (star).

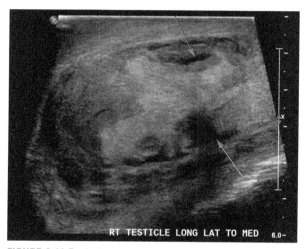

FIGURE 9-11 Testicular ultrasound after trauma. In addition to the heterogenous echo texture consistent with hematoma, there is frank disruption of the testicle (arrows).

When the appearance on ultrasound of a palpable intrascrotal structure is that of tortuous tubular structures within which blood can be seen, the diagnosis of varicocele is established (Fig. 9-14).

Extratesticular intrascrotal masses are almost always benign lesions, either the very common finding of an epididymal cyst, often multiple (Fig. 9-15), spermatocele or one of several uncommon benign solid masses.

In contrast to extratesticular masses, any solid mass found within the testicle is treated as a malignancy. Seminomas tend to be well-circumscribed masses that are hypoechoic to the normal surrounding testicular tissue and usually show a relatively homogeneous echo texture or only mild heterogeneity. The classic appearance of testicular seminoma is shown in Figure 9-16. A more complex ultrasound appearance with a great deal of heterogeneity of the

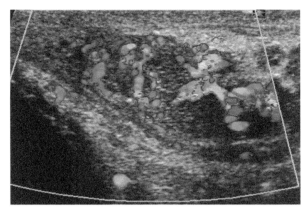

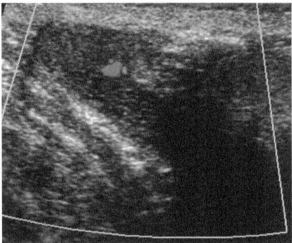

FIGURE 9-12 **Top:** Image from scrotal sonography with color flow Doppler that shows increased flow in the epididymis on the symptomatic side. **Bottom:** Contralateral epididymus with same color flow gain setting for comparison.

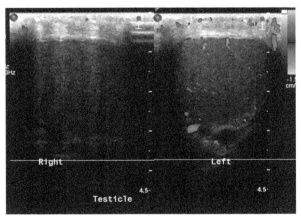

FIGURE 9-13 Duplex sonography that shows normal blood flow in the left testicle but no foci of color Doppler signal within the symptomatic right testicle.

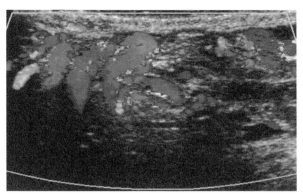

FIGURE 9-14 Image from scrotal sonography with color flow Doppler that shows a collection of discrete, dilated veins characteristic of a varicocele.

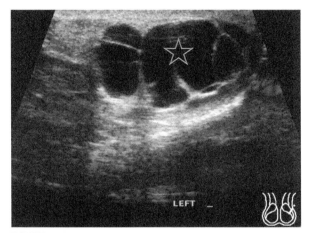

FIGURE 9-15 Image from scrotal sonography demonstrates that a palpable mass consists of multiple epididymal cysts/septated cyst or spermatocele (star).

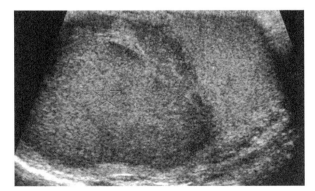

FIGURE 9-16 Testicular ultrasound shows a relatively homogeneous hypoechoic intratesticular mass (red star). This appearance is more consistent with seminoma than with other types of testicular malignancy. Normal testicular echo level and texture is indicated by the blue star.

echo texture makes it more likely that the lesion is a non-seminomatous tumor such as a mixed germ cell tumor or teratocarcinoma. When a testicular mass is found, chest radiography and CT of the abdomen and pelvis are usually done for staging.

When testicular microlithiasis (Fig. 9-17) is found on sonography, there may be an increased risk for the subsequent development of testicular cancer, although this relationship is uncertain. (See Patient Communication Box 9-1.)

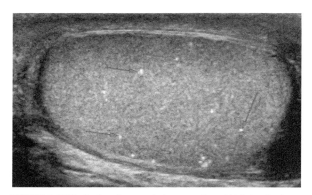

FIGURE 9-17 Testicular ultrasound shows scattered high-level echoes (arrows) indicating microlithiasis.

Patient Communication   Box 9-1

In many cases of testicular cancer, the imaging characteristics of the mass can provide a realistic measure of optimism to offer your patient. Although you must be careful to not offer a false promise, when a testicular mass is found that has imaging characteristics highly consistent with a pure seminoma, it is realistic for the patient to be very hopeful that surgery will reveal early disease with no metastases, in which case the long-term survival rate for this cancer is at least 95%.

 The location of an undescended testicle can be found with ultrasonography if the testis is relatively superficial. Otherwise, MRI is used to locate the testicle in cases of cryptorchidism.

CASE UPDATE

Your 49-year-old patient with a left ureteral calculus calls you to report little relief and that he has not found a calculus in the urine strainer. You arrange for him to have a supine radiograph to determine if the calculus has moved, but you caution the patient that a 3 mm calculus may not be visible on an "x-ray" and that it might be necessary to repeat CT. When the patient expresses concern about repeating the CT, you advise the patient that current CT scanning protocols, especially the "renal stone protocol," use techniques that result in exposure to a very low dose of ionizing radiation. On your order for the radiograph, you indicate to the imaging center to "hold patient and call report."

HEMATURIA AND RENAL MASSES

The classic clinical presentation of renal cortical cancer is painless hematuria. However, most renal masses are now discovered as incidental asymptomatic findings on imaging done for other reasons; this issue is discussed further in Chapter 12.

Cancers of the uroepithelium—transitional cell carcinomas—usually present with hematuria, although some transitional cell cancers of the ureter may be asymptomatic or cause slowly progressive obstruction of the ureter, with vague and delayed symptoms related to the slow onset of hydronephrosis. These can be clinically silent cancers until they present in the late stages with weight loss and back pain.

Hematuria can occur with pyuria in severe urinary tract infections. Non-obstructing urolithiasis can cause painless hematuria, clinically distinct from the hematuria associated with flank pain in patients with ureteral calculi.

Modalities

Gross painless hematuria is first evaluated with cystoscopy to rule out transitional cell cancer of the urinary bladder. If such a cancer is found and cystoscopic findings suggest that the cancer could involve the ureterovesical junction, ultrasonography of the kidneys may be done to rule out hydronephrosis. Ultrasound images can also reveal masses that arise from the bladder mucosa.

The classic radiographic procedure for evaluation of the upper urinary tract is the intravenous urogram (IVU): a series of radiographs obtained after the IV injection of contrast material. Linear radiographic tomography should always be done with this procedure to improve visualization of renal cortex and the renal collecting structures. However, the IVU is increasingly being replaced by CT urography: abdominal and pelvic CT using an injection and scan timing protocol optimized for demonstrating the urinary system. The transition to CT urography can be attributed to the vastly more specific depiction of renal cortical lesions on CT when compared with radiographs. CT of the abdomen and pelvis is important in staging patients who have urinary tract cancer, and PET scanning may be needed in patients under treatment for advanced urinary tract cancers.

Many renal masses have indeterminate features on ultrasound and CT; these are commonly evaluated further with MRI, as shown in Table 9-1.

Interpretation

As noted earlier, most bladder cancer diagnosis in patients with hematuria is achieved during cystoscopy and does not require imaging. However, polypoid mucosal lesions of the bladder mucosa may be seen as filling defects within the bladder when surrounded by opacified urine during IVU or CT, or as echogenic polypoid mucosa projections on ultrasonography, as shown in Figure 9-18.

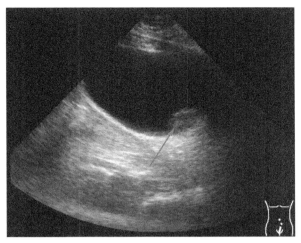

FIGURE 9-18 Urinary bladder ultrasound showing a mucosal polyp (arrow) that was subsequently proven to be a transitional cell carcinoma by cystoscopic biopsy.

The most common renal mass is a simple cyst (often multiple in the same patient) that may, depending upon the body habitus of the patient, be confidently diagnosed as a benign cyst by sonography (Fig. 9-19). These almost always have no clinical significance, unlike complex cystic and solid masses that may cause hematuria and/or metastasize. When ultrasonography does not provide a definitive diagnosis, cysts can be accurately evaluated by CT or MRI. Patients with adult polycystic kidney disease (APKD) will have enlarged kidneys with multiple cysts, shown well on CT, ultrasound (Fig. 9-20), or MRI (Fig. 9-21). Patients with APKD often also have multiple hepatic cysts (see Fig. 9-20).

The Bosniak classification system is widely used to describe the range of imaging findings, from the simple unilocular renal cyst (category I) with no perceptible wall thickness, through various degrees of septated cystic lesions, to complex partially cystic and partially solid masses (category IV). This system is used to provide guidance for imaging follow-up and intervention such as nephrectomy, partial nephrectomy

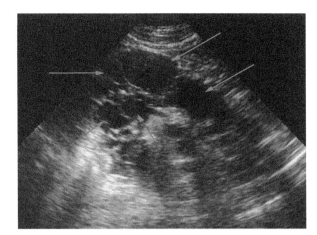

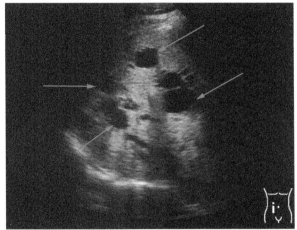

FIGURE 9-20 **Top:** Renal ultrasound in a patient with APKD shows an enlarged kidney distorted by numerous cysts (arrows). **Bottom:** Hepatic ultrasound on the same patient shows numerous hepatic cysts (arrows).

(often minimally invasive laparoscopic procedures), or minimally invasive percutaneous ablation of the lesion with cryotherapy or radiofrequency ablation.

A CT of a patient with both Bosniak categories I and III lesions is shown in Figure 9-22. Bosniak I and II renal cysts are reliably benign and require no further follow-up. In the case shown in Figure 9-22, the lesion on the left side (Bosniak III) is likely to be excised or ablated because a significant percentage of these lesions are malignant. However, if the patient is elderly or has comorbidities, the risk of intervention may be greater than the risk of malignancy when renal lesions have this appearance. Therefore, it may be categorized as a IIIF lesion, with recommendation for 6-month imaging follow-up, and intervention only if the lesion shows significant growth or other interval change that indicates a possibly aggressive malignancy.

Solid renal masses, as shown in Figure 9-23, are all considered malignant, except for those that contain macroscopic fat. A renal mass that contains macroscopic fat is likely to be a renal angiomyolipoma, as shown in Figure 9-24.

In addition to renal cortical tumors that may cause hematuria, transitional cell cancers of the renal collection system

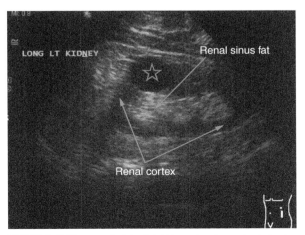

FIGURE 9-19 Ultrasound of the left kidney showing a simple benign renal cortical cyst (star).

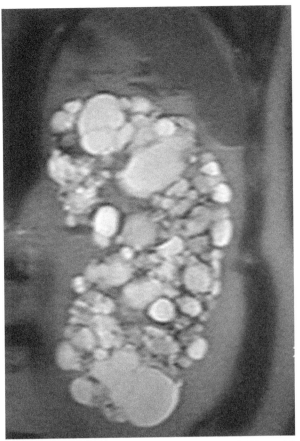

FIGURE 9-21 Coronal T2 MRI showing an enlarged left kidney with innumerable cysts in a patient with known APKD.

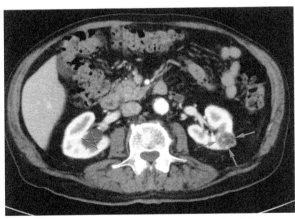

FIGURE 9-22 Axial contrast-enhanced CT showing a Bosniak category I simple benign cyst (star) in the right kidney and a Bosniak category III complex cyst in the left kidney (arrows).

and ureter may present with hematuria. Non-obstructive calculi may also present with painless hematuria. This may occur when a calculus has a very irregular shape and does not cause symptomatic obstruction. The maximum intensity projections (MIPs) shown in the top and bottom images in Figure 9-25 demonstrate how CT urography depicts these calculi as well as providing a comprehensive examination of the urinary system.

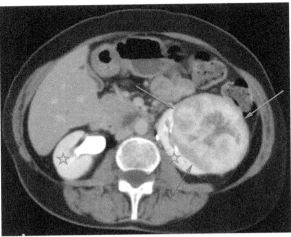

FIGURE 9-23 Axial contrast-enhanced CT showing that a large left renal mass (arrows) is hypoenhancing when compared with the residual normal medial left renal cortex and the contralateral kidney (stars).

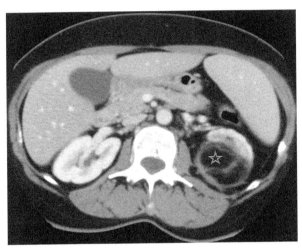

FIGURE 9-24 Axial contrast-enhanced CT showing a left renal mass; specifically an angiomyolipoma because of the fat density (star) within the tumor.

CASE UPDATE

The radiologist at the imaging center calls you with a report on your patient with the left ureteral calculus. A definite calculus is not evident in the expected location of the proximal or mid left ureter. There are several small calcifications in the pelvis, several of which are clearly phleboliths, but to the left of midline in the pelvis are at least three uncertain calcifications. You and the radiologist agree that a repeat CT is appropriate. This shows the calculus to have moved distally since the first study: It is now at the left ureterovesical junction. You advise the patient to continue with "pushing" fluids. The next day he calls to report relief of symptoms and retrieval of the calculus. You tell the patient that some more follow-up is needed because of an incidental finding in his right kidney. You order a contrast-enhanced abdominal and pelvis CT scan to evaluate the possible mass in the right kidney.

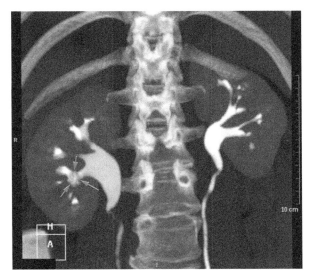

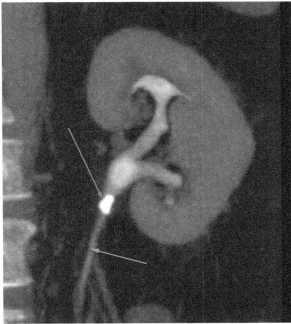

FIGURE 9-25 **Top:** MIP image from CT urography. The "filling defect" (arrows) in the right renal collecting system could be a calculus (depending upon degree of calcification) or uroepithelial tumor. **Bottom:** MIP image from CT urography. A calcified calculus at the left UPJ (red arrow) causes no significant obstructive dilatation of the renal collecting system; its irregular surface allows passage of opacified urine into the ureter distal to the stone (blue arrow).

DIFFICULTY VOIDING

A thorough history and physical examination are needed to differentiate mechanical bladder outlet obstruction from neurogenic bladder, which would lead to appropriate neurologic and spine imaging examination.

 Although congenital urethral deformities rarely present to primary care after infancy, a pediatric male patient may present after infancy with enuresis, urinary frequency, difficulty with aiming the urinary stream, and dysuria caused by meatal stenosis or phimosis.

Urethral strictures occur in adolescent and adult males secondary to trauma and infections. The primary cause of stricture of the short female urethra is iatrogenic. There is poor clinical correlation between reported urinary symptoms and measured bladder outflow.

Bladder outlet obstruction is rarely the presenting cause of prostate carcinoma (discussed later) but very commonly occurs secondary to benign prostatic hyperplasia (BPH). The medical significance of BPH may extend far beyond the inconvenience of frequent voiding; urinary retention may result in complications of infection and upper tract obstructive uropathy that in severe cases can result in renal failure.

Modalities

Ultrasonography of the urinary bladder and prostate is done pre- and post-voiding with estimate of bladder volume and completeness of bladder emptying.

Especially if there is significant post-void bladder residual volume, ultrasonography of the kidneys is appropriate to exclude the presence of obstructive dilatation of the upper urinary tract that can occur secondary to chronic bladder outlet obstruction.

Radiographic evaluation of the urethra, done with voiding cystourethrography, is used to identify urethral strictures.

Interpretation

Prostate size and bladder volumes can be estimated from measurements done during transabdominal sonography of the urinary bladder. Interpretation of sonography of the renal collecting system requires awareness of one common variant that could be misinterpreted as hydronephrosis: The extrarenal pelvis is a medially positioned renal pelvis that is sometimes quite capacious and can look "dilated." When there is distention of the renal pelvis in continuity with infundibula and calyces of the renal collecting system, as shown in Figure 9-26, then the diagnosis of hydronephrosis is confidently made.

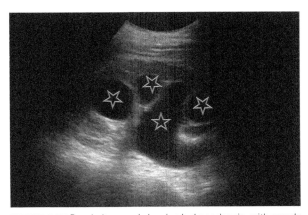

FIGURE 9-26 Renal ultrasound showing hydronephrosis, with grossly dilated renal pelvis and calyces (stars).

During any renal imaging study, hydronephrosis may be found secondary to UPJ obstruction, although this entity is usually not found with complete obstruction but rather with a stenosis of the junction of the renal pelvis with the ureter, as shown in Figure 9-27. Patients with this condition may be asymptomatic or have a history of intermittent flank pain.

URINARY TRACT INFECTION

There is great difference in the clinical presentations of lower urinary tract infections (UTIs) in males and females. Cystitis, uncomplicated by structural abnormalities or diabetes, is very common in females and very rare in males. Infectious disease in the male lower urinary tract usually involves prostatitis and urethritis, which may present with dysuria, or epididymitis or orchitis, which present with hemiscrotal pain that is evaluated with ultrasonography (see Acute Scrotal Pain and Scrotal Masses section above).

Pyelonephritis, infection in the kidneys, usually has clinical features that differentiate it from simple cystitis. The most common route of infection in the kidneys is retrograde via the lumen of the urinary tract from the urinary bladder, although hematogenous spread does occur.

Modalities

In both males and females, ultrasonography can be very useful for screening to rule out excessive urinary bladder residual volume, hydronephrosis, and renal or perirenal

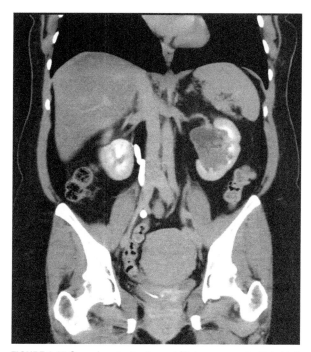

FIGURE 9-27 Coronal contrast-enhanced CT shows a greatly dilated left renal pelvis (star), consistent with congenital UPJ obstruction in the absence of another explanation for the obstruction, such as tumor or calculus.

abscess. However, accuracy of sonography is not high for renal disease; false negative findings for renal abscess occur in up to one third of patients.

In patients with recurrent UTIs, **voiding cystourethrography (VCUG)** may be important to rule out incomplete bladder emptying, vesicoureteral reflux, or structural abnormalities such as duplication of the ureters. (See Patient Communication Box 9-2.)

An alternative to VCUG in the evaluation of vesicoureteral reflux is a radionuclide cystogram.

 Vesicoureteral reflux is more common in children than in adults. The degree of reflux found is critical in determining treatment.

If there is clinical suspicion that UTI is a complication of renal stone disease and there is no concern for renal abscess or other advanced disease, then unenhanced urinary tract CT is appropriate to identify calculi, just as in the patient who presents with symptoms of an acute ureteral calculus.

In females, routine imaging is not done for uncomplicated UTIs, including pyelonephritis, because uncomplicated cystitis is so common that you are not likely to find important structural abnormalities in a female with pyelonephritis. Only with frequent recurrence or clinical features of complications such as renal abscess is imaging of the upper urinary tract done in females. In males, however, pyelonephritis is often an indication for imaging because cystitis in the male is uncommon and there is a high degree of suspicion of complicated disease. For comprehensive evaluation of the urinary tract, CT scanning without and with contrast enhancement (CT urography) is ideal (see Fig. 9-22).

 Renal scintigraphy (radionuclide renogram) is preferred over CT in children because of its lower radiation dose, although focal renal defects found on scintigraphy are less specific than with CT. Such defects are almost certainly inflammatory when there has been a clinical diagnosis of pyelonephritis.

There is relatively little experience in using MRI for diagnosis in complicated pyelonephritis. However, it may be an excellent choice in a patient with allergy to iodine-based contrast agents.

Interpretation

During VUCG, the finding of reflux is graded. Low-grade reflux (I and II) into non-dilated ureters (Fig. 9-28, top) and the renal collecting systems usually resolves spontaneously. Even grade III reflux into mildly dilated collecting systems (Fig. 9-28, top) often resolves. These grades of reflux are treated medically with long-term antibiotics to suppress infection. Grade IV reflux, with moderate dilatation of the collecting system and grade V reflux with severe hydronephrosis (Fig. 9-28, bottom), are often treated surgically.

A renal abscess is shown on CT as a well-defined, thick-walled cystic mass (Fig. 9-29). Gas density within such a mass virtually ensures that the lesion is an abscess and not a tumor. There is often perirenal fluid and inflammatory changes in perirenal fat.

Although medullary sponge kidney (renal tubular ectasia) is familial, it is frequently found as a previous undiagnosed condition during radiographic or CT urography done for pyelonephritis. CT urography is well suited to display the characteristic blush of contrast material in the renal pyramids, as seen in Figure 9-30. These patients frequently

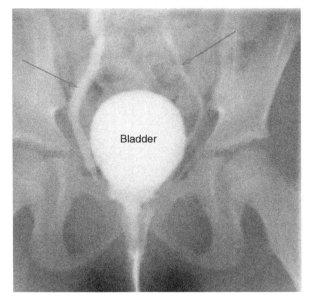

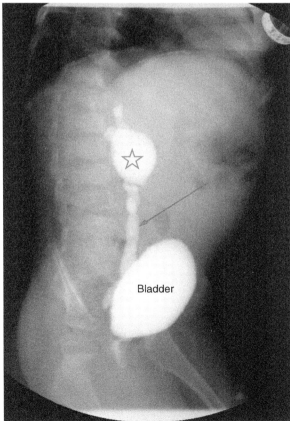

FIGURE 9-28 **Top:** VCUG with reflux into both ureters (arrows). The left ureter is normal in diameter (grade I reflux); the right ureter is mildly dilated (grade III reflux). **Bottom:** VCUG (lateral projection) showing grade V reflux resulting in a dilated and tortuous left ureter (arrow) and dilated renal pelvis (star).

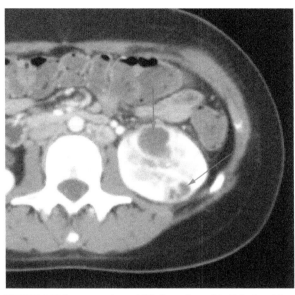

FIGURE 9-29 Contrast-enhanced CT of a patient with clinically evident severe pyelonephritis showing two areas of renal abscess formation (arrows).

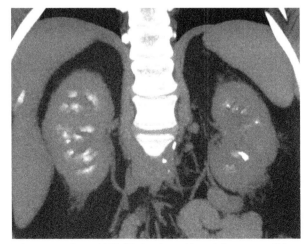

FIGURE 9-30 Coronal MIP CT of patient with medullary sponge kidney showing numerous intra-renal calculi and the characteristic blush of contrast enhancement in the renal pyramids. Note that it is difficult to visually distinguish between the contrast-enhanced tubules and calcifications, but the calcifications are higher density (whiter).

develop numerous small calculi in their dilated renal tubules.

RENAL FAILURE/INSUFFICIENCY

When a patient presents with an elevated creatinine level, it is frequently unclear if the azotemia is acute or chronic. When renal failure presents acutely, it is imperative to rule out obstructive uropathy that could be reversible. Chronic kidney disease is not commonly secondary to structural disease that is diagnosed by imaging, but most cases are secondary to hypertension, diabetes, and glomerulonephritis. However, imaging is done to rule out chronic obstructive uropathy or vascular insufficiency, and to exclude previous undiagnosed adult polycystic kidney disease.

Chronic kidney disease is graded into five stages, according to the measured glomerular filtration rate (GFR). These stages are important in radiology not only to provide consistent perspective on severity of disease to all of the medical professionals involved in a patient's care, but also as a guide for the safety of, or contraindication to, the use of IV contrast media, especially gadolinium-based contrast agents used in MRI for patients in advanced renal failure. That is why you may be asked to write an order for creatinine clearance when you request MRI on patients who meet certain criteria (varies by facility, but criteria may include patients above a specific age, all diabetic patients, and all patients with history of renal disease of any kind).

Modalities

Renal and bladder sonography are indicated to rule out obstructive uropathy. This should be done with Doppler imaging of the renal arteries to assess for possible arterial insufficiency.

Radionuclide imaging with the agent Tc-99m MAG3 is often used for evaluation of renal function and can help distinguish acute from chronic renal insufficiency. If renal artery Doppler sonography is not definitive, renal arterial insufficiency can be ruled out with MRA, either with or without contrast enhancement, depending upon the stage of renal disease. Patients with mild to moderate renal insufficiency are at greater risk from the nephrotoxicity of iodine-based contrast media used in CT than from the very low incidence of nephrogenic systemic sclerosis after the administration of gadolinium-based contrast agent in MRI. Therefore, CTA is not highly recommended for many of these patients. In some cases, however, patients with mild renal insufficiency may be safely studied with CTA if the patient is kept well hydrated and the dose of injected contrast material is minimal. As with any such complex medical situation, consultation with specialists, including radiologists, is beneficial to patient care.

Interpretation

When severe obstructive uropathy (bilateral hydronephrosis, or hydronephrosis in a patient with a solitary kidney) is demonstrated with imaging in a patient with azotemia, renal function often improves when drainage is established.

When it is clinically unclear if renal failure is acute or chronic, the imaging finding of small kidneys with hyperechoic cortices without dilatation of the collecting systems suggests that the patient has had previously undiagnosed chronic kidney disease, as shown in Figure 9-31.

THE PROSTATE GLAND

Prostate cancer is usually diagnosed by physical examination, the finding of an elevated prostate specific antigen (PSA), and less commonly (but not rarely) when a male patient presents with blastic skeletal metastatic disease. In fact most radiologists have had the experience of being the first medical professional to suspect prostate cancer in a patient while viewing a chest or skeletal radiograph, an abdominal CT scan, or any other imaging exam in which skeletal abnormalities may be appreciated (see Fig. 6-6). BPH causing obstructive voiding symptoms is very common. This is discussed earlier in this chapter, in the section on difficult voiding.

Modalities

Urologists use transrectal prostate ultrasound to guide needle biopsy. In major medical research centers, prostate MRI is sometimes used for staging of a known malignancy. After biopsy, patients who have a high Gleason (histologic grade of the tumor) score and/or high PSA levels often undergo

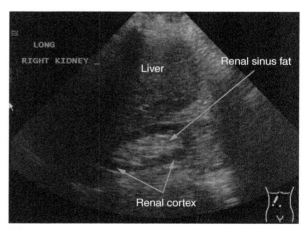

FIGURE 9-31 Ultrasound of the right kidney in a patient with chronic renal insufficiency. Note that the renal cortex is relatively thin when compared with the brightly echogenic fatty renal hilus. Atrophy of the kidney was documented by its very small size when measured on the sonogram.

radionuclide bone scanning to search for metastatic disease. When a urologist has suspicion of invasive metastatic disease in the pelvis, CT or MRI of the abdomen and pelvis may be used for evaluation.

In the primary care setting, the most common imaging on prostate cancer patients is done for suspected metastatic disease. This may occur when a patient has a very high PSA level suspicious for metastatic disease or a patient with a history of prostate carcinoma develops symptoms of metastatic skeletal disease.

Interpretation

A radionuclide bone scan that shows multiple foci of increased uptake is suspicious for metastatic disease. Occasionally, very widespread skeletal metastases from prostate cancer result in a "superscan," as shown in Figure 9-32, in which there is markedly increased diffuse uptake without distinguishable focal disease. The clue to the diagnosis is the remarkable degree of skeletal uptake of the radiopharmaceutical, with virtually no soft tissue activity.

When a bone scan is positive, selective radiographs are often done to ascertain whether there is radiographically visible blastic disease. CT scans can be viewed with bone windows to display the characteristic prostatic cancer bone changes, as shown in Figure 9-33. False negatives do occur, however, and it is estimated that micrometastasis may reside in the skeleton for up to 5 years before the bone scan is positive in some cases. Although blastic disease is most characteristic of metastatic prostate disease, lytic bone lesions are occasionally seen.

CASE CONCLUSION

Your male patient who passed a solitary left ureteral calculus has had a contrast-enhanced CT to follow up on the possible mass in the right kidney. This shows a 1.8 cm solid renal cortical mass along the lateral margin of the lower pole of the right kidney. The left kidney is normal. There is no adenopathy or liver lesion. You refer the patient to a urologist, who perform a minimally invasive laparoscopic partial nephrectomy.

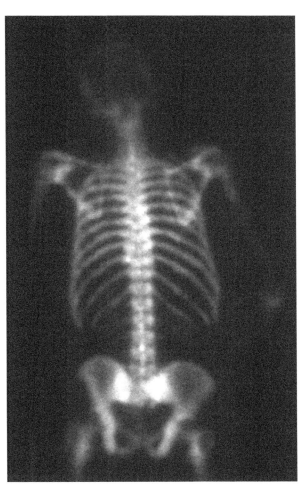

FIGURE 9-32 Radionuclide bone scan on a patient with diffuse metastatic prostate carcinoma. Note the high level of activity in bones and the absence of renal or soft tissue activity.

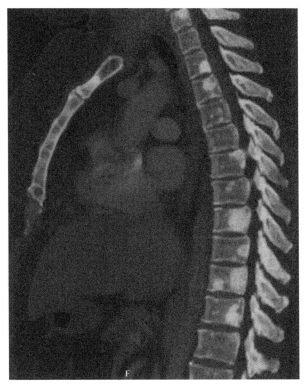

FIGURE 9-33 Blastic bone disease shown on a sagittal MIP CT. Note the areas of abnormally increased bone density in the spine and in the sternum in a patient with a markedly elevated PSA.

Chapter Review

Chapter Review Questions

1. When a patient has painless hematuria that is not associated with UTI and cystoscopy is normal, which of the following is correct?

   A. There is nothing to worry about

   B. Ultrasonography is definitive

   C. CT urography is the best exam

   D. A radionuclide renal study should be done

   E. Unenhanced CT (renal stone protocol) should be done immediately

2. The procedure of choice for suspected acute ureteral calculus is:

   A. KUB.

   B. CT urography with IV contrast.

   C. MRI.

   D. Unenhanced CT.

   E. VCUG.

3. For diagnosis of renovascular hypertension in an obese patient with severely compromised renal function, the preferred procedure would likely be:

   A. ultrasonography.

   B. MRA.

   C. CTA.

   D. radiography.

   E. ACE-inhibitor renal scintigraphy.

4. Which of the following is correct pertaining to the imaging of ureteral stones?

   A. They are always visible on KUB (abdominal) radiographs

   B. On a renal stone CT they may be distinguished from a phlebolith by a much higher density

   C. Ultrasound may be helpful, but only if there is significant obstructive dilatation of the affected renal collecting system

   D. IVU is a currently acceptable imaging modality for the diagnosis of ureterolithiasis

   E. MR is never useful for the diagnosis of ureterolithiasis

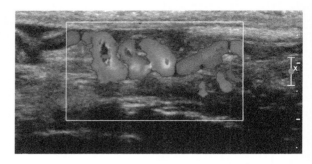

5. Your diagnosis based on the testicular Doppler ultrasound shown here is:

   A. varicocele.

   B. hydrocele.

   C. testicular torsion.

   D. testicular tumor.

   E. epididymal cyst.

6. Adult polycystic kidney disease may be diagnosed with all of the following EXCEPT:

   A. ultrasound.

   B. CT.

   C. MRI.

   D. KUB.

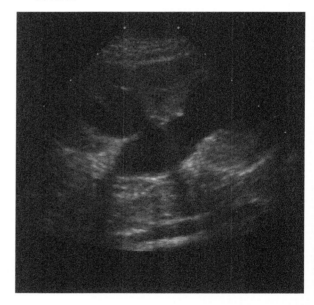

7. After an elderly male complained of difficulty voiding and has elevated serum BUN and creatinine, a renal ultrasound was done (see the image shown above). Your diagnosis is:

   A. renal calculi.

   B. renal tumor.

   C. renal cyst.

   D. hydronephrosis.

   E. polycystic kidney disease.

8. Which of the following is correct pertaining to imaging for UTIs?

   A. In females with suspected cases of uncomplicated UTI, imaging is routinely performed

   B. In males with UTI, imaging is appropriate in most cases

   C. MRI is the typical procedure of choice in UTI

   D. CT urography is the procedure of choice in children with UTI

   E. Ultrasonography is the procedure of choice for diagnosis of associated renal abscesses

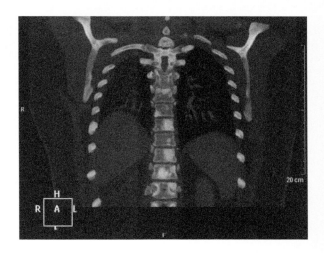

9. The coronal CT shown above if on a male, would most likely be associated with:

   A. azotemia.

   B. medullary sponge kidney.

   C. prostate cancer.

   D. angiomyolipoma.

   E. cortical renal tumor.

10 FEMALE PELVIC IMAGING

CASE STUDY

A 55-year-old female complains of pelvic pain and pressure. Pelvic examination reveals an enlarged uterus. You order pelvic sonography.

FUNDAMENTALS OF FEMALE PELVIC IMAGING

Ultrasonography has been and is likely to remain the most fundamental and useful imaging modality for the female pelvis and gravid uterus. All ultrasound machines that are appropriate for use in obstetric sonography include software that can generate graphical representation of fetal growth.

 COST-EFFECTIVE MEDICINE
Sonography is the most cost-effective and complete imaging evaluation of pelvic disease for patient management.

MRI is now the second most important modality for imaging the female pelvis because of its superior soft tissue resolution when compared with CT.

Ultrasound and MRI do not use ionizing radiation, often a significant concern with respect to possible radiation effects on the ovaries and/or a fetus. Therefore, there is a patient safety issue for selection of the ideal modality in imaging of the female pelvis, in addition to technical and cost issues. In specific clinical situations, however, radiography and CT are appropriate, as tabulated in Table 10-1 and discussed in detail in the following sections of this chapter.

Clinical findings relevant to optimum image acquisition and interpretation should be stated concisely on your imaging orders for suspected pelvic conditions, as exemplified in Table 10-2.

CASE UPDATE

The report from pelvic sonography on your 55-year-old patient with the enlarged uterus indicates no adnexal mass or endometrial thickening. The uterus is moderately enlarged and contains several fibroids, ranging in size up to 6 cm. The patient, who has been researching her treatment options on the Internet, asks you for your recommendation. She is pleased with your referral to see both a gynecologist, who advises hysterectomy, and an interventional radiologist, who offers her the option of uterine artery embolization (UAE).

TABLE 10-1 Imaging Modalities for the Female Pelvis

Primary Modality	Specific Exam	Uses	Comment
Ultrasound (US)	Transabdominal and transvaginal pelvic sonography	Baseline exam of uterus and adnexa, including obstetric examinations	Widely available and cost effective
	Sonohysterography (hysterosonography)	Detailed examination of endometrium	Requires insertion of HSG catheter (see below) for saline infusion during transvaginal sonography
MRI	Pelvis, unenhanced	Uterine anomalies associated with infertility	Excellent intrinsic soft tissue contrast resolution
	Pelvis, without and with contrast enhancement	Uterine and adnexal masses	Ideal exam for uterine fibroids and identifying local extent of pelvic malignancies
Radiography	Hysterosalpingography (HSG)	Examine endometrial cavity and assess tubal patency	Small balloon-tipped catheter is inserted into endometrial cavity through cervical canal
CT	Abdomen and pelvis with contrast enhancement	Large pelvic masses that extend into the abdomen	Ionizing radiation; avoided in pediatric patients and younger women of reproductive age—negative beta HCH required for CT of female in reproductive years

TABLE 10-2 **Sample Requisition Information for Female Pelvic Imaging**

Modality	Clinical Data/History
Pelvic ultrasound (transabdominal and transvaginal)	Dysfunctional uterine bleeding; uterine enlargement on pelvic exam
Third trimester limited obstetric sonography	Marginal placenta previa on prior exam; assess placenta, fetal position
Hysterosalpingography (HSG)	Infertility workup; assess tubal pregnancy Patient has history of endometriosis
CT abdomen and pelvis without and with contrast (CT urography)	Large pelvic mass and abdominal distention, elevated CA-125 (lab results forwarded)
MRI pelvis without and with contrast enhancement	Fibroids seen on office sonogram; patient candidate for uterine artery embolization

FERTILITY IMAGING

The complexities of infertility have led to the emergence of a subspecialty of gynecology dedicated to navigating the web of medical and anatomical issues discussed later in this chapter, which may prevent successful pregnancy. Infertility specialists often begin the complex process by ordering imaging exams with the hope that a structural problem can be found and corrected, leading to a successful pregnancy.

Modalities

Transabdominal and transvaginal sonography of the pelvis provides a basic examination of the uterus and ovaries that may identify major uterine abnormalities, ovarian pathology, or hydrosalpinx, any of which may explain infertility. For a detailed look at the endometrium and myometrium, a more advanced ultrasound procedure, called sonohysterography (hysterosonography), is used. In this exam, transvaginal sonography is done while the endometrial cavity is filled with saline via an HSG catheter (see below).

Hysterosalpingography (HSG) is a radiographic procedure used to assess the endometrial cavity and tubal patency in which a small balloon-tipped catheter is passed through the cervical canal into the endometrial cavity. The balloon is then inflated to hold the catheter in place, and radiographic contrast material is injected into the endometrial cavity and fallopian tubes, while radiographs are obtained that may exclude or reveal pathology, such as fallopian tube obstruction, endometrial disease, or developmental uterine abnormalities.

Interpretation

Pelvic pathology found on imaging may result in fertility problems related to ovulation, fertilization, implantation, or repeated pregnancy loss. For discussion of ovarian cysts and masses and uterine fibroids, see Imaging of Abnormal Vaginal Bleeding and Pelvic Masses in the next section.

Tubal patency is evaluated on HSG by the passage of injected contrast material into the fallopian tubes. Free spill of the contrast material into the peritoneal cavity indicates

patency, as shown in Figure 10-1. If both tubes are obstructed, with or without hydrosalpinx, then a cause of infertility has been established.

Round or ovoid filling defects within the contrast-filled endometrial cavity in an HSG are suspicious for endometrial polyps, as shown in Figure 10-2. Focal deformity of the contour of the endometrial cavity may be caused by a submucosal fibroid. Irregularity of the endometrial contours and linear filling defects in the contrast-filled endometrial cavity suggest post-inflammatory changes.

Developmental abnormalities such as a bicornuate uterus, with a Y-shaped endometrial cavity as shown in Figure 10-3, may be seen on HSG and may interfere with fertility, cause higher incidence of spontaneous abortion, and cause difficulties with delivery. Because classification of a uterine anomaly may require visualization of the external contours of the myometrium, which is not visible on an HSG, MRI may be necessary, as illustrated by the uterine didelphys shown in Figure 10-4. Ultrasound may also be used to examine the myometrium, but it can be almost impossible in many cases to obtain a cross-sectional view in the ideal plane

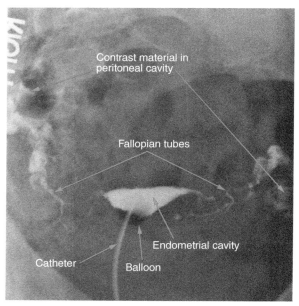

FIGURE 10-1 Normal hysterosalpingogram (HSG).

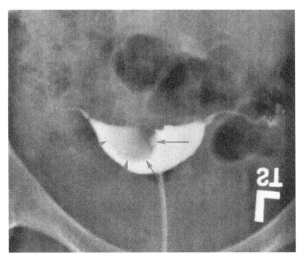

FIGURE 10-2 HSG showing a large round filling defect (arrows) within the endometrial cavity that is suspicious for endometrial polyp.

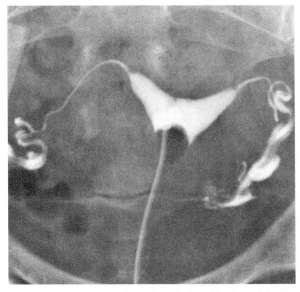

FIGURE 10-3 HSG showing the typical "Y-shaped" endometrial cavity configuration of a bicornuate uterus.

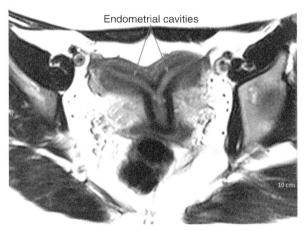

FIGURE 10-4 Oblique axial (tangent to the long axis of the uterus) T2 MRI of a uterine didelphys.

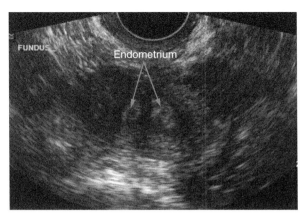

FIGURE 10-5 Transverse transvaginal ultrasound image of the uterus with brightly echogenic endometrium (arrows) in two distinct endometrial cavities separated by hypoechoic tissue.

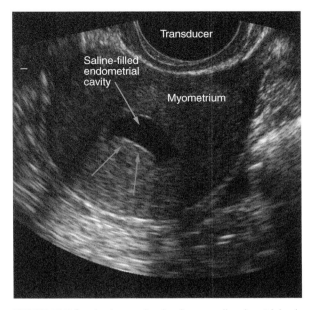

FIGURE 10-6 Sonohysterography showing a small endometrial polyp (red arrows).

for depicting the contours needed for classification of the anomaly. The ultrasound image shown in Figure 10-5 depicts two separate foci of increased echogenicity representing endometrium, but this could be either a septate uterus or a uterine didelphys.

Sonohysterography clearly shows endometrial pathology that may interfere with implantation, such as endometrial hyperplasia, submucosal fibroids, and endometrial polyps (Fig. 10-6).

OBSTETRIC IMAGING

Routine imaging during pregnancy, including assessing fetal growth and development, has become standard. Imaging is also done in the evaluation of clinical problems that may develop during pregnancy, such as vaginal bleeding.

Modalities

Ultrasound is the primary imaging modality in obstetrics, with occasional use of MRI in major medical centers for evaluation of some fetal abnormalities. In all three trimesters, transabdominal sonography, with as full a bladder as tolerated by the pregnant patient, may be sufficient for a complete exam. The full bladder acts as an acoustic "window" for clearly visualizing the lower uterine segment and cervix. However, especially in the earliest stages of pregnancy, transvaginal sonography is often needed for higher spatial resolution of the smaller structures present during an early pregnancy.

Most obstetric sonography is done as a basic or screening (level 1) procedure. When needed, more advanced and detailed examinations (level 2 or higher) are performed by qualified personnel.

First trimester obstetric sonography is done with the basic goals of the following:

- Determining if the pregnancy is intrauterine and viable
- Determining whether single or multiple
- Obtaining an accurate gestational age
- Ascertaining whether there are any abnormalities of the uterus, such as fibroids or adnexal abnormalities, that might interfere with pregnancy

In addition, during the first trimester, when the patient has pelvic pain or vaginal bleeding, or when there is clinical suspicion of ectopic gestation or trophoblastic disease, sonography may be focused on detection of those specific pathologies. In patients at high risk for fetal chromosomal abnormality, the ultrasound exam, done ideally between 10 and 14 weeks gestational age, includes a measurement of fetal nuchal translucency, which is very accurate for detection of trisomy 21.

During the second trimester, it is the expectation of even routine level 1 ultrasound exams to be comprehensive and to detect any major fetal abnormalities such as neural tube, abdominal wall, or cardiac defects, as well as determine position of the placenta and fetus, amniotic fluid volume, and appearance of the uterine cervix. Second trimester ultrasound studies are also used to determine gestational age or check for normal growth of the fetus by comparing with a first trimester ultrasound.

When there is suspicion of a fetal defect on routine second trimester obstetric sonography, a level 2 ultrasound exam should be done by trained and experienced personnel using state-of-the-art equipment capable of advanced sonographic

diagnosis, such as definitive diagnosis of fetal cardiac abnormalities or neural tube defects. As mentioned earlier, MRI is sometimes also used at the most advanced level of fetal evaluation.

Third trimester sonograms are largely focused upon evaluating fetal growth because most fetal weight is gained during the latter half of pregnancy. When a fetus is small for established gestational age or has low volume or absent amniotic fluid, a fetal biophysical profile is indicated. This includes fetal breathing movements, cardiac reactivity, fetal movements and tone, and determination of amniotic fluid volume.

A "limited" obstetric ultrasound procedure is done for a specific purpose, such as confirming fetal cardiac activity, measuring fetal growth, and determining fetal position when a patient is in labor. Such limited exams should only be done after a complete obstetric sonogram has been obtained previously.

Interpretation

When the beta human chorionic gonadotropin (β-hCG) is 1,000 to 2,000 mIU/mL, an intrauterine sac should be visible if there is a normal pregnancy. An intrauterine gestational sac as small as 3 mm in diameter is visible on ultrasound at a gestation of about 4 to 5 weeks.

When there is first trimester bleeding, a suspected ectopic gestation, or missed spontaneous abortion, or if the viability of an early pregnancy is uncertain, ultrasound imaging is used; it is most effective if imaging personnel are aware of serial β-hCG levels. Because the normal gestational sac grows quickly, repeat sonography after only a few days may be appropriate if an initial exam is not definitive.

The yolk sac should be visible in a normal pregnancy when the gestational sac has reached a diameter of 8 mm and if the β-hCG is greater than 5,000 mIU/mL, as shown in Figure 10-7. The earliest sonographic visualization of the embryo is an indistinct thick linear echo, often referred to as a fetal pole. Dating of a pregnancy after this stage is done by measuring the crown-rump length (CRL) of the fetus, as shown in Figure 10-8. When this length is equal to or greater than 5 mm, fetal cardiac activity should be visible, as shown in Figure 10-9, and the rate should be measured using M-mode sonography, which graphs cardiac activity against time.

Poor outcome of pregnancy can be predicted by ultrasound findings that include the following:

- Slow or absent growth in the size of the gestational sac or CRL
- Abnormal shape of the gestational sac or yolk sac
- Abnormally low position of the gestational sac
- Fetal bradycardia

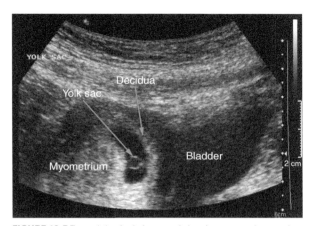

FIGURE 10-7 Transabdominal ultrasound showing a normal-appearing, simple round ring-shaped yolk sac.

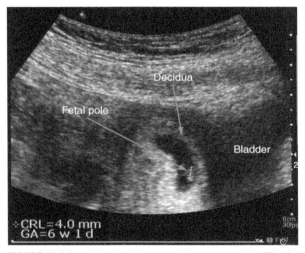

FIGURE 10-8 Transabdominal ultrasound that measured the CRL of a fetal pole at 4 mm. This length is equal to a mean gestational age of 6 weeks and 1 day.

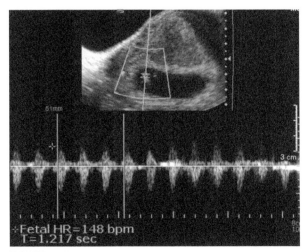

FIGURE 10-9 Transabdominal ultrasound using color Doppler and M-mode measurement of cardiac rate of the fetus.

The diagnosis of a blighted ovum is made when an empty gestational sac is identified, as shown in Figure 10-10.

Up to 25% of all pregnancies are associated with some vaginal bleeding early in pregnancy. The most common finding in women with vaginal bleeding and a viable pregnancy is subchorionic hemorrhage (or hematoma), identified as a fluid collection between the chorionic membrane and the uterine wall. Small subchorionic hemorrhages, as shown in Figure 10-11, usually have a good outcome, but larger hemorrhages, especially in older pregnant patients, increase the risk of pregnancy loss. When no visible hemorrhage is seen on ultrasound exam on a pregnant patient with vaginal bleeding, there is usually an excellent outcome and the bleeding is typically self-limiting.

If you suspect an ectopic pregnancy because of pelvic pain, the sonographic finding of a definite intrauterine gestational sac will almost always rule out ectopic gestation because simultaneous intrauterine and ectopic pregnancies are very rare.

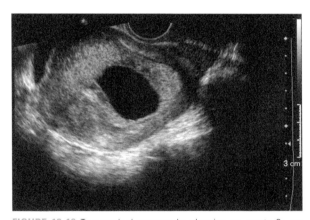

FIGURE 10-10 Transvaginal sonography showing an empty 2+ cm gestational sac, indicating a blighted ovum.

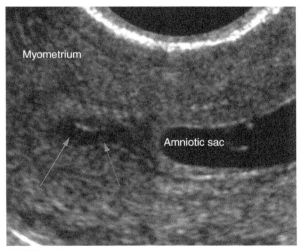

FIGURE 10-11 Transvaginal sonography of an early gestation showing a small hypoechoic subchorionic hemorrhage (arrows).

Under the hormonal influence of either a normal or ectopic pregnancy, there is a decidual response that results in the sonographic appearance of a thickened, hyperechoic endometrium, as shown in Figure 10-12. The diagnosis of an ectopic gestation is firmly established by identifying a gestational sac and its contents outside the uterus. Figure 10-13 shows the ectopic pregnancy in the same patient as in Figure 10-12. (See Patient Communication Box 10-1.)

Anencephaly, the failure of development of the cranium clearly seen on ultrasound as the absence of the normal echogenic skull, as shown in Figure 10-14, is an example of a major fetal structural defect that in this case was discovered during routine obstetric sonography in a radiology facility.

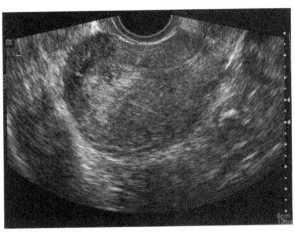

FIGURE 10-12 Transvaginal sonography showing decidual reaction (arrows) but no intrauterine gestational sac in a pregnant patient with pelvic pain and β-hCG greater than 5,000 mIU/mL.

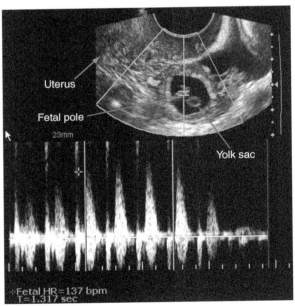

FIGURE 10-13 Transvaginal sonography (different image from the same examination shown in Figure 10-12) showing well developed early gestation in the adnexa with documentation of fetal cardiac activity.

Patient Communication Box 10-1

Upon finding a fetal defect, an ultrasound technologist should ask his or her medical supervisor, typically an obstetrician or radiologist, to observe or participate in additional scanning to confirm the finding. The subsequent interaction with the patient becomes extremely sensitive because the patient is immediately aware of a possibly devastating situation. It is imperative that the obstetrician or radiologist, while performing additional sonography to confirm the technologist's finding, be honest with the patient, explaining the situation and expressing concern. He or she should never simply just tell the patient that a report will be sent to her primary care provider. When the ultrasound exam is done in a radiology facility, ideally a radiologist should contact you immediately. The patient will want to speak with her primary care provider, with whom there is an established relationship of trust, as soon as possible. If an obstetrician is performing the procedure, he or she will likely be prepared to manage this difficult situation but should also contact you as soon as possible.

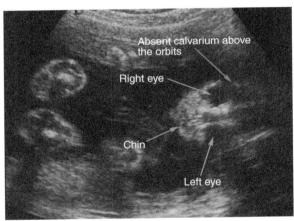

FIGURE 10-14 Image from the first routine obstetric sonography done during this pregnancy that by menstrual history was early in the second trimester. No fetal structures were visible above the orbits indicating absence of the calvarium (red arrow), and therefore a fetus with anencephaly.

The radiologist immediately discussed the emotionally devastating ultrasound finding with the patient and called the patient's primary care provider to report the finding. The primary care provider then, after talking with the patient on the phone, arranged for the patient to immediately see an obstetrician subspecializing in high risk and difficult obstetric cases. This is an example of shared professional interaction with a patient.

Serial obstetric ultrasound exams are used to determine fetal growth rates from measurements of the fetal head, abdomen, and femur length. Graphical representations of the growth of a fetus clearly show either fetal growth retardation or macrosomia.

As mentioned earlier, serial obstetric ultrasound exams are used to measure fetal growth rates; additionally, they are used to determine the position and appearance of the placenta, abnormalities of which can lead to fetal distress, bleeding, or difficulty with delivery. An example of a second trimester sonogram that revealed a placenta previa is shown in Figure 10-15, in which the placenta covers the internal cervical os.

The amount of amniotic fluid is estimated during obstetric sonography, either subjectively or using a semi-quantitative method, the Amniotic Fluid Index (AFI). Figure 10-16 shows obviously excessive amniotic fluid indicating polyhydramnios,

which raises suspicion of a fetal abnormality that prevents the fetus from swallowing amniotic fluid such as esophageal atresia. Figure 10-17 shows the virtual absence of amniotic fluid, indicating oligohydramnios that could be seen with premature rupture of the membranes or can occur with renal agenesis or other major fetal urinary tract malformations.

ACUTE PELVIC PAIN IN PATIENTS OF REPRODUCTIVE AGE

Patients who are of reproductive age experiencing acute pelvic pain include a special group of patients because of the initial clinical concern that the pain may be related to a gestation.

Many causes of acute pelvic pain in the reproductive-age female also have non-specific associated symptoms of nausea and vomiting, and leukocytosis. Imaging in this group of patients is based on the following:

- Determining if the patient is pregnant by obtaining a serum β-hCG
- Deciding if the history, physical exam, and laboratory studies suggest that the cause of pelvic pain is likely to be gynecologic, or related to the GI or urinary tract

Modalities

For patients who have a positive serum β-hCG and for those women with a negative serum β-hCG test but whose clinical evaluation strongly suggests gynecologic disease, ultrasonography is performed. Although transvaginal sonography usually provides higher spatial resolution of the adnexa and uterus than transabdominal sonography, important

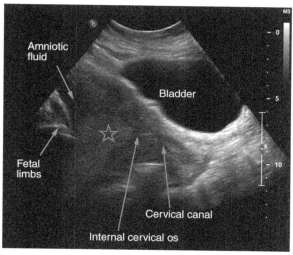

FIGURE 10-15 Routine second trimester obstetric sonography showing a posterior placenta previa star.

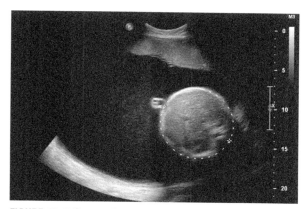

FIGURE 10-16 Sonography done at 32 weeks' gestation because the patient was "large for dates" demonstrates the presence of polyhydramnios and the absence of the normally expected fluid-filled fetal stomach. Note the dashed line along the circumference of the fetal abdomen, placed by the technologist while measuring the fetus.

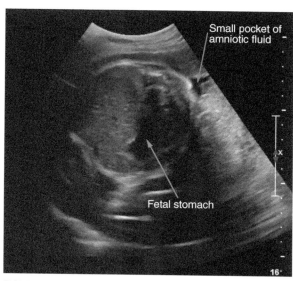

FIGURE 10-17 Sonography near term showing an almost complete absence of amniotic fluid (red arrow).

structures and significant pathology may be outside the field of view of the transvaginal transducer. Therefore, whenever practical, both transabdominal (done with a full urinary bladder) and transvaginal pelvic sonography should be performed in these patients.

For the pregnant patient with clinical suspicion of appendicitis, ultrasonography may be used but is often not definitive. Unenhanced MRI done in this clinical situation is very accurate and poses no threat to the fetus. Gadolinium-based contrast agents are usually avoided because they cross the placenta, although there are no published data currently that suggest a specific risk. CT is avoided because the developing fetus should never be exposed to ionizing radiation unless there is no other choice.

When a pregnant patient has symptoms of a ureteral calculus, sonography is done initially, but there is a wide reported range of sensitivity of sonography for documenting the presence of an obstructing ureteral calculus (see Chapter 9). MR urography (done without contrast enhancement) has been shown to be very useful in these cases, although sensitivity and specificity are only moderately high for ureteral calculus. When uncertainty persists, repeat ultrasonography and/or MR urography may be needed.

If the patient is not pregnant, ultrasonography may be preferred in adolescent and thin young adult female patients with suspected GI and urinary tract pathology, for whom it is appropriate to avoid ionizing radiation. However, CT is otherwise appropriate in most cases of suspected GI and urinary tract pathology because it is a more accurate examination than ultrasound, as discussed and illustrated in Chapters 8 and 9.

Interpretation
The Pregnant Patient

For the first trimester pregnant patient, sonography for detection or exclusion of ectopic pregnancy is discussed in the Obstetric Imaging section earlier. Spontaneous abortions may present with pelvic pain as well as bleeding, and pelvic sonography documents the loss of the pregnancy by the absence of an intrauterine gestation in a previously established pregnancy. Later in pregnancy, abruptio placentae presents with abdominal pain, premature contractions, and bleeding. Sonographic evaluation of the position and size of the retroplacental hematoma may be helpful, but because the hematoma may be organized, all or part of it may be isoechoic with the placenta. Therefore, sonography is not definitive and other clinical parameters are more important for clinical decisions in managing these patients.

As noted in Chapter 9, the hormonal environment of pregnancy causes reduced ureteral tone. Because of this and the extrinsic pressure on the distal ureters by the gravid uterus, the presence of dilated ureters does not establish the presence of an obstructing distal ureteral calculus. However, frank hydronephrosis shown by sonography, as in Figure 9-26, in a pregnant patient with flank pain and hematuria strongly suggests the presence of a calculus impacted in the associated ureter, even without direct visualization of that calculus.

When MR urography shows an edematous kidney, hydronephrosis, and perirenal fluid, the findings are consistent with a dilated ureter resulting from a distal obstructing calculus. The images may show the abrupt termination of the fluid-distended ureter at the level of the impacted calculus, as shown in Figure 10-18.

The Non-pregnant Patient

Mittelschmerz is a benign and common cause of pelvic pain, affecting up to 20% of women during their reproductive years. It is caused by fluid released when the dominant ovarian follicle ruptures at ovulation. This diagnosis is usually established by a history of repeated monthly episodes that are more intense on one side than the other. No imaging is required for the majority of these patients. However, occasionally the pain is severe enough to raise clinical concern, leading to ultrasonography. If the only sonographic finding is a modest amount of free fluid in the pelvis, as shown in Figure 10-19, then the pelvic pain can be attributed to the normal physiologic event of ovulation rather than any significant pathology.

In the patient who is not pregnant, gynecologic causes for acute pelvic pain include pelvic inflammatory disease (PID),

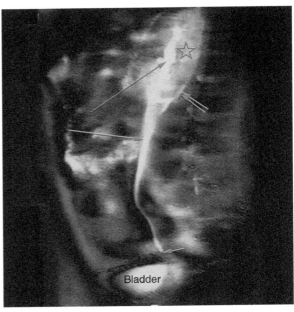

FIGURE 10-18 Sagittal MR urogram showing an edematous, enlarged kidney (star), perirenal fluid (double arrow), distended renal collecting system and ureter (long arrows), and the abrupt termination of the ureter at the level of an impacted calculus (short arrow).

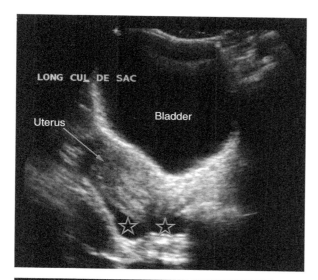

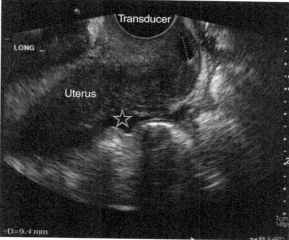

FIGURE 10-19 *Top:* Transabdominal sonogram showing a small amount of free fluid in the retrouterine cul-de-sac (stars) that is a normal physiologic finding in a female who has just ovulated. *Bottom:* Similar incidental small amount of cul-de-sac fluid (star) shown on transvaginal sonography. Note that the ultrasound technologist has measured a small Nabothian cyst to be 9.4 mm in diameter.

The ovarian follicle is a cyst up to 2.5 cm in diameter. When the follicle fails to ovulate due to abnormal levels of follicle stimulating hormone and/or luteinizing hormone, a large (>2.5 cm) follicular or "functional" cyst results, sometimes as large as 15 cm! An example of a follicular cyst of the ovary is shown in Figure 10-20. A corpus luteum cyst is a sonographically more complex cyst that forms from a follicle after ovulation.

A hemorrhagic ovarian cyst is initially hyperechoic, as shown in Figure 10-21. Later, the hemorrhage within a cyst may organize into hematoma or result in fibrinous septations within the cyst that may result in a complex structure on sonography.

Pelvic pain in a patient with an intrauterine device (IUD) to prevent pregnancy raises concern for displacement of the IUD that can cause bleeding and infection if it perforates the uterine wall. Confirmation of IUD position within the endometrial cavity is easily accomplished with sonography, as shown in Figure 10-22.

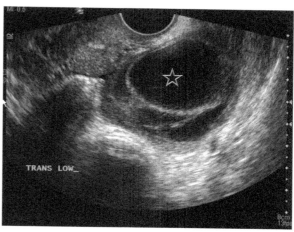

FIGURE 10-20 Pelvic sonography showing a small unilocular follicular or "functional" cyst (star) of an ovary.

ovarian torsion, and hemorrhagic cysts. Most PID does not show specific imaging findings, often showing only prominent adnexa, enlarged ovary, and some free pelvic fluid, but complications of PID may be evident as more discreet findings. For example, a tubo-ovarian abscess may be seen as a partially solid and partially cystic mass. Hydrosalpinx, a common complication of PID, may be evident as a tubular fluid-filled structure on ultrasound.

Ovarian torsion diagnosis is not as straightforward a sonographic diagnosis as testicular torsion because of more complicated anatomy and less reliable Doppler imaging findings for the ovary. However, conspicuously reduced Doppler flow in an edematous, enlarged ovary strongly suggests the diagnosis of ovarian torsion.

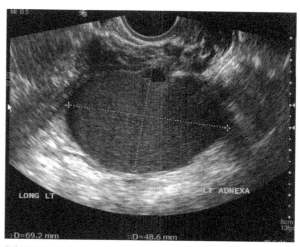

FIGURE 10-21 Pelvic sonography showing a hemorrhagic ovarian cyst, measured by the ultrasound technologist as 69.2 × 48.6 mm.

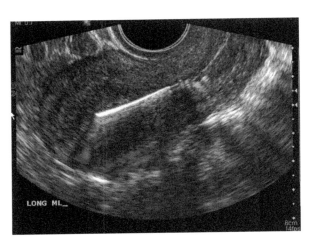

FIGURE 10-22 Pelvic sonography documenting that an IUD, seen as a very bright linear echo, is centrally placed within the uterus, thus properly positioned with the endometrial cavity.

IMAGING OF ABNORMAL VAGINAL BLEEDING AND PELVIC MASSES

Pelvic masses in the female include ovarian cysts and tumors, uterine fibroids, and masses that originate from outside of the reproductive system, such as colon masses or enlarged iliac chain lymph nodes.

CASE UPDATE

Your 55-year-old patient with fibroids has decided upon UAE. While arranging for this procedure, you are informed by the interventional radiologist that pre-procedure pelvic MRI is part of their routine protocol so that any needed follow-up MRI can be compared to a baseline study, and therefore you order that procedure for the patient. She has the MRI and then undergoes successful UAE.

A 6-month follow-up pelvic MRI shows dramatic reduction in the size of fibroids, and the patient's symptoms have improved. No special follow-up is recommended, other than routine yearly medical visits. For several years after UAE she remains asymptomatic and has normal physical examinations.

Modalities

The initial imaging modality used whenever there is clinical concern about a gynecologic mass is ultrasound, except in the case in which there is a very large mass that clinical exam suggests extends beyond the pelvis into the abdomen in a woman who is past reproductive age. In that case, it may be more efficient to proceed directly to contrast-enhanced CT of the abdomen and pelvis as a first study.

For postmenopausal vaginal bleeding, ultrasonography is initially used to measure endometrial thickness. In some cases, sonohysterography may be used for more detailed evaluation than provided by routine sonography. When a diagnosis of endometrial carcinoma has been established based on endometrial biopsy, MRI without and with contrast enhancement is important for staging purposes, including determination of the depth of myometrial invasion by the endometrial tumor. When the disease is advanced, CT of the chest is recommended to rule out pulmonary metastases. PET-CT is also useful for evaluating the extent of advanced metastatic disease.

For evaluation of the extent of locally invasive cervical carcinoma, MRI of the pelvis without and with contrast enhancement is done, often along with PET-CT for staging related to the presence or absence of distant metastatic disease.

CASE UPDATE

Seven years after UAE, your now 62-year-old patient reports the recent onset of postmenopausal bleeding. Ultrasonography reveals a thickened endometrium. You refer the patient to a gynecologist who performs an endometrial biopsy.

Interpretation

Abnormal menstrual bleeding may be the result of hormonal problems that are not explained by pelvic imaging. Also, endometrial pathology can exist that does not have macroscopic changes seen on imaging. In these cases, imaging is useful in ruling out gross pathology in the pelvis. As is often the case with imaging, pelvic sonography may be a triage tool in differentiating between disease that can be treated medically and disease that may require surgery.

Imaging findings of masses in the pelvis are often nonspecific with respect to histology. For example, a complex partially cystic and partially solid mass could be an abscess or tumor. Below we present some imaging findings that are strongly associated with specific pathology.

Young women with the classic clinical presentation of polycystic ovarian syndrome (i.e., hirsutism and insulin resistance) have bilateral enlarged ovaries with many tiny follicles. The numerous small follicular cysts may be difficult to distinguish on transabdominal ultrasound scanning, and transvaginal sonography may not be appropriate in the adolescent who is not sexually active. When only transabdominal scanning can be done in an adolescent with polycystic ovarian syndrome, the sole sonographic finding may be that the ovaries are about the same size as the uterus.

When an adolescent female with an imperforate hymen presents with a history of amenorrhea, and physical examination reveals an enlarged uterus, ultrasound may reveal a fluid-distended endometrial cavity, as shown in Figure 10-23.

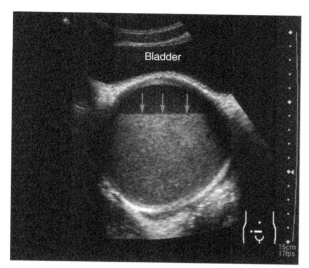

FIGURE 10-23 Pelvic sonography shows a distended endometrial cavity with a fluid–fluid level (arrows) that can be seen when any fluid collection contains cellular debris or old products of hemorrhage that "settle out" of the fluid, similar to the laboratory finding of a hematocrit level.

Endometriosis may present with very small endometrial implants that can be found in a wide range of extra-uterine locations. Occasionally, such an implant may become a moderately large endometrioma. The characteristic sonographic appearance is that of an adnexal cystic mass, within which there is a fluid–fluid level similar to that shown in Figure 10-23. MRI is more specific than ultrasound because of the hypointensity of the chronic heme products within the cyst, as shown in Figure 10-24.

Uterine fibroids are commonly diagnosed by sonography, with MRI or sonohysterography used when sonography is not definitive. Figure 10-25 is an example of sonohysterography showing the relationship between a fibroid and the endometrial cavity. In this case, a hypoechoic myometrial mass that is typical of a fibroid is not immediately submucosal and thus does not cause a focal endometrial deformity, but this fibroid is very large and has displaced the endometrial cavity caudally.

MRI is a valuable imaging tool for pre-treatment planning for patients with fibroids (Fig. 10-26)—for example, before myomectomy or UAE.

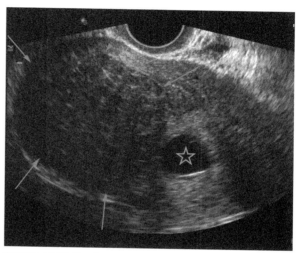

FIGURE 10-25 Sonohysterography showing a large mural fibroid (arrows) displacing, but not focally deforming, the saline-filled endometrial cavity (star).

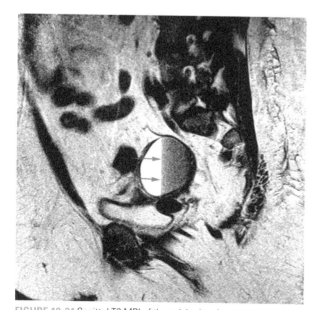

FIGURE 10-24 Sagittal T2 MRI of the pelvis showing an endometrioma with a fluid–fluid level (arrows) that was horizontal in the patient who was scanned while supine. The chronic heme products are hypointense in the dependent portion of the cyst posteriorly, and the serous fluid in the non-dependent portion of the cyst is T2 hyperintense.

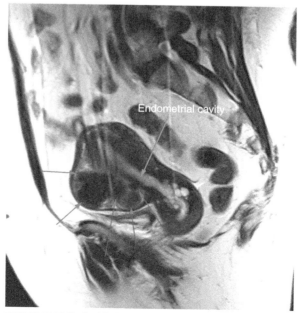

FIGURE 10-26 Sagittal T2 MRI of the pelvis showing multiple fibroids in the anterior uterine wall (red arrows) and incidental Nabothian cysts seen as the small round T2 hyperintense lesions of the uterine cervix.

Pelvic masses that are complex on sonography, including not only cystic and solid components but also components that cause acoustic shadowing, are suspicious for dermoid cysts (teratomas) of the ovary. The sonographic shadowing is caused by the variety of tissues that can be found in such lesions, such as lipids, hair, and teeth. Large dermoids may be missed because the shadowing is assumed to be from air-filled bowel loops adjacent to the adnexa. When sonography suggests a dermoid, CT can easily show the calcified structures, as well as the lipid contents, as shown in Figure 10-27. Radiography may be also useful to demonstrate the occasional presence of well-formed teeth, as shown in Figure 10-28.

The likelihood of malignancy of complex, septated ovarian cystic tumor increases with the amount of solid tissue of the lesion. Pelvic sonography provides excellent visualization of the architecture of ovarian lesions, but is limited in field of view for larger lesions. CT can be excellent for large lesions that extend into the abdomen, as shown in Figure 10-29. However, for pelvic lesions that do not extend into the abdomen, the higher intrinsic tissue contrast of MRI makes it a better study of pelvic pathology in most cases. Figure 10-30 is an example of an ovarian cystic lesion shown on MRI. Figure 10-31 shows a partially cystic but mostly solid T2 ovarian tumor.

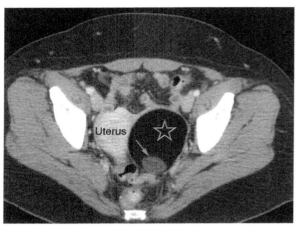

FIGURE 10-27 Axial CT showing a hypodense lipid-filled ovarian cyst (star) with a soft tissue mural nodule (arrow). Such a lipid-filled cyst is found in ovarian teratomas.

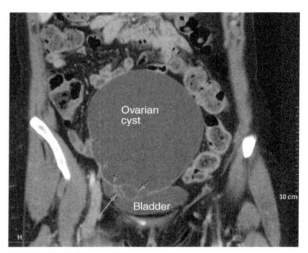

FIGURE 10-29 Coronal CT showing a large ovarian cyst with thin septations (arrows).

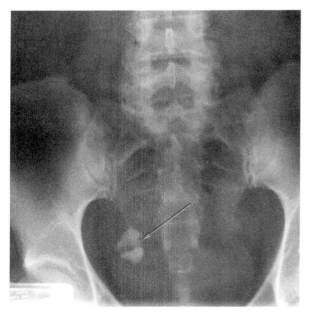

FIGURE 10-28 Radiograph showing teeth (arrow) that are within an ovarian teratoma.

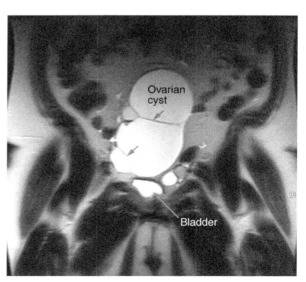

FIGURE 10-30 Coronal T2 MRI showing a large ovarian cyst with thin septations (red arrows).

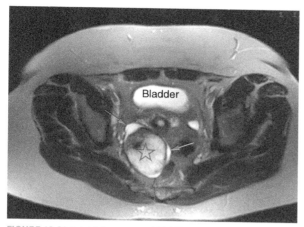

FIGURE 10-31 Axial fat-suppressed T2 MRI showing an ovarian tumor, within which there is a large solid mass (star) surrounded by thin crescent-shaped collections of fluid (arrows).

Ovarian malignancy commonly presents with peritoneal metastases. These may form soft tissue masses that are referred to as omental caking, as shown in Figure 10-32.

CASE CONCLUSION

The endometrial biopsy on your 62-year-old patient reveals endometrial carcinoma, and the gynecologist has ordered a pelvic MRI and referred the patient to a gynecologic oncologic surgeon. The MRI reveals no evidence of deep myometrial invasion by the tumor. Prior to scheduled surgery, she asks to speak with you about her current situation. She has been informed about test results by her surgeon, but she does not feel secure about what she has heard; she has been a patient of yours for a long time and needs to hear from you. You assure her that the MRI strongly suggests that the cancer is early stage and the outcome is very hopeful.

Hysterectomy and regional lymph node biopsy of this patient with endometrial carcinoma went well. All nodes were negative for disease, and her long-term prognosis is excellent.

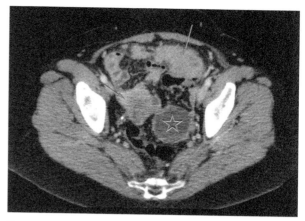

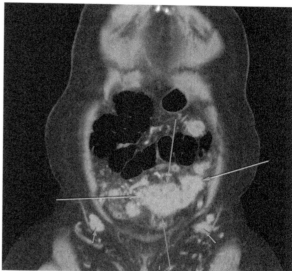

FIGURE 10-32 **Top:** Axial CT showing a portion of a partially cystic and partially solid ovarian tumor (star) and omental caking (arrows) indicating peritoneal metastatic disease. **Bottom:** Coronal CT showing omental caking (long arrows) and some prominent inguinal lymph nodes (short arrows).

Chapter Review

Chapter Review Questions

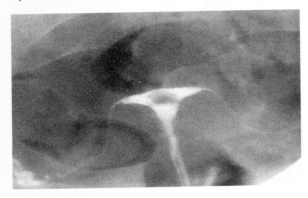

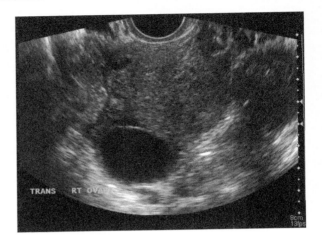

1. Which of the following is correct for the above image?
    A. It is a sonohysterogram with a filling defect caused by a fibroid
    B. It is a sonohysterogram and shows a filling defect caused by an endometrial polyp
    C. It is an HSG and shows a filling defect caused by a fibroid
    D. It is an HSG that shows a filling defect caused by an endometrial polyp
    E. It is a transabdominal ultrasound and shows an ovarian tumor

2. An ectopic pregnancy:
    A. commonly occurs simultaneously with an intrauterine pregnancy.
    B. can be excluded by the finding of a hyperechoic endometrium on ultrasound.
    C. can be firmly diagnosed by the presence of a gestational sac external to the uterus on ultrasound.
    D. is diagnosed by the absence of filling defects on HSG.
    E. must be diagnosed by CT of the abdomen.

3. Your diagnosis based on the ultrasound image shown above is:
    A. hemorrhagic ovarian cyst or endometrioma.
    B. simple ovarian cyst.
    C. ectopic gestation.
    D. free fluid in the pelvis.
    E. evidence of ovarian torsion.

4. Which of the following is incorrect about ureteral calculi during pregnancy?
    A. Hormonal changes during pregnancy greatly reduce the likelihood of the development of calculi
    B. Ureteral dilatation is common during pregnancy
    C. Frank hydronephrosis shown by sonography in a pregnant patient with flank pain and hematuria strongly suggests the presence of a calculus in the associated ureter
    D. MR urography may be conducted in a pregnant patient
    E. Renal stone protocol CT scanning is avoided in pregnant patients

5. In a patient with fever, pelvic pain, and leukocytosis, the finding on an ultrasound exam of prominent adnexa, enlarged ovary, and free pelvic fluid is consistent with:
    A. ovarian torsion.
    B. PID.
    C. Mittelschmerz.
    D. ovarian hemorrhagic cysts.
    E. blocked fallopian tube.

6. Omental caking is associated with:

    A. ovarian cancer.

    B. ectopic pregnancy.

    C. Mittleschmerz.

    D. PID.

    E. endometriosis.

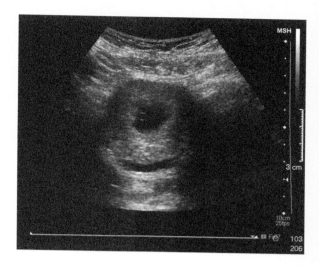

7. Ultrasound is usually definitive for diagnosis of:

    A. advanced stage ovarian cancer.

    B. development utereine anomalies.

    C. simple ovarian cysts.

    D. endometriosis.

    E. ureteral calculus in the pregnant patient.

11 IMAGING OF BONE DISEASE AND ENDOCRINE DISORDERS

CASE STUDY

A 35-year-old female, who is new to your practice, has hypertension and relates to you that she has been taking antihypertensive medications for several years. These were prescribed for her at community health clinics. The records that you acquire include a report from renal CTA that had been ordered to rule out renovascular hypertension. No renovascular cause for her hypertension was found.

FUNDAMENTALS OF IMAGING OF BONE DISEASE AND ENDOCRINE DISORDERS

Diagnosis of hormonal disorders depends upon clinical evaluation and laboratory studies. Imaging is usually used to select among the various possible causes of an endocrine dysfunction, which are associated with different treatment options. Once the biochemical status of endocrine disease is established, imaging can be specifically tailored to identify the cause.

The most common bone disease in your practice will be bone mineral loss in post-menopausal women and in some elderly males. A variety of screening and diagnostic tests for this condition are widely used, and they are discussed later in this chapter.

 Osteopenia and osteoporosis are major public health issues that may affect half of American adults older than age 50. Medical care of fractures related to osteoporosis costs billions of dollars each year in the United States. Only one third of hip fracture patients regain pre-fracture functional status, and approximate 20% of elderly patients will die within 1 year of suffering a hip fracture from minor trauma that would not have fractured normal bone.

OSTEOPOROSIS AND PAGET DISEASE

As your female patients pass through menopause (or have post-surgical menopause), part of your clinical responsibility as primary care provider will be to ensure that they undergo appropriate surveillance for loss of bone mineral density.

Some of your patients may undergo a heel ultrasound screening for bone mineral density at health screening "fairs." However, this screening test is not sufficiently accurate to determine whether medical treatment for bone mineral loss is needed.

Alcoholism, smoking, and the long-term use of corticosteroids increase the risk for osteoporosis in both men and women. Similar to women, elderly males may lose significant bone mineral, but because their baseline bone mineral density is so much higher than in women, the risk of insufficiency fracture remains relatively low in men until a later age.

Regional or focal bone disease may be secondary to tumor or infection. A relatively uncommon but important primary bone disease that you may encounter, especially in older patients, is Paget disease, which is a localized bone disorder that results in derangement of osteoclastic and osteoblastic activity. In affected bone, there is excessive bone mineral resorption and abnormal remodeling resulting in thickened but abnormal trabeculae and cortices, with weakening of bone that seems paradoxical when there is conspicuous bone thickening.

Modalities

Unless there is profound osteoporosis, diagnosis of osteopenia or osteoporosis is not possible by viewing radiographs. The only reliable radiographic diagnosis of bone mineral status is for localized bone changes—for example, the periarticular demineralization caused by hyperemia related to an inflammatory arthritis. Specific localized bone changes can also be clues to metabolic and endocrine disease, such as renal failure and hyperparathyroidism.

The most widely used and validated test for systemic bone mineral density is dual energy x-ray absorptiometry, usually called a **DEXA (or DXA)** scan. Another accurate method of quantifying bone mineral density in the spine is **quantitative CT (QCT),** but this is less widely available than DEXA scanning and exposes the patient to a higher dose of ionizing radiation.

For older patients, lateral spine radiography may be recommended to screen for vertebral insufficiency fracture(s) in addition to DEXA scanning.

When the clinical presentation of non-traumatic or minimally traumatic acute back pain, especially in a post-menopausal woman or elderly man, suggests that an insufficiency fracture has occurred, radiography is the most appropriate exam.

Although radiography may establish the diagnosis and provide sufficient information for conservative treatment, it may not show all vertebral fractures, and it can be difficult to distinguish old from new vertebral compression fracture deformities on radiographs. When there is a clinically acute symptomatic vertebral insufficiency fracture, particularly when partial vertebral collapse is shown radiographically, MRI is recommended if the patient is a candidate for verte-broplasty or kyphoplasty. MRI and/or CT are also indicated if needed after radiography to differentiate benign insufficiency fracture from a pathologic fracture (fracture of bone weakened by tumor or infection) of a vertebral body.

When musculoskeletal radiography is done as the initial evaluation for a painful bone or joint in the non-trauma situation, findings may indicate an arthritis, as discussed in Chapter 2. Lytic or blastic bone disease, cortical bone erosion that is not related to an arthritis, or periosteal reaction (as shown in Figure 2-47) raises concern for an infectious or oncologic process affecting the bone. Occasionally, the still poorly understood Paget disease of bone is found to be the underlying pathology. A markedly elevated serum alkaline phosphatase level may be found on routine blood chemistries in patients with minimal or no symptoms who have not come to clinical attention for Paget disease.

Interpretation

DEXA scan reports include bone mineral density in the lumbar spine and femoral necks. The Z-score indicates how the patient's mineral density ranks in standard deviations above or below the mean for his or her age and sex-match cohort. The T-score ranks the patient's bone mineral density in standard deviations above or below that of mean for young adult women.

A T-score between −1 and −2.5 indicates the presence of osteopenia. T-scores below −2.5 are diagnostic of osteoporosis. These T-scores (and Z-scores) are statistically related to risk of insufficiency fracture.

Depending upon a patient's underlying risk factors, results of bone densitometry, and any current medical treatment affecting bone mineral status, repeat DEXA scanning

is commonly done at intervals that range from yearly to several year intervals.

Paget disease of bone progresses from excess osteoclastic to excess osteoblastic activity and is diagnosed radiographically by the characteristic findings of thickened cortices and trabeculae and altered bone density, as shown in Figure 11-1. The original name for this disease, osteitis deforms, addresses the often bizarre appearance of bone affected by this disease. Although most areas within bone affected by Paget disease are hyperdense, areas where the thickened trabeculae are widely spaced can be hypodense. This altered bone architecture may sometimes be difficult to distinguish from mixed lytic and blastic malignant bone disease. In this case, CT is valuable for more detailed assessment of bone architecture, as shown in Figure 11-2. To assess activity of Paget disease, as with any bone disease, a radionuclide bone scan visually indicates the level of bone mineral turnover, as shown in Figure 11-3.

Deafness may occur if Paget disease affects the bones of the middle ear. High resolution temporal bone CT will demonstrate this involvement. When this disorder affects the spine, the

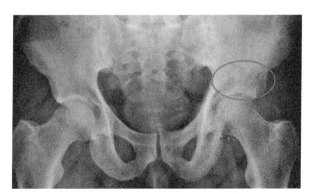

FIGURE 11-1 AP radiograph of the pelvis showing diffusely increased bone density, thickened and disorganized trabeculae, and thickened cortices throughout the entire left hemi-pelvis in a patient with Paget disease of bone. Look carefully at the abnormal trabeculae within the oval area above the left acetabulum and compare with the normal bone on the contralateral side.

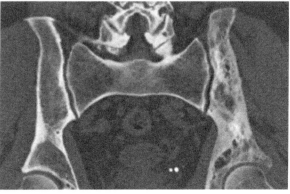

FIGURE 11-2 Coronal CT of the same patient as in Figure 11-1. Note the abnormal spacing and orientation of thickened trabeculae in the left hemi-pelvis.

thickened bone may cause spinal canal stenosis, which is evaluated with MRI or CT myelography. Other complications include stress fractures, as shown in Figure 11-4; congestive heart failure (CHF) secondary to arteriovenous shunting within severely affected bone; and the development of bone sarcomas.

THYROID AND PARATHYROID DYSFUNCTION

In Chapter 5, appropriate imaging of a patient who presents with an enlarged thyroid gland or thyroid mass is discussed. In this section we discuss those thyroid and parathyroid diseases that present with systemic symptoms that are biochemically characterized as thyroid or parathyroid dysfunction. Some overlap in clinical presentation of thyroid disease exists because patients with thyroid dysfunction may have enlarged thyroids. Hyperthyroidism is most commonly due to Graves disease, which results in goiter and enlargement of the thyroid and may be associated with thyroid ophthalmopathy and thyroid dermopathy. Less common causes of hyperthyroidism include solitary hyperfunctioning ("autonomous") nodules and toxic multinodular goiter. Hyperthyroidism also occurs transiently during the early phase of Hashimoto thyroiditis and subacute thyroiditis. Imaging of the thyroid is part of the evaluation of these conditions, and imaging of the orbits is appropriate when there is clinical concern for thyroid ophthalmopathy (see Chapter 5).

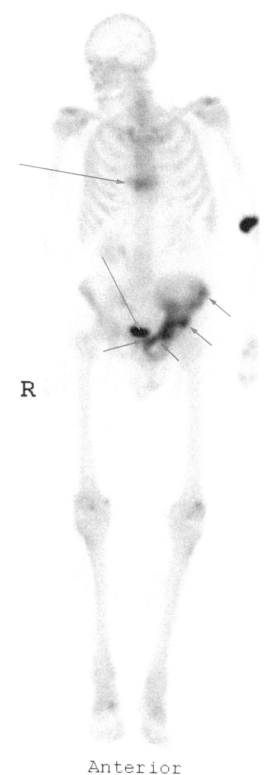

FIGURE 11-3 Anterior view, radionuclide bone scan showing increased activity in a subacute thoracic vertebral compression fracture (long arrow) and abnormally increased uptake in areas of Paget disease in the left hemi-pelvis (short arrows). Note the expected activity in the urinary bladder (blue arrow) and the intense activity in the left antecubital fossa from extravasation around the vein that occurred with a difficult IV injection.

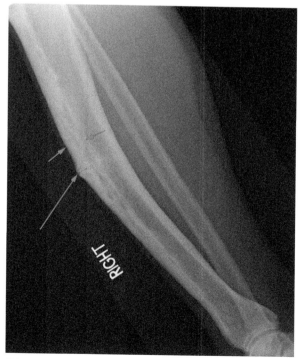

FIGURE 11-4 Lateral radiograph of the right lower leg showing an incomplete fracture (long arrow) from stress injury that occurred within the thickened (but structurally abnormal, weakened) cortex (short arrows) in a patient with Paget disease of the tibia.

Hyperthyroidism with high serum thyroid stimulating hormone (TSH) levels secondary to a hyperfunctioning pituitary adenoma is rare, but when it does occur, pituitary imaging should be done to identify such an adenoma and to guide treatment planning.

Hypothyroidism is less likely to require imaging for evaluation than hyperthyroidism. When the serum TSH is very low in the presence of depressed thyroid function, imaging of the pituitary may be appropriate to search for a cause of pituitary hypofunction. When clinical and laboratory studies point to Hashimoto thyroiditis as the cause of hypothyroidism, thyroid imaging may be appropriate.

Medullary carcinoma of the thyroid gland may result in elevated calcitonin levels, is often hereditary, and may occur with one of the multiple endocrine neoplasia (MEN) syndromes, in which case the clinical presentation may first be from an associated pheochromocytoma or parathyroid adenoma. Patients with MEN syndromes often require extensive imaging of multiple organ systems.

In patients without malignancy, hypercalcemia is most commonly caused by primary hyperparathyroidism, and imaging is done to search for a parathyroid adenoma. Although a solitary parathyroid adenoma is the cause of 80% to 85% of cases of primary hyperparathyroidism, the existence of many ectopic parathyroid glands, multiple adenomas, and parathyroid hyperplasia can make it very difficult to localize the cause of an elevated parathyroid hormone (PTH) level.

COST-EFFECTIVE MEDICINE

Skilled EENT surgeons have a very high operative success rate in identifying and removing parathyroid adenomas without imaging. Therefore, it is debatable if an aggressive and expensive imaging workup is always needed. However, post-operative recurrence or persistence of an elevated PTH level does require thorough imaging evaluation.

Hypercalcemia may also be associated with advanced malignancy, with imaging directed to finding malignant masses.

Modalities

As discussed in Chapter 5, ultrasonography is the primary modality for imaging of thyroid morphology, with Doppler imaging used to assess thyroid vascularity. Radionuclide thyroid scanning, usually done with the oral administration of a very small dose of I¹²³, along with measurement of radioiodine thyroid uptake, is often a key part of the functional evaluation of the thyroid.

In patients with hyperparathyroidism, thyroid ultrasonography is appropriate in the initial search for a parathyroid adenoma. When there is an elevated PTH and no parathyroid adenoma is found in the neck, there may be an ectopic parathyroid gland with an adenoma that is in the mediastinum. MRI may be helpful in this situation.

Radionuclide scanning using the radiopharmaceutical ⁹⁹ᵐTc sestamibi has high sensitivity and specificity for parathyroid adenomas. When the source of elevated PTH remains elusive, thoracic MRI is recommended to search for a mediastinal ectopic parathyroid adenoma.

Interpretation

When the normal thyroid gland is imaged by a gamma camera, most but not all of an orally administered dose of I¹²³ is taken up by the thyroid gland, and this uptake is conspicuous on the scan. However, some minimal "background" activity is commonly seen in soft tissues of the neck outside the thyroid gland itself. When there is a hyperactive thyroid gland, it shows avid uptake of the radioiodine and little or no background activity is seen, even on scans done as early as 4 to 6 hours after administration of I¹²³, as shown in Figure 11-5. More specific and informative is the measured thyroid uptake of radioiodine that is done along with the scanning. Typically, I¹²³ uptake is measured at 6 hours after oral administration, as shown in Figure 11-6, and often also at 24 hours.

In the case of an autonomous hyperfunctioning thyroid nodule, the "hot" nodule may so avidly take up the orally administered radioiodine that there is little activity in the adjacent normal thyroid tissue. Careful correlation of a nuclear scan showing a hyperfunctioning nodule with thyroid sonography can identify the responsible lesion.

Ultrasonography in Graves disease shows thyromegaly and may show some non-specific alteration in thyroid

I–123 SCAN

FIGURE 11-5 Anterior view, radionuclide thyroid scan, 6 hours after the oral administration of I¹²³. Note the absence of activity external to the thyroid. Depending upon exposure settings, one usually sees some background activity in soft tissues; not all of an administered dose of a radiopharmaceutical is taken up by the "target tissue." For comparison, the bone scan in Figure 11-3 shows normal background soft tissue activity.

Standard: 59021.11 cts

Thyroid: 33451.00 cts

Background: 2231.00 cts

Thyroid Uptake: 56.68 %

FIGURE 11-6 Result of the measured 6-hour uptake of I¹²³ in the same patient as in Figure 11-5. The 56.65% uptake is well above normal and is consistent with the markedly elevated T3 and T4 and depressed TSH levels in this hyperthyroid patient.

echogenicity, as shown in Figure 11-7, but otherwise no distinct imaging features. Doppler sonography in Graves disease may show hyperemia. Incidental thyroid nodules may be seen that are not related to the hyperthyroidism.

Patients with subacute thyroiditis and acute severe hyperthyroidism ("thyroid storm") may have the sonographic finding of dramatic hyperemia on Doppler imaging.

In the patient with hyperparathyroidism, thyroid sonography may demonstrate the presence of a lesion consistent with parathyroid adenoma as a solid or cystic nodule at the posterior margin of the thyroid gland. Ultrasound-guided fine-needle aspiration may establish the diagnosis by revealing markedly elevated PTH levels in fluid that is aspirated from cystic components of a parathyroid adenoma.

ADRENAL DYSFUNCTION AND NEUROENDOCRINE TUMORS OF THE PANCREAS

Imaging of the adrenal glands and pancreas is done specifically to explain the biochemical evidence of functioning neuroendocrine tumors. Functioning tumors of the pancreas are often referred to as islet cell tumors, and these may be

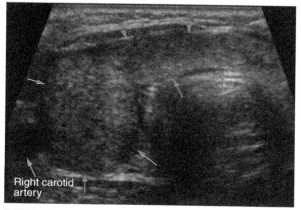

FIGURE 11-7 Transverse thyroid ultrasound image in a hyperthyroid patient shows some mild diffuse irregularity in the echo texture of the thyroid, which by measurement was nearly twice the volume of a normal thyroid gland.

well-differentiated tumors with little risk for metastatic disease or may be malignant endocrine-producing cancers. Islet cell tumors are very different from the malignant adenocarcinomas of the pancreas that make up 95% of pancreatic malignancies (see Chapter 8).

A rare cause of hypertension is a catecholamine-secreting tumor called a pheochromocytoma. Most of these are found in an adrenal gland. Extra-adrenal pheochromocytomas are often called paragangliomas.

A functioning adrenal adenoma may result in Cushing syndrome; however, 85% of patients with Cushing syndrome have either ectopic ACTH production (most common from small cell lung carcinoma), or an ACTH-producing pituitary adenoma.

Patients with hypoglycemia caused by hyperinsulinism are often found to have functioning beta-cell tumors of the pancreas called insulinomas. Patients with Zollinger-Ellison syndrome usually have a gastrin-secreting tumor that may be found in the pancreas or the wall of the duodenum.

Incidental non-functioning adrenal adenomas are found frequently on abdominal CT and MRI done for a wide variety of non-endocrine conditions. These are discussed further in Chapter 12 in the discussion of "incidentalomas."

CASE UPDATE

The detailed medical history that you obtain from your 35-year-old patient includes repeated episodes of symptoms that may be related to her hypertension: headache, palpitations, and diaphoresis. These episodes have been progressively more severe and more frequent. You order abdominal and pelvic CT without and with contrast enhancement, after laboratory studies showed high serum and 24-hour urine catecholamine levels.

Modalities

When there is biochemical evidence of a pheochromocytoma (elevated serum metanephrines and elevated 24-hour urine metanephrine and catecholamine levels), CT scanning of the abdomen and pelvis is recommended to identify an adrenal pheochromocytoma or an extra-adrenal pheochromocytoma (called paraganglioma).

Whenever CT is done for a suspected adrenal tumor, it is important to order CT to be done without and with contrast enhancement. The CT density of an adrenal lesion that is not altered with intravenous contrast enhancement is important because adrenal adenomas are homogeneous low-density (lipid-containing) lesions, while adrenal carcinomas and pheochromocytomas are soft tissue density or complex lesions.

In some cases in which CT is not definitive, abdominal MRI without and with gadolinium enhancement is appropriate for further study. There are also special nuclear medicine procedures that can localize an elusive

---

pheochromocytoma. Consultation with a radiologist may be needed to find out which of these is locally available.

If a patient with Cushing disease has suppressed ACTH levels, CT or MRI of the adrenal glands without and with contrast enhancement should be done. In a Cushing syndrome patient with no oncologic history and elevated ACTH, imaging of the pituitary gland is required, as discussed in the next section.

When there is biochemical evidence of a neuroendocrine pancreatic tumor, contrast-enhanced CT scanning is indicated. Because many of these tumors are hypervascular, the timing of a typical pancreatic protocol CT may be altered if radiology is alerted to this specific clinical concern. Abdominal MRI without and with contrast enhancement is also excellent for detecting these tumors.

Interpretation

Carcinomas of the adrenal are rare; most adrenal masses are benign adenomas that have the characteristic imaging finding of high lipid content that can be documented with special MRI sequences (or by low density on an unenhanced CT scan as discussed earlier), as shown in Figure 11-8.

Pheochromocytomas are adrenal masses that are usually less homogeneous in density on non-contrast CT or intensity on MRI images than adenomas, although there may be some overlap.

Neuroendocrine pancreatic tumors are visible within the pancreas on MRI or CT as distinct lesions, as shown in this case of an islet cell tumor of the pancreas that has a rim of hyperenhancing tissue and central low density (Fig. 11-9).

CASE UPDATE
The CT scan on your 35-year-old hypertensive female patient showed a mass in the left adrenal gland consistent with pheochromocytoma. Adrenalectomy cured her hypertension.

PITUITARY DYSFUNCTION

By convention, tumors of the pituitary that are 1 cm or less in diameter are called microadenomas and tumors larger than 1 cm are called macroadenomas. Up to 20% of the clinically normal adult population has non-functioning pituitary microadenomas. This highlights the importance of thorough laboratory evaluation of endocrine status with respect to imaging findings in the pituitary.

The most common anterior pituitary endocrine dysfunction related to excess production of a hormone is a prolactinoma, which is suspected by the finding of hyperprolactinemia. Less common functioning pituitary adenomas are those that secrete ACTH, resulting in Cushing syndrome, and those that

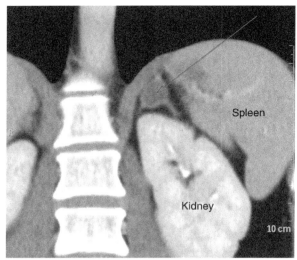

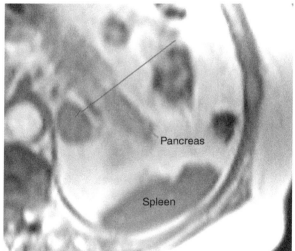

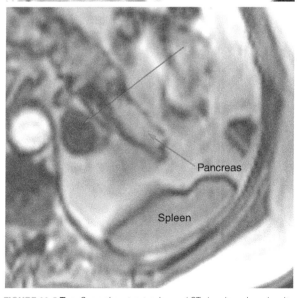

FIGURE 11-8 **Top:** Coronal contrast-enhanced CT showing a low-density left adrenal adenoma. **Middle:** Axial "in-phase" T1 MR image of a left adrenal mass. **Bottom:** Axial "out-of-phase" T1 MR image of the same left adrenal mass (red arrow), showing decreased signal (darker) in the mass when compared with the "in-phase" image, indicating the presence of intracellular lipid, consistent with adrenal adenoma.

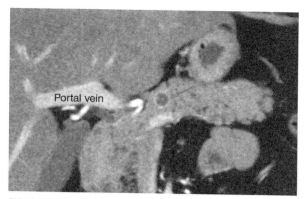

FIGURE 11-9 Coronal contrast-enhanced CT showing a functioning islet cell (neuroendocrine) tumor (arrow) in the body of the pancreas that has central low density and a rim of hyper-enhancing tissue, a finding not characteristic of pancreatic adenocarcinoma.

secrete growth hormone (GH), resulting in gigantism. Functioning pituitary adenomas that secrete TSH, follicle stimulating hormone (FSH), or luteinizing hormone (LH) are rare. Antidiuretic hormone (ADH) is secreted by the posterior pituitary, but most cases of the syndrome of inappropriate ADH secretion (SIADH) are the result of ectopic ACH production, not a pituitary lesion.

Non-functioning pituitary adenomas, as well as other destructive lesions such as hemorrhage, may result in hypopituitarism.

The most common cause of hypopituitarism in pediatric and young adult patients is a craniopharyngioma. Other causes include primary CNS tumors that involve the hypothalamus.

Pituitary tumors are rarely malignant, but histologically benign pituitary macroadenomas can cause serious complications from mass effect on adjacent structures, such as the optic chiasm and nerves in cavernous sinus, and can be difficult or impossible to completely remove surgically. Therefore, large pituitary tumors may present clinically with headache or visual disturbances rather than endocrine disease.

Modalities

MRI of the brain and pituitary without and with contrast enhancement is the appropriate imaging procedure for either endocrine dysfunction related to the pituitary or neurologic symptoms secondary to a suspected hypothalamic or pituitary mass. MRI is the procedure of choice for suspected craniopharyngioma, but CT is often done as a supplementary study because many of these lesions are partially calcified; the calcifications are better seen and characterized on CT than on MRI.

Interpretation

Although the blood–brain barrier prevents gadolinium from entering the brain's interstitium, the pituitary gland lacks this

blood–brain barrier and therefore enhances intensely after an injection of a gadolinium-based contrast agent. Pituitary microadenomas are seen as hypo-enhancing lesions surrounded by brightly enhancing normal pituitary tissue, as shown in Figure 4-27 of Chapter 4, Brain.

A pituitary macroadenoma is usually seen as an enhancing mass that may involve the cavernous sinuses if expansion is lateral, or the optic chiasm if expansion is suprasellar, as shown in Figure 11-10.

Craniopharyngiomas are usually complex lesions with cystic and solid components that are well seen on MRI, as shown in Figure 11-11, as well as calcifications that are best seen on CT.

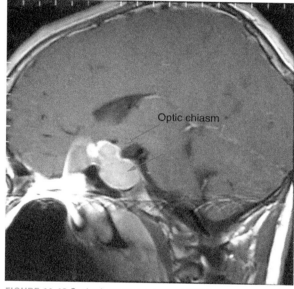

FIGURE 11-10 Sagittal contrast-enhanced MRI in a teenage patient (note distortion of the image anteriorly because of metallic dental braces) who had bitemporal hemianopsia because of a pituitary macroadenoma (red arrow).

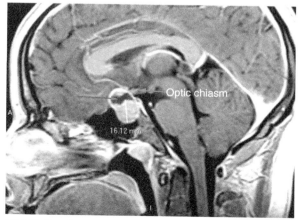

FIGURE 11-11 Sagittal contrast-enhanced MRI in which the solid portion of a craniopharyngioma has been measured (solid line with measurement on image), and in which there is a T1 hypointense cystic portion (red arrow).

Chapter Review

Chapter Review Questions

1. An ultrasound heel screening test for bone mineral density:
   A. is available in hospital settings and provides the highest level of diagnostic accuracy.
   B. is comparable to DEXA in its level of diagnostic accuracy.
   C. can be used to diagnose Paget disease.
   D. is not sufficiently reliable or accurate to use as the basis for treatment of osteoporosis.
   E. should be used in all patients with suspected vertebral insufficiency fractures.

   Answer the following questions based on the image below:

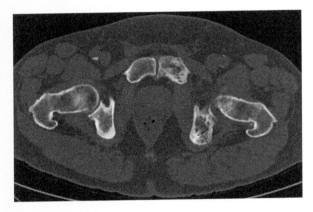

2. Your diagnosis based on the image above is:
   A. osteopenia.
   B. Paget disease.
   C. hypercalcemia.
   D. insufficiency fracture.
   E. multiple endocrine neoplasia (MEN).

3. In a patient with elevated PTH and in whom ultrasonography failed to reveal an adenoma in the neck, you might:
   A. order a radiograph of the mediastinum.
   B. order an MRI of the brain.
   C. order a CT of the brain.
   D. order a I^{123} nuclear medicine scan.
   E. order a ^{99m}Tc sestamibi nuclear medicine scan.

4. Ultrasound-demonstrated thyromegaly and diffuse hyperemia is consistent with:
   A. multinodular goiter.
   B. subacute thyroiditis with thyroid storm.
   C. hyperparathyroidism.
   D. pituitary microadenoma.
   E. suppression of TSH secretion because of pituitary macroadenoma.

5. For a patient with Cushing syndrome with elevated ACTH and no oncologic history, you would order:
   A. CT of the abdomen.
   B. MRI of the abdomen.
   C. MRI of the pituitary.
   D. thyroid ultrasound.
   E. DEXA scan.

6. Adenomas of the adrenal gland are typically demonstrated on:
   A. abdominal radiographs.
   B. unenhanced abdominal CT.
   C. nuclear medicine scans.
   D. ultrasound scans.
   E. DEXA scans.

12 CLINICAL PRACTICE ISSUES IN MEDICAL IMAGING

Your patients and your practice will benefit from your careful consideration of the issues discussed in this chapter that relate to the wise *use* of radiologic knowledge. Not every finding on medical images is clinically significant; the fantastically detailed look at your patients' interior structures now provided by today's technologically advanced medical imaging instruments may sometimes be "too much information." This assertion may seem paradoxical when the care we provide often depends upon gathering as much clinical, laboratory, and imaging information as possible. However, the quality of medical care is ultimately measured by clinical outcome, and some of the many bits of information that emerge from medical imaging may have very little or no clinical significance. This issue of potentially superfluous information from radiologic studies is one that you will deal with frequently.

The selection of an ideal medical imaging procedure for each clinical problem is not always straightforward. Although we have in these chapters presented our best advice for making imaging choices, the ideal imaging procedure for each clinical problem is sometimes contentious, as advocates for one type of imaging procedure compete with those who promote an alternative modality as more accurate, or safer, or more cost effective.

The potential risks and discomforts of radiologic procedures are widely discussed on the internet and in print media, sometimes becoming front-page news items. This very public issue is one that you will confront when making decisions about ordering procedures and when discussing procedures with your patients.

In a large and complex medical system, communication among caregivers is not always ideal, and this can negatively impact upon patient care. This issue deserves special attention in a medical system in which many specialists often share responsibility for patient care.

Finally, while the issues of efficacy and cost-effectiveness of medical care are being widely discussed for economic and political reasons, the quality of medical care you provide is still largely determined by medical professional ethics.

"INCIDENTALOMAS"

The CT of your 75-year-old patient, which you ordered for diverticulitis, shows a small adrenal mass. In a patient of this age with an acute illness and perhaps other comorbidities, do you follow up this unexpected finding? It may be entirely reasonable for you not to act upon this imaging finding in this particular patient. In contrast, for the same finding in a much younger patient who has some cushingoid features, you would likely order an endocrine laboratory workup and a follow-up adrenal-specific imaging study.

The finding of this mass in your 75-year-old patient is an example of an incidental imaging finding, commonly referred to as an *incidentaloma*—findings that are not related to the clinical concern associated with the requested imaging study. These surprise findings may require your immediate attention or may pose little or no risk to your patient.

The report you receive from the radiologist will describe any incidentalomas identified during the imaging evaluation and should include general guidance for acting (or not) on these unexpected results. Whether you decide to follow up on incidentalomas cannot be based on a flow chart but on thoughtful clinical judgment as to what is best for your patient.

When you discuss incidentalomas with your patient you must provide him or her with an appropriate context to understand your recommendations. Inappropriately alarming a patient by saying that a "tumor was found in your left adrenal" without careful explanation about why it is likely to be a trivial finding could lead to patient-driven unnecessary and expensive imaging follow-up studies and excessive biopsies, and of course avoidable patient distress.

Furthermore, you should keep foremost in your mind that the whole question of incidentalomas can often be avoided if you only order imaging studies when the results of such studies will affect the clinical management of your patient.

The problematic finding of incidentalomas is a potential adverse consequence of imaging studies, along with the small risks from diagnostic radiation and nephrotoxicity or allergic reaction from intravenous contrast agents.

Next we discuss common incidental findings that you will likely see on the radiology reports on the radiologic examinations performed on your patients.

Incidental Findings on Chest CT

Among the common unsuspected findings on chest CT is a thoracic aortic aneurysm, the clinical significance of which depends principally upon size; aneurysms only slightly above normal in diameter may have little current clinical significance and may only need to be followed with imaging at appropriate intervals. When a chest CT report indicates that your 65-year-old male patient, who is 6 feet 6 inches tall, has a 4.1 cm aneurysm of the ascending aorta (tall people have relatively large aortas), you should choose your words carefully when discussing this finding with the patient: Instead of telling the patient that he has an "aneurysm," consider tempering the issue by telling him that his aorta is slightly larger than normal and needs to be followed up on but is not currently affecting his health. It may be prudent to seek an opinion from a cardiothoracic surgeon, but you can provide reassurance to your patient that the surgeon is unlikely to recommend immediate surgery, and that the visit is providing a "baseline" in case the aorta enlarges significantly in the future.

In contrast to that 65-year-old male patient, the surprise finding of an asymptomatic 7 cm aortic aneurysm on a coronary calcium score in virtually any patient needs prompt surgical attention. In this situation, it is certainly appropriate to communicate to the patient the potential danger of such a large aneurysm and the need for urgent attention. For many incidental findings, size matters.

Screening chest CT scans for detection of early lung cancer on high-risk patients (smokers) frequently reveal previously undiagnosed coronary artery disease and emphysema, which are variable in clinical significance. For example, the incidental finding of a few scattered coronary calcifications may result in nothing more than a recommendation that the patient undergo a coronary calcium score, while the finding of extensive and severe coronary calcifications should result in an urgent coronary evaluation that may include cardiology consultation, CCTA, or coronary catheterization.

CT is very sensitive to detecting minimal centrilobular emphysema that may not require more "care" than cessation of smoking, and this should be communicated to the patient and followed up much differently than the finding of extensive panlobular emphysema in a patient previously not under care for severe lung disease.

Pulmonary nodules are often found on chest CT ordered for a variety of clinical concerns. Only a small percentage of these will be malignant. There are well-established guidelines (e.g., by the Fleischner Society) that all radiologists should refer to for their recommendation as to whether and how an incidental pulmonary should be followed up. Furthermore, because of the high frequency of incidental pulmonary nodular findings, the risk/benefit and cost/benefit ratios of screening CT scans for lung cancer have been controversial.

Incidental Hepatic Lesions

Cystic hepatic findings are common and are almost always benign and clinically insignificant. Characteristically simple hepatic cysts and similar benign bile duct hamartomas do not need to be reported to patients.

Within generalized hepatic steatosis, there may be a small region of the liver that is spared from this process, referred to as focal sparring. This can have a mass-like appearance. When this finding has characteristic features, such as the absence of mass effect on intrahepatic vessels, no further evaluation is needed. However, when the nature of this finding is not clear, it is sometimes necessary to get another imaging study to document the absence or presence of a true mass.

The most common incidental mass found in the liver on routine CT is the benign cavernous hemangioma. Definitive hepatic mass evaluation cannot always be expected from a routine abdominal CT scan, and the radiologist may only report the presence of a nonspecific mass. When explaining to patients why a more focused abdominal imaging procedure is now needed, you can reassure them that in the absence of a history of cirrhosis or cancer, a malignant hepatic mass is not likely.

Incidental Pancreatic Cysts

Unfortunately, definitive histologic characterization of pancreatic cystic tumors by imaging is difficult. Depending upon patient factors (age and comorbidities) and size of the lesion, the radiologist may recommend imaging surveillance rather than biopsy or resection.

Incidental Adrenal Masses

The adrenal gland can be the site of primary malignancy and is often the target of metastatic disease. However, when a small adrenal mass in found in a patient with no oncologic history, the overwhelming likelihood is that the lesion is an incidental benign nonfunctioning adrenal adenoma that has no clinical significance. Adrenal-specific imaging studies are often recommended on radiology reports to evaluate incidental adrenal masses. You can reassure your patient that malignancy is very unlikely.

Incidental Renal Masses

Simple renal cysts are very common incidental findings that can be ignored. Chapter 9 discussed the evaluation of more complex cysts that may have malignant potential.

Greater than 50% of all renal tumors are now found as incidental findings on abdominal CT or MRI. Many of these are renal carcinomas that must be treated. However, nearly 50% of renal tumors less than 1 cm are found to be benign.

Incidental Bone Findings

Benign vertebral cavernous hemangiomas are often seen as incidental findings on spinal imaging studies and can be ignored.

A bone island, also called an enostosis, is a focus of compact bone within medullary or cancellous bone. These are visible on radiographs and are often found on CT and MRI; they have no significance but may need to be differentiated from a blastic metastatic lesion.

Incidental Thyroid Nodules

Two thirds of adults have incidental thyroid nodules! These are found on carotid ultrasound, cervical spine MRI, chest CT, or any study that may include the thyroid gland in the field of view. Only a small number of these are found to be malignant. A careful search for benign imaging characteristics, follow-up sonography to document stability, and fine-needle aspiration are recommended to limit the number of surgical biopsies of these common incidental findings.

THE AMERICAN COLLEGE OF RADIOLOGY ACR APPROPRIATENESS CRITERIA®

A major theme of this text has been the optimal selection of imaging procedures for many clinical conditions. Once you have learned the information provided in the book, we recommend you refer to the outstanding, up-to-date, and concise Internet resource provided by The American College of Radiology (http://www.acr.org/). These "Appropriateness Criteria" consists of numeric ratings of appropriateness for imaging procedures that might be considered for a large number of specific clinical situations. The tabulated ratings include brief comments about those procedures and the relative radiation level to which a patient is exposed during each procedure. The tables are followed by an excellent "Summary of Literature Review" that a multi-specialty expert panel (radiologists, internists, and surgeons) used to establish the appropriateness ratings. These summaries are not just discussions of the technology involved in imaging but also review the pathology involved in these clinical situations. A list of references is also provided, should you want to dig deeper into the topic.

The ACR example shown on the next page was found by clicking on "Musculoskeletal Imaging" and then on "Chronic Neck Pain." Note the clinical variants that focus recommendations on highly specific clinical situations.

TALKING TO PATIENTS ABOUT THE RISKS OF IMAGING PROCEDURES

In Chapter 1 we provided data on the relatively low exposure doses associated with contemporary radiography and CT. Guided by the primary medical dictate of "do no harm," the medical community and equipment manufacturers, along with federal and state regulatory agencies, continually strive to further reduce these exposures following the principle of using radiation doses "as low as reasonably achievable (ALARA)" while maintaining adequate image quality.

For example, all or most chest and abdominal CT studies once typically involved two scans: prior to and after the injection of iodinated IV contrast material. Now, only a single contrast enhanced scan is usually done for "routine" cases.

The Alliance for Radiation Safety in Pediatric Imaging has initiated an Image Gently™ campaign to minimize pediatric exposures. More information about this campaign can also be found on the website of the ACR.

While as a matter of principle no patient should ever be exposed to radiation for even a single radiographic image unless absolutely needed for diagnosis, the risk from diagnostic exposure to radiation is extremely low. It has been estimated that a CT examination that exposes the patient to 10 mSv might be associated with an increased risk of fatal cancer of 1 in 2,000. This compares with the natural risk of fatal cancer of 1 in 5. With newer scanners and CT protocols, the radiation exposure and risk cited earlier are becoming even smaller.

Some patients may harbor exaggerated perception about the risk of radiation. When talking to patients about this risk, it is more important to discuss relative risks rather than to cite statistics. Some patients need to be reminded that *not* having a definitive diagnosis (because of a scan not performed) poses other risks. Taking medications, even over-the-counter "supplements," is associated with some risk. Driving to a medical clinic exposes one to a slight risk. Sometimes you need to remind patients that you are aware of these risks and are using sound medical judgment in balancing risks when ordering imaging procedures.

Some of your patients have an exaggerated perception of risks from contrast agents used in radiologic procedures, and this may emerge during your clinical encounter with a patient when you explain to them about a procedure you are ordering that will involve an intravenous injection.

When addressing risks in medical imaging procedures other than the radiation issue with your patients, it is helpful to keep in mind some of the information presented earlier in this book. For example, severe allergic reactions to contrast agents are very rare. Another issue that has been promoted publicly is the risk of developing nephrogenic systemic sclerosis (NSF) after the use of gadolinium-based contrast agents. In any discussion about this issue that you may have with a patient, use your new knowledge that it is a risk limited to a select group of patients, and that your

American College of Radiology
ACR Appropriateness Criteria®

__Clinical Condition:__   Chronic Neck Pain
__Rating Scale:__   1,2,3 usually not appropriate; 4,5,6 may be appropriate; 7,8,9 usually appropriate

Variant 1: Patient without or with a history of previous trauma, first study.

Radiologic Procedure	Rating	Comments	Relative Radiation Level
X-ray cervical spine	9	AP, lateral, open mouth, both obliques.	☢☢
X-ray myelography cervical spine	2		☢☢☢
CT cervical spine without contrast	2		☢☢☢
Myelography and post myelography CT cervical spine	2		☢☢☢☢
MRI cervical spine without contrast	2		0
Tc-99m bone scan neck	2		☢☢☢
Facet injection/arthrography cervical spine selective nerve root block	2		☢☢

Variant 2: Patient with history of previous malignancy, first study.

Radiologic Procedure	Rating	Comments	Relative Radiation Level
X-ray cervical spine	9	AP, lateral, open mouth, both obliques.	☢☢
CT cervical spine without contrast	2		☢☢☢
MRI cervical spine without contrast	2		0
Tc-99m bone scan neck	2		☢☢☢

Variant 3: Patient with history of previous neck surgery, first study.

Radiologic Procedure	Rating	Comments	Relative Radiation Level
X-ray cervical spine	9	AP, lateral, open mouth, both obliques.	☢☢
CT cervical spine without contrast	2		☢☢☢
MRI cervical spine without contrast	2		0
Tc-99m bone scan neck	2		☢☢☢

Variant 4: Radiographs normal. No neurologic findings.

Radiologic Procedure	Rating	Comments	Relative Radiation Level
X-ray myelography cervical spine	2		☢☢☢
CT cervical spine without contrast	2		☢☢☢
Myelography and post myelography CT cervical spine	2		☢☢☢☢
MRI cervical spine without contrast	2		0
Tc-99m bone scan neck	2		☢☢☢
Facet injection/arthrography cervical spine selective nerve root block	2		☢☢

Variant 5: Radiographs normal. Neurologic signs or symptoms present.

Radiologic Procedure	Rating	Comments	Relative Radiation Level
MRI cervical spine without contrast	9		0
Myelography and post myelography CT cervical spine	5	If MRI contraindicated.	☢☢☢☢
X-ray myelography cervical spine	2		☢☢☢
CT cervical spine without contrast	2		☢☢☢
Tc-99m bone scan neck	2		☢☢☢
Facet injection/arthrography cervical spine selective nerve root block	2		☢☢

Clinical Condition: Chronic Neck Pain
Rating Scale: 1,2,3 usually not appropriate; 4,5,6 may be appropriate; 7,8,9 usually appropriate

Variant 6: Radiographs show spondylosis. No neurologic findings.

Radiologic Procedure	Rating	Comments	Relative Radiation Level
X-ray myelography cervical spine	2		
CT cervical spine without contrast	2		☢☢☢
Myelography and post myelography CT cervical spine	2		☢☢☢
MRI cervical spine without contrast	2		☢☢☢☢
Tc-99m bone scan neck	2		0
Facet injection/arthrography cervical spine selective nerve root block	2		☢☢☢
X-ray discography cervical spine	1		☢☢

Variant 7: Radiographs show spondylosis. Neurologic signs or symptoms present.

Radiologic Procedure	Rating	Comments	Relative Radiation Level
MRI cervical spine without contrast	9		0
Myelography and post myelography CT cervical spine	5	If MRI contraindicated.	☢☢☢☢
X-ray myelography cervical spine	2		☢☢☢☢☢
CT cervical spine without contrast	2		☢☢☢
Tc-99m bone scan neck	2		☢☢☢
Facet injection/arthrography cervical spine selective nerve root block	2		☢☢
X-ray discography cervical spine	1		☢☢

Variant 8: Radiographs show old trauma. No neurologic findings.

Radiologic Procedure	Rating	Comments	Relative Radiation Level
X-ray myelography cervical spine	2		☢☢☢
CT cervical spine without contrast	2		☢☢☢
Myelography and post myelography CT cervical spine	2		☢☢☢☢
MRI cervical spine without contrast	2		0
Tc-99m bone scan neck	2		☢☢☢
Facet injection/arthrography cervical spine selective nerve root block	2		☢☢
X-ray discography cervical spine	1		☢☢

Variant 9: Radiographs show old trauma. Neurologic signs or symptoms present.

Radiologic Procedure	Rating	Comments	Relative Radiation Level
MRI cervical spine without contrast	9		0
Myelography and post myelography CT cervical spine	5		☢☢☢☢
X-ray myelography cervical spine	2		☢☢☢
CT cervical spine without contrast	2	If MRI contraindicated.	☢☢☢
Tc-99m bone scan neck	2		☢☢☢
Facet injection/arthrography cervical spine selective nerve root block	2		☢☢
X-ray discography cervical spine	1		☢☢

Variant 10: Radiographs show bone or disc margin destruction.

Radiologic Procedure	Rating	Comments	Relative Radiation Level
MRI cervical spine without contrast	9		0
CT cervical spine with contrast	5	CT with contrast should be performed if MRI is unavailable or cannot be performed for any suspected disc space infection.	☢☢☢
X-ray myelography cervical spine	2		☢☢☢
CT cervical spine without contrast	2		☢☢☢
Myelography and post myelography CT cervical spine	2		☢☢☢☢
Tc-99m bone scan neck	2		☢☢☢

Adapted from American College of Radiology ACR Appropriateness Criteria.

ordering of a laboratory study to check renal function can exclude them from that high-risk group.

CLAUSTROPHOBIA AND MRI

Approximately 15% of patients are too claustrophobic to undergo MRI without some assistance. When discussing your plan to order MRI with a patient, you should always ask the patient if they "have trouble with tight spaces." If the patient is claustrophobic, you must inform the imaging facility or department to which you are referring the patient for MRI that this is the case because extra time may need to be scheduled.

Some MRI facilities are much better than others in handling claustrophobic patients, whether through "verbal sedation," hand-holding, or allowing for short breaks during a lengthy procedure, or with intravenous conscious sedation. Claustrophobic patients should be referred to such facilities if available in your community.

COMMUNICATION AND COLLABORATION AMONG MEDICAL PROFESSIONALS

Throughout this book we have indicated the kind of concise but critical clinical information that should be shared on imaging requisitions between the medical practitioners who order radiologic studies and the imaging facilities/departments and radiologists responsible for those examinations.

In some modern medical practices a tendency has developed to only use diagnostic codes to provide "information" on radiology orders. Such codes are appropriate for the process of seeking approval or authorization from third party payers for imaging exams. However, these codes are not designed to provide the kind of information that might make a difference in the implementation or interpretation of an imaging study.

The information you provide on an imaging order or requisition is the beginning of the cooperative process between members of the health care team that improves patient care.

Imaging diagnosis can be difficult. Imaging findings can be subtle, complex, and confusing. Imaging procedure protocols sometimes need to be modified for optimal results in difficult cases. Quality health care requires teamwork. *The team approach to good health care works only if there is good communication between those on the medical team.* This ideal team effort may sometime require direct personal communication, in person or by telephone.

The following true case illustrates the problems that arise when important information is not shared.

CASE STUDY

A patient with lung cancer fell and subsequently experienced pain in the shoulder, arm, and elbow. He was seen in the ED and radiographs were done. The radiologist was not informed about the lung cancer and that a radionuclide bone scan done the previous month at a different facility had shown metastatic disease in the patient's right mid-humeral shaft, and was also not informed about the location of point tenderness on physical exam. The radiologist did not detect a fracture, and the patient was discharged without treatment.

Three weeks later, the patient had swelling of the arm that led one of his physicians to order an upper extremity venous ultrasound to rule out venous thrombosis, based on the ED report that that patient did not have a fracture. No venous thrombosis was found.

Because of progressive pain in his arm that extended from his shoulder to his elbow, the patient had MRI of the right shoulder and of the right elbow. Again, no significant musculoskeletal pathology was identified.

Finally, 5 weeks after the initial trauma, repeat radiographs of the humerus, done because of persistent pain, showed a displaced pathologic fracture of the mid shaft. The radiologist who interpreted this final study then reviewed the original radiographs done on the day of the fall and discovered that there was a subtle fracture visible on one view in the original study.

Had the original radiologist been provided with complete and appropriate clinical information (evidence of metastatic bone disease in the humeral shaft on a bone scan done elsewhere and the location of point tenderness on physical exam), it is much more likely that he would have detected the subtle fracture and/or directed the radiology technologist to obtain additional views of the region where there was point tenderness and pain.

Even if that had not been done, when the patient's symptoms grew progressively worse and were "unexplained" by the original radiographs, there should have been a conference among his physicians. At the very least a radiologist should have been provided with all the appropriate information and asked to review the original radiographs. None of the patient's physicians put together the previous bone scan findings with the current chief complaint. Instead of a review (costing nothing) of the original x-rays, costly (and uncomfortable for a patient with a fracture) MR scans of the shoulder and elbow were ordered and an ultrasound exam was done.

Better professional communications would have resulted in earlier diagnosis and less patient pain and suffering, and would have avoided three additional procedures.

QUALITY PATIENT CARE IN IMAGING

There is currently a trend among third party payers in the United States to require accreditation of imaging facilities, resulting in a generalized improvement in the consistency and quality of radiologic procedures. An excellent example of improvement in the quality of imaging that results from accreditation is the legislative requirement for accreditation of mammography facilities found in the Mammography Quality Standard Act (MQSA).

However, such external controls on quality are limited and thus the quality and safety of diagnostic radiology procedures is still largely guided by the professional ethics and policies of those individuals and institutions providing such examinations. Unfortunately, grossly poor radiologic examinations get billed (and paid) the same as superb studies done on state-of-the-art equipment.

If you are in a position to select among several imaging providers, you should determine which of those providers will tailor imaging procedure protocols, when needed, for specific individual clinical concerns rather than always performing "routine" imaging on every case. Compare the image sequences used by each MRI facility to see which may use only a minimum number of sequences and which routinely offer more comprehensive procedures. You do not have to be a radiologist to form a basic judgment about the clarity of anatomic features visible on a CT or MR scan, or to judge if a patient had a cursory examination with just a few images recorded or if a comprehensive procedure was well documented with recorded images.

You should judge the clarity and completeness of radiologic reports you receive from different facilities and modify your referrals based on the clinical utility of those reports.

You can learn to be a good judge of proper positioning and exposure of radiographs. You can tell if fine bone or lung detail is visible on a radiograph or not. Just by consistently looking at the images from radiology exams done on your patients you can learn where you patients are more (or less) likely to have a good diagnostic examination.

When your referral options are limited, you can still be influential about the quality of imaging done on your patients just by discussing imaging policies with your radiologists. Most radiologists will listen to your clinical concerns and be responsive to inquiries about how imaging procedures are conducted.

If you are the medical professional who is supervising radiologic procedures, you must have high goals for quality and demand that suboptimally positioned or exposed radiographs be repeated. You must also adopt or campaign for policies that limit unnecessary radiation exposure.

Not every medical facility can afford "state-of-the-art" equipment, but every facility doing medical imaging has the same responsibility to strive for excellence. This is what every patient deserves.

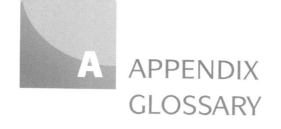

A APPENDIX
GLOSSARY

Term	Definition	Rad	CT	MR	US	NM
ACE-inhibitor renal scintigraphy	Radionuclide renal scan in which renal blood flow response to administration of an ACE inhibitor is used for detection of renal artery stenosis					X
Air bronchogram sign	The abnormal visibility of the contours of an air-filled bronchus when any pathologic process opacifies surrounding lung parenchyma	X	X			
Air–fluid level	Sharp, flat horizontal edge representing interface between gas and the surface of a fluid	X	X	X		
Alveolar infiltrate	Disease process that fills alveoli with fluid and/or cellular material; an older phrase used to describe pulmonary consolidation or opacification	X	X			
Angiography	Imaging procedure optimized for display of vessels	X	X	X		
Apical cap	Abnormal radiographic density appearing unilaterally or bilaterally over the apex of the lung	X	X			
Arterial Doppler sonography	Arterial ultrasonography in which a Doppler shift of the ultrasound beam is used to visualize arterial flow and measure its velocity				X	
Arthrography	Imaging of a joint after the intra-articular injection of a contrast agent	X	X	X		
Atelectasis	A complete or partial collapse of lung parenchyma	X	X	X		
Batwing (butterfly) configuration	Appearance of bilateral parahilar pulmonary edema	X	X			
Blowout fracture	Orbital wall fracture that occurs with sudden increase of intra-orbital pressure	X	X	X		
Bronchiectasis	Irreversible dilatation of bronchi	X	X			
Bulla (bullae)	Abnormal air space(s) in emphysematous lung; ranges in size from 1 cm to entire lung					
Cardiac catheterization	Interventional procedure in which catheters are passed into the heart and coronary arteries	X			X	
CCTA (coronary or cardiac CTA)	Contrast-enhanced CT optimized for visualization of cardiac structures		X			
Centrilobular emphysema	Type of emphysema affecting the proximal respiratory bronchioles, particularly of the upper lung zones; strongly associated with smoking	X	X			
Cephalization	Pathologic change in the diameter gradient of pulmonary veins, resulting in larger veins in upper lung zones than normally seen	X				
Cisternography	Nuclear medicine procedure in which CSF flow is evaluated after the injection of a radionuclide into the lumbar subarachoid space					X
Collimation	Restriction of the size and shape of an x-ray beam by fixed or variable shielding (typically lead shutters)	X	X			
Consolidation	Opacification of the pulmonary airspace associated with disease that replaces air in alveoli with fluid and/or soft tissue	X	X			
Coronary calcium score	Measure of calcified coronary artery atherosclerotic plaque; statistically correlates with risk of coronary stenosis and incidence of acute coronary events		X			
CTA (CT angiography)	Contrast-enhanced CT optimized for visualization of arteries		X			
CTPA (CT pulmonary angiography)	Contrast-enhanced CT optimized for visualization of pulmonary arteries		X			
Decubitus	Position of patient lying on side (right or left lateral decubitus) for radiologic examination	X				

Continued

Term	Definition	Rad	CT	MR	US	NM
DEXA (also DXA; dual photon x-ray absorptiometry)	Bone densitometry based on the attenuation of two x-ray beams that have different energy levels	X				
Diffusion weighted MRI sequence	MR pulse sequence that results in the depiction of degree of water diffusion in tissue; visualization of restricted diffusion with intracellular edema is important in identifying acute cerebral infarction			X		
Dynamic swallowing study	Fluoroscopic examination of pharyngeal function while patient is drinking barium contrast agent	X				
Echocardiography (cardiac ultrasound; cardiac ECHO)	Ultrasound evaluation of the heart; typically uses Doppler shift to measure cardiac blood flow				X	
Flail chest	Refers to segment of thoracic wall that moves paradoxically with respiration because rib segments are unstable after multiple fractures of a rib	X	X			
Functional MRI	Depiction of regional cerebral hemodynamics with varied external stimuli using special MRI sequences			X		
Gradient echo sequence	Refers to a group of MR pulse sequences that have a broad range of generic and proprietary names; sequences are usually very rapid image acquisitions, and can be T1 or T2* (equivalent of T2 in spin echo and fast spin echo sequences)			X		
Grashey view	Commonly used oblique radiographic projection of shoulder	X				
Ground glass opacity	Hazy increase in lung density in which underlying lung architecture remains visible		X			
Honeycombing	Radiologic appearance of lungs associated with advanced fibrosis	X	X			
HRCT (high resolution CT)	Thin section CT protocol used for diagnosis and assessment of interstitial lung disease		X			
Hyperdense vessel sign	Visualization of cerebral vessel on non-contrast CT scan because of increased density of acute intraluminal thrombus		X			
HSG (hysterosalpingography)	Procedure in which endometrial cavity and fallopian tubes are made visible by injection of contrast material through catheter placed into endometrial cavity	X				
Infiltrate	Commonly used term in pulmonary radiology that refers to an increase in lung density	X	X			
Insular ribbon sign	Loss of gray/white matter interface in the insula in acute strokes involving the middle cerebral artery		X			
Interstitial lung disease	Pulmonary disease that primarily involves the interstitial compartment of lung parenchyma, rather than air-space consolidation	X	X			
Intravenous urography (IVU)	Radiographic procedure in which kidneys, intrarenal collecting structures, ureters, and bladder are opacified by intravenous injection of iodinated contrast agent	X				
Kerley lines (A, B, C)	Thin, linear radiodense lines visible in lungs of patients with interstitial pulmonary edema	X	X			
KUB	Common term for supine AP radiograph of abdomen that classically includes kidneys, ureters, and bladder in the field of view	X				
Le Fort fractures	Specifically defined facial fractures; classification related to stability of involved osseous structures	X	X			
Lower extremity non-invasive testing	Doppler ultrasound procedure used to assess suspected arterial insufficiency				X	
Mass	Used radiologically to refer to any abnormal structure that takes up space (space-occupying lesion)	X	X	X	X	
Micronodular	Small spherical pulmonary opacities; this term currently recommended for lesions ≤3 mm diameter	X	X			
MRI brain spectroscopy	MR pulse sequence that maps distribution and concentration of various metabolic substances			X		
Nodule	Spherical abnormal structure that in the lung may be up to 3 cm diameter	X	X			
Opacity	Structure that is visible because of relatively higher radiographic density than normal or compared with surrounding tissue	X	X			
Panlobular (panacinar) emphysema	Type of emphysema that is more advanced than centrilobular; involves acinus and secondary pulmonary lobule		X			

Term	Definition	Rad	CT	MR	US	NM
Panorex	Panoramic x-ray of mandible and maxillary alveolar ridge using special dental radiographic equipment	X				
Paraseptal emphysema	Emphysema characterized by involvement of subpleural distal alveoli; often associated with bullae (air spaces >1 cm diameter)	X	X			
Parenchymal opacity	Lung tissue with abnormally increased radiographic density	X	X			
Pedicle sign	Loss of visibility of vertebral pedicle on AP or PA radiograph because of erosion or destruction of cortex of the pedicle	X				
Peribronchial cuffing	Thickening of bronchial walls usually caused by an inflammatory process	X				
Pulmonary airspace	Air-containing lung parenchyma, including alveoli and respiratory bronchioles	X	X			
Pulmonary function test	Nonimaging procedure evaluating lung function, primary using spirometer to measure lung capacity and air flow					
Quantitative CT (QCT)	CT bone densitometry		X			
Radionuclide myocardial perfusion	Procedure in which regional myocardial perfusion is depicted by distribution of intravenously injected radiopharmaceutical; usually done at rest and after stress					X
Reticular	Pulmonary pattern of lace or net created by many fine linear densities	X	X			
Reticulonodular	Pulmonary appearance characterized by a combination of reticular and micronodular patterns	X	X			
Rib series	Set of radiographs that usually include PA chest and multiple rib radiographs including oblique views	X				
Salter-Harris classification	System of classifying fractures involving the physis or growth plate of a bone	X	X	X		
Scapular Y view	Lateral radiographic projection of shoulder and scapula	X				
Silhouette sign	Loss of visibility of border between structures that normally have different radiographic densities	X				
Skin marker	Radiopaque indicators that are placed on skin to identify location of underlying radiographic areas of interest	X	X	X		
Spatial resolution	Measurement of image detail; usually described by smallest element visible on the image	X	X	X	X	X
Spondylolisthesis	Abnormal alignment of vertebral segments	X	X	X		
Syndesmophytes	Marginal osteophytes of a vertebral body	X	X	X		
Tram tracks	Abnormal visibility of parallel lines that represent thickened bronchial walls	X				
Transillumination	Nonradiographic examination of any structure by transmission of visible light through that structure					
Ventilation/perfusion (V/Q) lung scans	Nuclear scan that images both airflow (ventilation) and blood flow (perfusion) in lungs; used to diagnose pulmonary emboli when techniques that provide direct visualization of such emboli cannot be used					X
Venous Doppler sonography	Venous ultrasonography in which Doppler shift of the ultrasound beam is used to visualize venous flow and measure its velocity				X	

B APPENDIX
ANSWERS TO CHAPTER
REVIEW QUESTIONS

CHAPTER 1

1. D	**2.** A	**3.** C	**4.** E
5. B	**6.** B	**7.** C	**8.** B

CHAPTER 2

1. B	**2.** A	**3.** E	**4.** C
5. C	**6.** D	**7.** A	**8.** B
9. E	**10.** C	**11.** C	**12.** D
13. A	**14.** B		

CHAPTER 3

1. C	**2.** B	**3.** A	**4.** A
5. C	**6.** E	**7.** C	

CHAPTER 4

1. C	**2.** B	**3.** C	**4.** D
5. A	**6.** B	**7.** A	**8.** A
9. E	**10.** B		

CHAPTER 5

1. B	**2.** D	**3.** C	**4.** E
5. A	**6.** A	**7.** B	**8.** D
9. A	**10.** B	**11.** D	

CHAPTER 6

1. B	**2.** C	**3.** E	**4.** C
5. C	**6.** B	**7.** E	**8.** A
9. E	**10.** E		

CHAPTER 7

1. B	**2.** C	**3.** D	**4.** B
5. D	**6.** B	**7.** C	

CHAPTER 8

1. B	**2.** C	**3.** C	**4.** A
5. D	**6.** C	**7.** A	**8.** C
9. B			

CHAPTER 9

1. C	**2.** D	**3.** E	**4.** C
5. A	**6.** D	**7.** D	**8.** B
9. C			

CHAPTER 10

1. D	**2.** C	**3.** B	**4.** A
5. B	**6.** A	**7.** C	

CHAPTER 11

1. D	**2.** B	**3.** E	**4.** B
5. C	**6.** B		

INDEX

Note: Page numbers followed by "b" denote boxes, page numbers followed by "f" denote figures, and page numbers followed by "t" denote tables.